T0289394

Reducing Risks in Surgical Facial Plastic Procedures

Editors

DAVID B. HOM
DEBORAH WATSON

FACIAL PLASTIC SURGERY CLINICS OF NORTH AMERICA

www.facialplastic.theclinics.com

Consulting Editor
ANTHONY P. SCLAFANI

May 2023 • Volume 31 • Number 2

ELSEVIER

1600 John F. Kennedy Boulevard • Suite 1800 • Philadelphia, Pennsylvania, 19103-2899

http://www.theclinics.com

FACIAL PLASTIC SURGERY CLINICS OF NORTH AMERICA Volume 31, Number 2
May 2023 ISSN 1064-7406, ISBN-13: 978-0-323-93879-2

Editor: Stacy Eastman
Developmental Editor: Ann Gielou M. Posedio

Facial Plastic Surgery Clinics of North America (ISSN 1064-7406) is published quarterly by Elsevier Inc., 360 Park Avenue South, New York, NY 10010-1710. Months of issue are February, May, August, and November. Business and Editorial Offices: 1600 John F. Kennedy Blvd., Suite 1800, Philadelphia, PA 19103-2899. Periodicals postage paid at New York, NY, and additional mailing offices. Subscription prices are $428.00 per year (US individuals), $728.00 per year (US institutions), $477.00 per year (Canadian individuals), $904.00 per year (Canadian institutions), $568.00 per year (foreign individuals), $904.00 per year (foreign institutions), $100.00 per year (US students), $100.00 per year (Canadian students), and $255.00 per year (foreign students). Foreign air speed delivery is included in all *Clinics* subscription prices. All prices are subject to change without notice. POSTMASTER: Send address changes to *Facial Plastic Surgery Clinics*, Elsevier Health Sciences Division, Subscription Customer Service, 3251 Riverport Lane, Maryland Heights, MO 63043. **Customer service: 1-800-654-2452 (US and Canada); 1-314-447-8871 (outside US and Canada); Fax: 314-447-8029; E-mail: journalscustomerservice-usa@elsevier.com (for print support); journalsonlinesupport-usa@elsevier.com (for online support).**

Reprints. For copies of 100 or more of articles in this publication, please contact the Commercial Reprints Department, Elsevier Inc., 360 Park Avenue South, New York, NY 10010-1710. Tel.: 212-633-3874; Fax: 212-633-3820; E-mail: reprints@elsevier.com.

Facial Plastic Surgery Clinics of North America is covered in *MEDLINE/PubMed* (*Index Medicus*).

Contributors

CONSULTING EDITOR

ANTHONY P. SCLAFANI, MD, MBA, FACS
Professor of Otolaryngology, Department of
Otolaryngology–Head and Neck Surgery, Weill
Cornell Medicine, Director of Facial Plastic
Surgery, NewYork-Presbyterian/Weill Cornell
Medical Center, New York, New York, USA

EDITORS

DAVID B. HOM, MD, FACS
Professor of Surgery, Co-Director, Facial
Plastic and Reconstructive Surgery, Professor
of Clinical Surgery, Department of
Otolaryngology–Head and Neck Surgery,
University of California San Diego School of
Medicine, Administrative Assistant III, San
Diego, California, USA; Professor of Facial
Plastic and Reconstructive Surgery,
Department of Otolaryngology–Head and Neck
Surgery, University of California San Diego, La
Jolla, California, USA

DEBORAH WATSON, MD, FACS
Professor of Surgery, Program Director,
Department of Otolaryngology–Head and Neck
Surgery, Co-Director, Facial Plastic and
Reconstructive Surgery, University of
California San Diego School of Medicine, San
Diego, California, USA; Department of
Otolaryngology–Head and Neck Surgery,
University of California San Diego, La Jolla,
California, USA

AUTHORS

JEFFREY D. BERNSTEIN, MD
Resident Physician, Department of
Otolaryngology–Head and Neck Surgery,
University of California San Diego, San Diego,
California, USA

JESSICA BLACK, MD
Assistant Professor, Department of
Anesthesiology, University of California San
Diego School of Medicine, San Diego,
California, USA

KENDRA BLACK, MD
Clinical Instructor and Acute Care Surgery
Fellow, Division of Trauma, Surgical Critical
Care, Burns and Acute Care Surgery,
University of California San Diego, San Diego,
California, USA

DONN R. CHATHAM, MD
Clinical Instructor, Department
Otolaryngology, University of Louisville
Medical School

KAYVA L. CRAWFORD, MD
Department of Otolaryngology–Head and Neck
Surgery, University of California San Diego, La
Jolla, California, USA

NÉHA DATTA, MD
Department of Otolaryngology–Head and Neck
Surgery, Upstate Medical University, State
University of New York, Syracuse, New York,
USA; Department of Plastic and
Reconstructive Surgery, Johns Hopkins
School of Medicine, Baltimore, Maryland,
USA

MORGAN E. DAVIS, MD
Resident Physician, Department of
Otolaryngology–Head and Neck Surgery,
University of California San Diego School of
Medicine

SARAH M. DERMODY, MD
Division of Facial Plastic and Reconstructive
Surgery, Department of Otolaryngology–Head
and Neck Surgery, University of Michigan
Medical Center, Ann Arbor, Michigan, USA

JAY DOUCET, MD, MSc, FRCSC, FACS, RDMS
Professor and Chief, Division of Trauma,
Surgical Critical Care, Burns and Acute Care
Surgery, University of California San Diego,
San Diego, California, USA

ALBERT J. FOX, MD, FACS
Private Practice, Dartmouth, Massachusetts,
USA

SAPIDEH GILANI, MD, FACS
Associate Professor, Department of
Otolaryngology, University of California San
Diego, San Diego, California, USA

JACQUELINE J. GREENE, MD
Department of Otolaryngology–Head and Neck
Surgery, University of California San Diego
Health, La Jolla, California, USA

DAVID B. HOM, MD, FACS
Professor of Surgery, Co-Director, Facial Plastic
and Reconstructive Surgery, Professor of
Clinical Surgery, Department of Otolaryngology–
Head and Neck Surgery, University of California
San Diego School of Medicine, Administrative
Assistant III, San Diego, California, USA;
Professor of Facial Plastic and Reconstructive
Surgery, Department of Otolaryngology–Head
and Neck Surgery, University of California San
Diego, La Jolla, California, USA

STEVEN G. HOSHAL, MD
Department of Otolaryngology–Head and Neck
Surgery, University of California Davis,
Sacramento, California, USA

JACLYN A. KLIMCZAK, MS, MD
Facial Plastic and Reconstructive Surgery
Fellow, Rousso Adams Facial Plastic Surgery,
Birmingham, Alabama, USA; Nose and Sinus
Institute of Boca Raton, Boca Raton, Florida,
USA

BOBBY S. KORN, MD, PhD, FACS
Division of Oculofacial Plastic and
Reconstructive Surgery, Viterbi Family
Department of Ophthalmology, UC San Diego
Shiley Eye Institute, Division of Plastic Surgery,
UC San Diego Department of Surgery, La Jolla,
California, USA

TYLER MARION, MD, MBA
Department of Dermatology, University of
Florida College of Medicine, Gainesville,
Florida, USA

SARA MEITZEN, MD
UCSD Advanced Airway Management
Program, Assistant Professor, Department of
Anesthesiology, University of California San
Diego School of Medicine, San Diego,
California, USA

MEGAN V. MORISADA, MD
Department of Otolaryngology–Head and
Neck Surgery, University of California
Davis, Sacramento, California,
USA

JEFFREY S. MOYER, MD
Collegiate Professor of Facial Plastic and
Reconstructive Surgery, Professor and
Division Chief, Division of Facial Plastic and
Reconstructive Surgery, Department of
Otolaryngology–Head and Neck Surgery,
University of Michigan Medical Center, Ann
Arbor, Michigan, USA

BENJAMIN T. OSTRANDER, MD, MSE
Department of Otolaryngology–Head and Neck
Surgery, University of California San Diego, La
Jolla, California, USA

TAMMY B. PHAM, MD
Department of Otolaryngology–Head and
Neck Surgery, University of California San
Diego Health, La Jolla, California,
USA

DANIEL E. ROUSSO, MD
Rousso Adams Facial Plastic Surgery,
Birmingham, Alabama, USA

SHERARD A. TATUM, MD
Department of Otolaryngology–Head and Neck
Surgery, Upstate Medical University, State
University of New York, Syracuse, New York,
USA

MICHELLE TING, MA (Cantab), MBBS (AICSM), FRCOphth
Division of Oculofacial Plastic and Reconstructive Surgery, Viterbi Family Department of Ophthalmology, UC San Diego Shiley Eye Institute, La Jolla, California, USA; Royal Free Hospital London NHS Foundation Trust, London, United Kingdom

TRAVIS T. TOLLEFSON, MD, MPH, FACS
Division of Facial Plastic and Reconstructive Surgery, Department of Otolaryngology–Head and Neck Surgery, University of California Davis, Sacramento, California, USA

ABEL TORRES, MD, JD, MBA
Department of Dermatology, University of Florida College of Medicine, Gainesville, Florida, USA

WILLIAM H. TRUSWELL IV, MD, FACS
Immediate Past President of the American Board of Facial Plastic and Reconstructive Surgery, Past President of the American Academy of Facial Plastic and Reconstructive Surgery, Senior Advisor to the European Board for Certification in Facial Plastic and Reconstructive Surgery, Senior Advisor to the International Board for Certification in Facial Plastic and Reconstructive Surgery, Westhampton, Massachusetts, USA

DEBORAH WATSON, MD, FACS
Professor of Surgery, Program Director, Department of Otolaryngology–Head and Neck Surgery, Co-Director, Facial Plastic and Reconstructive Surgery, University of California San Diego School of Medicine, San Diego, California, USA; Department of Otolaryngology–Head and Neck Surgery, University of California San Diego, La Jolla, California, USA

TYLER WERBEL, MD, MS
Department of Dermatology, University of Florida College of Medicine, Gainesville, Florida, USA

ALISA YAMASAKI, MD
Division of Facial Plastic and Reconstructive Surgery, Department of Otolaryngology–Head and Neck Surgery, University of Michigan Medical Center, Ann Arbor, Michigan, USA

Contents

This review summarizes common risk factors for poor surgical healing on the face and neck and a generalized approach to treating a delayed healing wound. During the preoperative evaluation patients should be screened for prior irradiation, cigarette or e-cigarette use, chronic steroid use, alcoholism, diabetes, malnutrition, and other chronic medical conditions and medications. Despite the surgeon's best efforts to prevent poor surgical healing, some wounds may display signs of persistent inflammation. The facial plastic surgeon should be astute in recognizing delayed healing and identifying intrinsic and extrinsic risk factors so that timely intervention can be performed.

Patient selection in aesthetic surgery is the ultimate inexact science, a mixture of surgical judgment, expertise, ego, gut feelings, personality interactions, and a spin of the roulette wheel. Using our procedural skills as well as our interpersonal skills will enhance our professional satisfaction and improve the quality of life for others as we try to reduce the likelihood of dissatisfaction, both for our patients and ourselves.

Risk factors for the formation of facial scars include skin type, ethnicity, scar location, and certain medical conditions that contribute to poor or delayed healing. Risk of scar can be reduced with appropriate surgical planning, including proper placement and design of incisions, meticulous skin closure, aseptic technique, and wound care to improve healing. Common pathologic scars include hypertrophic scars and keloid scars, each of which has unique approaches to surgical revision and medical treatment due to their respective risks of recurrence. Topical scar therapies, medical therapies, and surgical revision techniques for improvement in final scar appearance are discussed.

Risks for Specific Procedures

Reducing complications after rhinoplasty is critical to ensuring optimal functional, aesthetic, and patient satisfaction outcomes. Many of the most frequent complications of rhinoplasty are technical in nature and can be prevented with meticulous attention to detail and preservation of critical nasal support structures. In this article, the authors review many of the common pitfalls of rhinoplasty and discuss preventative measures that can be used by the competent rhinoplasty surgeon.

Septoplasty is one of the most frequently performed procedures in otolaryngology. The procedure is also performed by oral and maxillofacial surgeons as well as plastic surgeons. Septal deviation is one of the most common findings on physical examination in the otolaryngologist's office. Nasal obstruction when caused by septal deviation may be addressed with septoplasty. Turbinate surgery may be performed in conjunction to further improve the airway.

Blepharoplasty is one of the commonest procedures performed for facial rejuvenation. The eyelids play a vital role in maintaining ocular surface integrity and visual functioning. Care must be taken to avoid complications that pose a risk to vision and ocular comfort. In addition, cosmetic complications can adversely affect patient satisfaction. Here the authors review the common complications encountered with blepharoplasty surgery and discuss how to minimize the risk of these and how to treat them if they do arise. With careful preoperative patient counseling, sound intraoperative technique, and appropriate postsurgical care, blepharoplasty remains a safe and well-tolerated procedure.

Complications after rhytidectomy will occur even in the best of circumstances. Establishing a good rapport with the patient, taking a thorough history and physical exam to elicit potential risk factors such as hypertension or a bleeding diathesis, enlisting staff members to help understand a patient's goals, psychology, and supports, as well as setting realistic expectations help both the surgeon and the patient navigate the journey of surgery toward a successful outcome. Lastly, understanding how to manage potential complications when they arise, in a supportive and caring manner, is vital to the patient relationship and end result: a happy and satisfied patient.

Prominauris is a common auricular deformity most often due to underdevelopment of the antihelical fold or overdevelopment of the conchal bowl. Significant psychosocial distress may result from prominent ears, leading to the development of a variety of surgical techniques over the years. A thorough understanding of the anatomy of both the normal and prominent ear is crucial for accurate analysis and surgical correction of the deformity. The procedure is well-tolerated and careful preoperative evaluation and adherence to meticulous cartilage-sparing techniques will lead to good results and low complication rates.

Hair loss is a common problem among men and women. Hair replacement surgery (HRS) has become increasingly popular as technological advancements have been made producing remarkably natural results when performed by a skilled surgeon. Although complications from HRS are low compared with other esthetic surgeries, they can still occur even with the best-trained and qualified surgeon or staff. The process of hair restoration can be a long road for some patients and active patient participation and education is key for successful results. In this article, we seek to discuss the surgical risks of HRS and discuss methods to prevent them in your practice.

Local tissue flaps are a fundamental technique in cutaneous reconstruction. Reducing the risk of flap failure is of critical importance. The intrinsic vascularity of a flap is the most important determinant of success. Good surgical techniques, including flap design, delicate tissue handling, and tension-less closure, help reduce the risk of flap compromise. Determining the etiology of compromise, including arterial, venous, hematologic, or infectious, is the first step in salvaging a failing flap. Common causes include pedicle kinking, hematoma, pressure/tension, systemic patient factors, and poor surgical technique. Swift action to restore perfusion or venous outflow through numerous strategies is required.

Facial skin defects pose unique challenges for the reconstructive surgeon. Aesthetically complex areas involving a free margin—such as the ear, eyelid, columella, columella–lobule interface, soft tissue triangle, alar rim, and internal nasal lining— are particularly demanding, as secondary soft tissue contracture in these locations can lead to a very poor cosmetic outcome. In these cases, composite grafts offer an ideal combination of soft tissue coverage and structural rigidity, all accomplished in a single-stage surgery. Composite grafts are often underused in facial reconstructive surgery due to the tenuous blood supply and high reported rates of graft failure.

introduces additional risks that should be considered by practicing facial plastic surgeons. Strategies should be implemented to protect yourself and your patients, which include an emphasis on informed consent as it relates to using photos on social media platforms, removing photos from social media, and addressing online reviews. By understanding the risks and using adequate strategies, facial plastic surgeons can minimize the risk of litigation when performing cosmetic procedures.

FACIAL PLASTIC SURGERY CLINICS OF NORTH AMERICA

Foreword: Risk

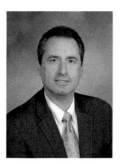

Anthony P. Sclafani, MD, MBA, FACS
Consulting Editor

If you know the enemy and know yourself, you need not fear the result of a hundred battles. If you know yourself but not the enemy, for every victory gained you will also suffer a defeat. If you know neither the enemy nor yourself, you will succumb in every battle.
— Sun Tzu, The Art of War

Risk, risk assessment, risk management, risk mitigation.... These are few of a collection of phrases about "risk" that we hear and read about on an almost daily basis, whether in our offices, on the evening news, or in the business section of the newspapers. We are acutely aware of risk as a threat to us, but do we ever consciously acknowledge that what we do as physicians, and indeed in most of our lives, is based on a calculation of risk and anticipated reward? While Sun Tzu wrote of actual war strategy, the quotation above can be applied to the practice of facial plastic surgery. The "enemy" is the possibility of an undesirable result, and the "battle" is the treatment we provide to patients. With risk such an ever-present part of our lives, it behooves us to develop evidence-based strategies, nuanced by personal experience, to identify, avoid, and manage risk.

David Hom, MD and Deborah Watson, MD have invited a range of thought-leaders in our field to discuss the risks inherent in our treatments and ways to reduce and manage that risk. This issue approaches risk management in facial plastic surgery by reviewing established foundational knowledge, delving into the specific risks inherent in particular procedures and then circling back to widely applicable concepts in reducing surgical risk.

As a military strategist, Sun Tzu points out that you, the general, must "know yourself"—as a surgeon; this means your training, your ability to properly assess the patient's needs, your mastery of surgical techniques, and your technical capacity to perform these. Knowing your enemy entails knowing the ways that techniques can fail and the complications that can occur. Elsewhere in *The Art of War*, Sun Tzu stresses the importance of knowing the terrain and anticipating the effects of the elements. Surgically, this means understanding the nuances of the landscape in which we work: understanding local tissue anatomy, how tissues handle, how wounds heal, and how wounds fail.

No field of medicine has higher patient expectations than facial plastic surgery. Understanding the risks we assume for ourselves and our patients is one of our greatest responsibilities. Enjoy this issue of *Facial Plastic Surgery Clinics of North America* and embrace your inner "general."

Anthony P. Sclafani, MD, MBA, FACS
Department of Otolaryngology
Weill Cornell Medicine
Weill Greenberg Center
1305 York Avenue, Suite Y-5
New York, NY 10021, USA

E-mail address:
ANS9243@MED.CORNELL.EDU

Facial Plast Surg Clin N Am 31 (2023) xiii
https://doi.org/10.1016/j.fsc.2023.01.018
1064-7406/23/

Preface
Reducing Risks in Facial Plastic Surgery

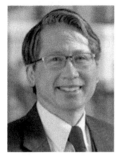 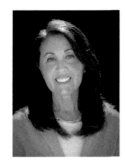

David B. Hom, MD, FACS   Deborah Watson, MD, FACS
Editors

Facial plastic and reconstructive surgeries encompass a wide variety of procedures to treat our patients. Despite their many favorable and positive outcomes for our patients, unfavorable occurrences and complications can happen even among experienced facial plastic surgeons.

Each type of surgical procedure has its own specific risks that can lead to complications or adverse effects. When perioperative complications do occur, disfigurement and compromise of quality of life can be apparent for all to see with public scrutiny. By understanding these risks, we need to be prepared with clinical responses that will help us either avoid or appropriately manage adverse events. This vigilance will serve to improve surgical outcomes as well as patient satisfaction.

This issue of *Facial Plastic Surgery Clinics of North America* highlights common risks and adverse events that may occur from common facial plastic surgical procedures; each article provides a discussion to help prevent, manage, and treat them.

The authors for this issue were selected for their national expertise on their respective topics. The first section of our issue provides an overview of generalized topics, such as wound healing, reducing scarring, salvaging compromised local skin flaps, and reducing risks for a dissatisfied cosmetic facial plastic surgical patient.

Our second section launches into our most common facial plastic surgeries (covering the cosmetic and reconstructive realms) with discussions that focus on reducing relevant risks and how to manage their unfavorable outcomes.

The last section of this issue highlights the importance of additional perspectives that relate to reducing adverse anesthesia outcomes, managing systemic conditions from panfacial injuries, and reducing legal and social media risks associated with facial plastic surgery.

We are very grateful for the insightful and superb contributions from our team of authors as they share their expertise in this issue. It has been a

Facial Plast Surg Clin N Am 31 (2023) xv–xvi
https://doi.org/10.1016/j.fsc.2023.01.001
1064-7406/23/© 2023 Published by Elsevier Inc.

pleasure and honor to be guest editors for this relevant topic on Reducing Risks in Facial Plastic Surgery. We hope it will be very informative to you.

David B. Hom, MD, FACS
Facial Plastic and Reconstructive Surgery
Department of Otolaryngology–
Head and Neck Surgery
University of California San Diego
School of Medicine
9300 Campus Point Drive
MC 7895
San Diego, CA 92037-7895, USA

Deborah Watson, MD, FACS
Facial Plastic and Reconstructive Surgery
Department of Otolaryngology–
Head and Neck Surgery
University of California San Diego
School of Medicine
University of California San Diego
9300 Campus Point Drive
MC 7895
San Diego, CA 92037-7895, USA

E-mail addresses:
dbhom@health.ucsd.edu (D.B. Hom)
dewatson@health.ucsd.edu (D. Watson)

Reducing Risks for Poor Surgical Wound Healing

David B. Hom, MD*, Morgan E. Davis, MD

KEYWORDS

- Wound healing • Delayed healing • Chronic wounds • Irradiation • Cigarette smoking • Vaping
- Malnutrition

KEY POINTS

- Poor surgical wound healing of the face and neck can lead to significant morbidity and dissatisfaction for patients.
- Preoperative evaluation should include a detailed history of chronic medical conditions, previous irradiation, diabetes, chronic steroid use, malnutrition, and smoking or e-cigarette use.
- Persistent inflammation for longer than 7 days is a common initial sign of delayed or poor surgical healing. If delayed healing persists, the wound can transform into a chronic healing wound.
- Clinical signs of decline in wound healing are increased odor, increased pain, increased exudate, dehiscence, and tissue necrosis.
- When poor wound healing does occur in this area, the primary goal is the identification of extrinsic and intrinsic factors contributing to poor wound healing and timely intervention.

INTRODUCTION

Normal wound healing of the face and neck is a commonly expected and assumed outcome from patients. However, when postsurgical wound complications occur, disfigurement and compromise of quality of life are clearly apparent for all to see with public scrutiny. The goals of this review article are to identify and understand common factors that contribute to poor surgical healing. By understanding these factors, one can help reduce surgical wound complications. Early recognition and clinical modification of variables that contribute to poor healing can assist in improved surgical wound outcomes.

OVERVIEW OF NORMAL WOUND HEALING

The wound healing process is made up of a highly orchestrated biological cascade of cell signaling and repair mechanisms via cytokines, growth factors, various cell types, and structural elements.

This process is divided into four main overlapping phases: hemostasis, inflammation, proliferation, and maturation or remodeling. Any delay or interruption in the phases of acute healing ultimately results in prolonged healing and an increased risk of developing a chronic or nonhealing wound. The four phases of normal wound healing are briefly described in the following section and are illustrated in **Fig. 1**.

Hemostasis

The first stage of wound healing is the hemostatic phase that begins within seconds to minutes of acute tissue injury. This is marked by vasoconstriction that reduces blood loss and the initiation of the extrinsic clotting cascade. Thrombocytes are activated by exposed collagen, and activated platelets adhere to the collagen and release cell signaling molecules resulting in the formation of a fibrin-platelet matrix.[1] The matrix serves a role in clot formation and acts as a scaffold for growth

Department of Otolaryngology Head and Neck Surgery, University of California San Diego School of Medicine
* Corresponding author. 9300 Campus Point Drive, La Jolla, CA 92037.
E-mail address: dbhom@health.ucsd.edu

Facial Plast Surg Clin N Am 31 (2023) 171–181
https://doi.org/10.1016/j.fsc.2023.01.002

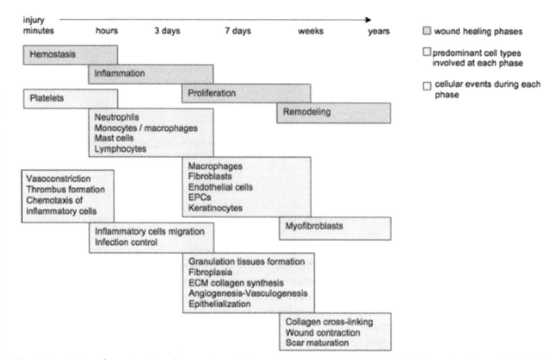

Fig. 1. Depiction of overlapping phases of repair in wound healing. Any disruption in the natural cascade of healing will ultimately delay healing and potentially lead to poor surgical healing, chronic wounds, and scarring. ECM, extracellular matrix; EPCs, endothelial progenitor cells. (*From* Baltzis D, Eleftheriadou I, Veves A. Pathogenesis and Treatment of Impaired Wound Healing in Diabetes Mellitus: New Insights. *Adv Ther.* 2014;31(8):817-836. https://doi.org/10.1007/s12325-014-0140-x with permission.)

factors and cytokines to signal the initiation of the healing process.

Inflammation

The inflammatory phase begins within 30 minutes and usually persists for several days. As a result of platelet degranulation and cytokine cascade, this phase is marked by 2 to 3 days of capillary vasodilation, which facilitates the migration of the characteristic inflammatory infiltrate to the wound.[2] Neutrophils are the initial cell type that phagocytose debris, kill bacteria, and secrete proteolytic enzymes. Monocytes then appear and transition to macrophages which are key for proper wound healing which phagocytize remaining debris and produce key cytokines that stimulate fibroblasts and regulate the production of collagen. A key point is that a wound remains in the inflammatory phase as long there is a persistent bacterial burden or other inflammatory nidus present such as a reactive foreign body. This is important to recognize as wounds that exhibit signs of persistent inflammation for more than 7 days are prolonging the inflammatory phase, a common initial sign of poor or delayed wound healing.[1]

Proliferation

The proliferative phase is marked by fibroplasia, neovascularization, and reepithelialization. Fibroblasts migrate to the wound and proliferate forming disorganized type III collagen during the formation of granulation tissue. Neovascularization allows new blood vessels to form to provide nutrients and oxygen for cells to sustain wound healing. After adequate granulation tissue has developed, reepithelialization initiated by keratinocytes and wound contraction by myofibroblasts should begin to occur within 2 to 3 weeks to complete the proliferative phase.

Maturation and Remodeling

The final stage of wound healing is the maturation or remodeling phase during which type III collagen is remodeled and replaced by stronger, more organized type I collagen. The remodeling phase begins at about 3 weeks and continues approximately 1 year. Although the maximum amount of collagen is present in the wound around 3 to 6 weeks, collagen is continuously remodeled by macrophages that secrete proteases and collagenases forming mature collagen and increasing the wound's tensile strength which plateaus at 80% of its original strength 3 months following injury.[2,3] The final appearance of the scar occurs 6 to 12 months after injury.

PREOPERATIVE CONSIDERATIONS AND PATIENT CHARACTERISTICS

Reducing the risk of poor surgical wound healing ultimately begins during the preoperative consultation when interviewing patients about their medical history and comorbidities that may affect their surgical outcome. This requires a thorough history and exam to look for extrinsic and intrinsic factors (Table 1) that may adversely impact wound healing. During this process, common conditions that affect tissue oxygenation such as pulmonary diseases, congestive heart failure, anemia, and cigarette smoking can be elicited. In addition, comorbid conditions such as malnutrition, diabetes, hypothyroidism, alcoholism, malignancy, and chronic conditions requiring certain medications can usually be identified during routine history and physical. In certain circumstances, additional workup may be indicated to diagnose or monitor chronic conditions including a complete blood count, metabolic panel, renal panel, serum glucose, hemoglobin A1c, nutritional panel, and/ or thyroid stimulating hormone level.

Surgical wounds on the face and neck generally are known to heal rapidly with few complications due to the robust blood supply in this area. As a result, when poor wound healing does occur, it can often be attributed to one of the following underlying extrinsic or intrinsic factors that impede healing.

EXTRINSIC FACTORS CONTRIBUTING TO POOR SURGICAL HEALING
Previous irradiation

Radiotherapy is a common modality used in the management of certain head and neck cancers either as primary treatment, adjuvant treatment (in addition to surgical resection with or without chemotherapy), or palliative therapy. Along with damaging tumor cells, however, radiotherapy also damages surrounding healthy tissue leading to complications such as skin atrophy, soft tissue fibrosis, desquamation, epithelial ulceration, and microvascular damage that overall contribute to poor healing of wounds.[4] Short-term reactions from radiotherapy occur in almost all patients due to the acute radiation injury to healthy epithelial cells resulting in radiation-induced DNA mutations, microvascular damage, and fibrosis. As consecutive radiation doses are applied, the cycle of normal cell regeneration is interrupted which may lead to delayed or nonhealing radiation ulcers. Cell damage is progressive and may continue for several years even after the course of radiotherapy resulting in long-term complications such as necrosis, atrophy, fibrosis, vascular damage, and carcinogenesis. Because of these detrimental effects on wound healing, subsequent surgical procedures on tissues that were previously irradiated heal poorly resulting in increased rates of delayed healing and complications such as flap failures, dehiscence, fistulas, wound necrosis, and infection.

Current strategies to reduce the risk of poor surgical healing in irradiated tissues are still very limited. Radiation oncologists are focusing on more precise targeting of radiotherapy to limit the dose of radiation to surrounding healthy, noncancerous cells and subsequent radiation-induced damage. For the surgeon, preoperative planning and a preventive approach to optimize conditions for wound healing and minimize potential complications are critical. The timing of radiotherapy in reference to surgery can also significantly affect the healing process. In patients receiving postoperative radiation, radiation can be initiated as early as 3 weeks following surgery without significantly impeding wound healing. According to Payne and colleagues,[5] wound healing is most affected when surgery is performed 6 months or more after completion of radiotherapy. Therefore in patients receiving preoperative radiation, the optimal time for surgery is 3 weeks to 3 months following completion of

Table 1	
Common factors contributing to poor surgical wound healing	
Extrinsic Factors	**Intrinsic Factors**
Previous irradiation	Malnutrition
Chronic steroid use	Obesity
Cigarette smoking	Diabetes
Vaping	Hypothyroidism
Medications[a]	Aging
	Ischemic conditions (ie, anemia, COPD, CHF, vascular disease, and renal failure)
	Alcoholism
	Immunodeficiency

[a] Medications listed below.

radiation therapy.[6] In cases with similar oncologic outcomes in patients treated with preoperative versus postoperative radiation therapy, postoperative radiation is preferred due to fewer wound healing complications.[5] Other proposed strategies to reduce the risk of surgical wound healing complications in irradiated head and neck cancer patients include adjunctive wound care modalities to reduce bacterial colonization, promote a moist environment, and stimulate granulation in addition to microvascular free tissue transfer.[7] Hyperbaric oxygen therapy (HBO) has also been used clinically in patients with wound healing complications after radiotherapy.

Chronic steroid use

Molecular studies have shown that corticosteroids affect all major phases of the wound-healing process. For example, during the inflammatory phase, treatment with dexamethasone has been shown to decrease the expression of important cytokines such as TGF-beta1, platelet-derived growth factor, tumor necrosis factor, and interleukin-1alpha thereby limiting the chemotactic and mitogenic stimulus for other inflammatory cells.[8,9] Dexamethasone use also causes decreased expression of intercellular adhesion molecules resulting in impaired cellular adhesion and migration.[10] Corticosteroids affect the second stage or proliferative phase of wound healing by reducing fibroblast proliferation and reepithelialization. Furthermore, during the final stage of wound healing, the collagen maturation process is adversely affected due to reduced wound tensile strength. A review of animal studies and the effect of steroids on wound strength shows an approximately 30% reduction in wound tensile strength at cortisone doses of 15 to 40 mg/kg/d (equivalent to 200 to 560 mg/d of prednisone in a 70-kg human).[11] In addition, patients chronically exposed to high levels of adrenocorticoids such as those with Cushing syndrome show the closest evidence that corticosteroid excess in humans decreases cutaneous wound tensile strength in a similar fashion by approximately 40%.

Although there are no formal recommendations regarding preoperative chronic steroid use in facial plastic surgery, data from other surgical specialties suggest that patients taking prednisone for at least 30 days preoperatively at doses of 40 mg/d or higher, may have increased wound complication rates by approximately two to five times compared with patients not taking corticosteroids.[11] In addition, a recent retrospective study of more than 94,000 plastic surgery cases from the American College of Surgeons National Surgical Quality Improvement Program database showed that chronic steroid users making up 1.8% of the study population were 1.25 times more likely to develop surgical complications and 1.77 times more likely to develop medical complications on multivariate analysis.[12] Limitations to the previously mentioned study include the inability to determine the dose or duration of chronic steroid use and the indication for which it was used; however, this information is still helpful in preoperative counseling of patients on steroid therapy.

Vitamin A plays an important role in wound healing due to its ability to stimulate epithelial growth, fibroblasts, granulation tissue, angiogenesis, collagen synthesis, epithelialization, and fibroplasia.[13] As a result, Vitamin A has been used to aid wound healing in steroid patients. In fact, studies have shown that dexamethasone significantly impairs the healing of both tracheal anastomoses and intestinal anastomoses in rats and rabbits, respectively, and Vitamin A has been used to counteract this inhibitory effect.[14,15] Unfortunately, the evidence for Vitamin A supplementation is limited due to the lack of human clinical trials; however, in wound patients, short-term vitamin A supplementation of 10,000 to 25,000 IU/day has been recommended.[16] Vitamin a toxicity can be a serious issue and even result in death; therefore, the use of vitamin A for counteracting corticosteroid use and optimization of wound healing should be carefully weighed against potential risks and side effects.

Medications

Certain medications are associated with poor wound healing and such medications should be elicited during the preoperative assessment. The patient should be informed that the risk of slow or poor surgical healing can occur with concurrent use of these medications (Box 1).

Smoking

The detrimental effects of cigarette smoke on wound healing were first reported in the late 1970s by Mosely and colleagues[17] and it is now widely accepted that smoking cessation may reduce the risk of postoperative wound complications. Although cigarette smoke contains more than 4,000 ingredients, nicotine, carbon monoxide, hydrogen cyanide, and nitric oxide are the main culprits for impaired wound healing. This involves multiple mechanisms working synergistically to decrease oxygen delivery to tissues, cause endothelial injury, reduce oxygen utilization, increase thrombogenesis, and impair the means of

---

Box 1
Common medications associated with poor wound healing

Steroids

Chemotherapeutic medications

Aspirin

NSAIDs (ibuprofen)

Penicillamine

Colchicine

Antirheumatic drugs (methotrexate)

Vasoconstrictive drugs (nicotine, adrenaline, and cocaine)

Anticoagulants (heparin and warfarin)

---

cellular repair. Nicotine, one of the most commonly studied cigarette components, is believed to cause local tissue ischemia due to its vasoconstrictive activity. One study showed that smoking one cigarette reduces tissue perfusion by 22% to 48% in 30 minutes.[18] Interestingly, gum containing nicotine did not affect tissue oxygenation with less nicotine serum peak levels compared with smoking.

Cigarette smoking also negatively impacts the inflammatory and proliferative phases of wound healing. For example, a randomized controlled trial in which smokers were randomized to continuous smoking or abstinence with a nicotine or placebo patch showed attenuated inflammation and fibroblast proliferation in smokers and restoration of inflammation following abstinence.[19] Smoking has also been associated with higher rates of wound infections and randomized trials have shown reduced incidences of infections following 4 weeks of smoking cessation.[20]

Facial plastics literature suggests that cigarette use is associated with increased severe surgical complications. Retrospective studies have shown increased nasal recovery time and increased rates of development of septal perforation in smokers following septoplasty compared with non-smokers[21] and almost three times the rate of skin slough in smokers following facelift procedures.[22] Parikh and Jacono[23] showed that a deep plan face-lifting technique can be used to decrease rates of skin slough even in smokers. Nevertheless, due to the electiveness of these procedures, some facial plastic surgeons have recommended mandatory smoking cessation before consideration of performing certain surgical procedures.

Although the evidence is clear that smoking adversely affects wound healing, established

guidelines to guide surgeons in reducing perioperative risk among smokers are lacking. The exact duration of perioperative abstinence before elective surgery is unknown. Studies suggest that at least 4 weeks is ideal; however, longer durations of smoking cessation, approximately 6 weeks have been shown to significantly reduce perioperative risk.[24] Nevertheless, all patients should be counseled on smoking cessation preoperatively with a goal of abstinence for at least 4 to 6 weeks before elective surgery.

Vaping (e-cigarettes)

Vaping is believed to be a detrimental risk factor for poor surgical wound healing, akin to cigarette smoking; however, the exact mechanism of tissue damage remains unknown. One study sought to identify the underlying molecular mechanism and found that both cigarette smoking and vaping were associated with decreased vascular endothelial growth factor expression, decreased microvessel density, and decreased areas of fibrosis in flap tissue of rodents exposed to vaping or cigarettes compared with controls.[25] Another animal study found that regular vaping within a month before surgery increases the risk of flap necrosis and that smoking and vaping were equally detrimental to wound healing.[26] As such, vaping should not be seen as a better alternative to cigarette smoking in the context of surgical wound healing and preoperative cessation should also be encouraged.

INTRINSIC FACTORS CONTRIBUTING TO POOR SURGICAL HEALING
Malnutrition

Adequate nutritional status is fundamental to the wound healing process. Malnutrition occurs when there is an imbalance between the nutrients that the body receives and the energy needed for the body to function properly. This imbalance may be undernutrition or overnutrition. For the purposes of this review, we focus on undernutrition and how nutrient deficiencies affect the wound healing process.

Undernutrition can be divided into macronutrient and micronutrient deficiencies. Macronutrients include proteins, fats, and carbohydrates. Protein malnutrition affects all four stages of wound healing. For example, inflammatory cell production depends on available protein and a deficiency results in an impaired immune response, which in turn will delay progression from the inflammatory to the proliferative phase. Protein deficiency also decreases fibroblast activity in the proliferative and remodeling phases, resulting in reduced angiogenesis and collagen formation.[27] Protein deficiency is associated with weight loss and decreased lean body mass. Although the body favors wound healing in patients who have lost approximately 20% lean body mass, this process is delayed while the body restores lean mass in patients who lose 30% lean body mass or more.[28] In addition, both carbohydrates and fats are important to support the inflammatory process, cellular formation and activity, angiogenesis, and collagen deposition. Specifically, carbohydrates are necessary for key events such as fibroblast production, leukocyte activity, and hormone and growth factor secretion. A depleted carbohydrate state also leads to protein catabolism which in turn depletes protein reserves essential to healing.[6] Fats are essential in building cell membranes and are also precursors to prostaglandins which are mediators of cellular inflammation and metabolism. Despite this evidence, formal recommendations for macronutrient supplementation are not well established.

Micronutrients involved in wound healing include amino acids, vitamins, and minerals. Arginine and glutamine are the key amino acids that play a role in the wound healing process and are involved in the inflammatory phase, collagen synthesis, antioxidation, and other essential enzymatic reactions. Kirk and colleagues[29] showed significantly higher amounts of total protein and improved reparative collagen synthesis in elderly patients treated with arginine supplementation for 2 weeks suggesting that arginine supplementation may enhance wound healing and immune responses in this patient population. Similarly vitamins such as vitamins A and C and B vitamins all significantly impact wound healing. Deficiencies in vitamin A result in impaired stimulation of fibroblasts, granulation tissue, angiogenesis, collagen synthesis, epithelialization, and fibroplasia.[13] Local (topical) and systemic supplementation with vitamin A has been proven to increase dermal collagen deposition and vitamin A has been shown to counteract delayed wound healing due to corticosteroid use. Patients with vitamin A deficiency should receive 25,000 IU/day of vitamin A supplementation.[5] Vitamin C and B1 (thiamine) are essential for cross-linking during collagen synthesis and deficiencies result in decreased wound strength.[6,30] Vitamin C is also involved in cell migration and transformation into macrophages during the inflammatory process and has key antioxidant properties that counteract the production of free radicals in damaged cells.[27] The current recommendation for vitamin C supplementation to reduce the risk of poor healing in noncomplicated wounds is 500 mg/d.[28] Supplementation should be increased to 1 to 2 g/d in patients with severe wounds. Chronic alcohol consumption is a known

risk factor for thiamine deficiency. Although thiamine deficiency is rare in other well-developed populations, it may also be seen in patients with a history of bariatric surgery, Crohn's disease, anorexia, kidney disease, or restrictive diets and should be corrected.

Zinc is an essential trace element in the human body and an important cofactor in numerous processes including cellular DNA replication, activation of lymphocytes, formation of antibodies, auto-debridement via matrix metalloproteinases, and stimulation of collagen production, fibroblast proliferation, and epithelialization. As a result, some experts recommend zinc supplementation in the perioperative period especially in high-risk populations such as head and neck cancer patients.[6] Current data support the use of oral zinc supplementation in zinc-deficient chronic leg ulcer patients[31]; however, the benefit of supplementation in non-zinc-deficient patients and surgical patients remains controversial. Topical zinc administration to surgical wounds and application of zinc-containing surgical bandages to surgical wounds, however, has been shown to improve the wound healing process.[31,32]

Malnourishment in surgical patients may be more common than one expects. One study showed that 12% of non-cancer, vascular, and abdominal surgery patients had preexisting malnutrition that adversely affected their postoperative outcome and increased their hospital stay.[33] Owing to the high incidence and significant implications of malnourishment on surgical healing, nutritional status should be considered during preoperative evaluation. Signs of malnutrition such as cachexia, muscle wasting, history of >20% weight loss, and gastrointestinal malabsorption (ie, history of gastric bypass or Crohn's disease) should be identified and corrected before surgery if possible. In addition, malnutrition can be shown in patients with low serum albumin (<3.0 mg/dL), prealbumin (<15 mg/dL), or transferrin (<200 mg/dL).[1] Common risk factors for malnutrition include low income, chronic illnesses, advanced age, and pediatric populations. Preoperative optimization of nutritional status with protein/multi-nutrient supplementation as early as possible is recommended for patients with preexisting malnutrition to reduce the risk of poor surgical healing. For those with poor nutritional status and decreased oral intake, enteral nutrition has been shown to significantly improve postoperative healing.[5]

Obesity

Obesity, referring to a body mass index (BMI) $\geq$ 30 kg/m^2, is a well-established risk factor for poor surgical outcomes, particularly poor wound healing; however, the exact mechanisms responsible are not well understood. Postulated mechanisms of obesity-associated impairments in wound healing are related to reduced perfusion of adipose tissue due to decreased capillary density and impaired angiogenesis and chronic aberrant low-grade inflammation which inhibits normal inflammatory responses that facilitate wound healing.[34] Animal studies have shown impaired reepithelialization, decreased fibroblast activity, reduced wound strength, and scar formation in rodents fed high-fat diets compared with nonobese control mice.[35,36]

Diabetes

Hyperglycemia (glucose >140 mg/dL) is a known independent risk factor for poor surgical outcomes including delayed wound healing, increased rates of infection, prolonged hospital stay, and higher postoperative mortality. The mechanisms of impaired wound healing are related to vascular dysfunction and neurologic impairment in addition to impaired inflammatory and cellular signaling processes affecting the inflammatory, proliferative, and remodeling phases of the healing cascade.[37] In diabetic patients, a detailed history of their medical condition including type of diabetes, anti-diabetic medications, current glycemic control, and related complications should be obtained during preoperative evaluation. In addition, a glycosylated hemoglobin A1c (HbA1c) should be checked on all patients if one has not already been obtained within the last 3 months as data suggests that the risk of wound healing complications is four times higher in diabetic patients with HbA1c greater than 7.8% compared with diabetic patients with HbA1c levels less than 7.8%.[38] As a result, surgeons should carefully weigh this risk and consider postponing elective or aesthetic surgeries until a patient's blood glucose levels are better controlled.

Aging

As we age, several age-related changes occur in normal skin, which negatively impact wound healing. These changes include decreased collagen density, fewer fibroblasts, macrophages, and mast cells, increased elastin fragmentation, and slower wound contraction.[6,39] Other notable changes in elderly skin are decreased epidermal growth rate, flattening of the dermal-epidermal junction, and reduced dermal cellularity and vascularity.[39,40] Morphologic alterations in elderly skin ultimately affect all phases in the wound healing process resulting in functional impairment and

temporal delay in wound healing; however, the quality of healing may be unaffected.[41] Similar to obese patients, delayed wound healing in the elderly is associated with an altered inflammatory response including increased secretion of inflammatory mediators, delayed infiltration of macrophages and lymphocytes, impaired macrophage function, and decreased secretion of growth factors. Other age-related alterations in the healing process are enhanced platelet aggregation, delayed reepithelialization, delayed angiogenesis and collagen deposition, reduced collagen remodeling, and decreased wound strength.[42] In addition, elderly patients have a higher susceptibility to comorbid chronic conditions, medication usage, and infection which may further impede wound healing. Aside from optimizing comorbid conditions and known risk factors, exercise has been reported to decrease the level of pro-inflammatory cytokines in healing tissue and improve wound healing in aged mice and humans.[43–45]

Chronic Conditions

Chronic medical conditions such as chronic obstructive pulmonary disease, congestive heart failure, peripheral vascular disease, and anemia impair tissue oxygenation placing patients at higher risk for poor surgical healing. In addition, hypothyroidism is an important factor for poor or delayed wound healing due to decreased collagen formation. Chronic kidney disease (CKD) is also known to affect wound healing and animal studies suggest that CKD impacts wound healing through disruption of normal reepithelialization and granulation tissue deposition rates, reduced cellular proliferation and angiogenesis, and a chronic dysfunctional inflammatory state.[46] Uremia from renal failure has also been associated with wound healing impairment. It is important to screen for these systemic comorbidities ideally before surgical intervention as these conditions can be optimized in collaboration with a primary medical physician to improve surgical wound outcomes.

GENERAL APPROACH TO DELAYED SURGICAL HEALING

Poorly healing wounds of the face and neck can be especially debilitating, both functionally and cosmetically, thus it is important that facial plastic surgeons not only be familiar with risk factors and prevention of poor surgical healing but also be well-informed about the signs and symptoms of at-risk wounds, treatment of delayed and chronic wounds, and adjuvant techniques to improve healing. Wound care nurses can also be very instructive in suggesting contemporary wound care

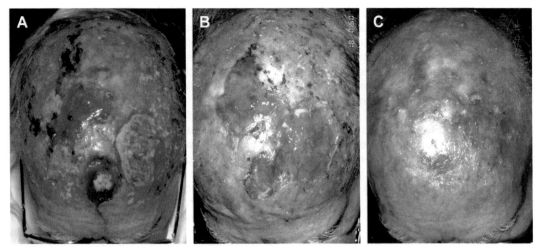

Fig. 2. (*A*) An 82-year-old man with a history of scalp postoperative radiation treatment 10 years previously and multiple excisions of squamous cell cancers on the scalp. He had a persistent 2 year history of an open nonhealing scalp wound down to calvarial bone. Multiple biopsies showed no evidence of neoplastic recurrence and CT scan showed no evidence of osteomyelitis. Over 2 years he saw multiple physician providers and despite multiple different aggressive daily dressings and antibiotic trials, no clinical healing or granulation tissue occurred. (*B*) He required "jump starting" this chronic wound to get it back to the acute wound healing state by burring down the outer calvarium to the diploic layer to stimulate granulation tissue growth along with moisture retentive dressings. Other possible options for treating this wound would be a vacuum-assisted closure (VAC) device or a synthetic dermal substitute, (ex. Integra, Integra Life Sciences, Plainsboro, NJ)to stimulate granulation tissue on the bone. (*C*) After adequate granulation tissue formation, a split thickness skin graft successfully covered most of the open wound so that he no longer required aggressive daily dressing changes. The chronic wound was transformed into an acute healing wound.

protocols and dressings available for slow-healing wounds.

A generalized approach to treating poorly healing wounds should be based on the principles of proper wound debridement, infection control, maintaining a moist environment while avoiding excessive exudates, and adequate wound edge reepithelialization. When wound healing is not proceeding normally over 2 to 4 weeks, the clinician must distinguish between an acute healing wound that is delayed versus a chronic healing wound based on physical characteristics such as size and depth of the wound, increased inflammatory changes, excessive exudate, purulence, necrotic tissue, wound edge epithelialization, and moisture balance.[47]

Clinical signs of a decline in wound healing are increased odor, pain, exudate, dehiscence, and tissue necrosis. If the wound is not healing, one can ask:

1. What is the most likely cause for poor healing?
2. What are the extrinsic or intrinsic factors contributing?
3. Is appropriate wound care being given?

A delayed healing wound usually responds to clinical intervention quicker than a chronic healing wound; however, if a delayed healing wound persists, it can transform into a chronic healing wound. Chronic healing wounds require a more comprehensive strategic approach involving wound bed preparation to achieve successful wound healing (**Fig. 2**).

If a wound fails to heal despite initial intervention, reevaluation of the current management and identification of the contributing factors that may be causing the poor healing should be reassessed. Wounds should be evaluated for the presence of foreign bodies, infection, tissue ischemia, and venous insufficiency. In addition, for a persistent nonhealing wound, a skin biopsy should be considered to rule out neoplasia. At the systemic level, metabolic conditions such as undiagnosed diabetes, anemia, or malignancy need to be ruled out. In addition, some patients may have concurrent factors playing a role in slower healing. One example is a poorly controlled insulin-dependent diabetic who is chronically on steroids for asthma. In this particular instance, as healing occurs over time, management of these comorbid conditions will have to be modified.[48]

Once the local and systemic tissue factors that contribute to poor wound healing are identified, the next step is to "jump-start" the tissues back into the acutely healing phases by removing necrotic tissue and eschar with effective debridement (**Table 2**).

Table 2
Methods of tissue debridement

Types of Debridement	Description
Surgical debridement	Removes necrotic tissues via sharp surgical excision, typically with cold instruments either at bedside or in the operating room. Most effective form of debridement but results in most underlying tissue damage.
Mechanical debridement	Removes debris by physical force. Most common type is wet-to-dry dressings that should also include wound irrigation with either normal saline or antibiotic irrigations. Results in moderate amount of tissue damage.
Autolytic debridement	Relies on innate proteolytic enzymes to break down and liquefy necrotic debris by placing an occlusive or semi-occlusive dressing over the wound for 2 to 3 d while the enzymatic process takes place. Less effective at wound debridement, but is the gentlest method for underlying tissues. This method is not appropriate for highly exudative, infected or deep wounds.
Enzymatic debridement	Exogenous enzymes such as papain-urea cream or collagenase ointment are applied topically to digest and break down necrotic debris. This method is slightly harsher than autolytic debridement, but debrides tissues slightly faster.

Once initial debridement is performed, the next step is recognizing and treating the infection. Infected wounds prolong the inflammatory phase and typically present with increased erythema, warmth, and induration that persists more than 5 to 7 days after the initial insult. When infection is present, wounds should be opened to allow an oxygenated environment to eliminate obligate anaerobic bacteria. Wound cultures should also be obtained so that antibiotic treatment can be tailored to culture results. Topical antibiotics and skin cleansing solutions are also beneficial during dressing changes during the acute period.

Moist environments enhance the rate of epithelial migration and promote wound healing. As such, moisture balance in the wound should be maintained by using moisture-retaining ointment and hydrogels to avoid desiccation while also preventing excessive fluid which may cause maceration and lead to poor wound healing.

Adjunctive treatments such as hyperbaric oxygen and vacuum-assisted closure devices, can be considered in the treatment of unsatisfactory surgical healing that is refractory to standard treatment and wound-bed preparation.

SUMMARY

Common risk factors for poor surgical healing on the face and neck can be divided into extrinsic and intrinsic factors. Extrinsic factors include prior irradiation, chronic steroid use, cigarette use, and vaping. Intrinsic factors include comorbid medical conditions that affect tissue oxygenation and vascularity, malnutrition, diabetes, obesity, and normal aging. These risk factors should be identified and optimized ideally before surgical intervention to improve surgical healing outcomes. The facial plastic surgeon should be cognizant of the signs and symptoms of poor wound healing so that at-risk wounds can be recognized quickly, local and systemic factors affecting proper wound healing can be identified, and early intervention can be made. The principles of treating a delayed or chronic healing wound include effective debridement, recognizing and treating infection, adequate moisture balance, and wound edge reepithelialization. Chronic wounds may require more comprehensive wound bed preparation in addition to adjunctive treatments such as HBO, vacuum-assisted closure devices, and consultation with wound care nurses for additional treatments.

CLINICS CARE POINTS

- The risk of poor surgical wound healing can be reduced preoperatively by optimizing chronic comorbid medical conditions (i.e. diabetes, ect.), ensuring adequate nutritional status, and encouraging weight loss in addition to smoking or vaping cessation.
- Postoperative radiation can be initiated as early as 3 weeks following surgery and is typically preferred over pre-operative radiation due to fewer wound healing complications.

- Patients with a history of irradiation may develop chronic nonhealing wounds that require extensive wound bed preparation to "jump start" the wound back into the acute healing process, in addition to adjunctive therapies such as HBO, dermal substitutes, specialized dressings including vacuum assisted closure devices, and/or even free flap reconstruction.
- Once a delayed healing wound is identified, appropriate care consists of identifying and removing risk factors, tissue debridement, infection control, maintaining a moist environment, and wound edge reepithelialization.

DISCLOSURE

The authors have nothing to disclose.

REFERENCES

1. Houlton JJ, Hom DB. Approaching Delayed-Healing Wounds on the Face and Neck. Facial Plast Surg Clin North Am 2013;21(1):81–93.
2. Ramirez AR, Mabrie, DC, Maas CS, et al. Wound Management and Suturing Manual; 2001, American Academy of Facial Plastic and Reconstructive Surgery, VA, USA.
3. Levenson SM, Geever EF, Chowley LV, et al. The Healing of Rat Skin Wounds. Ann Surg 1965; 161(2):293–308.
4. Dormand E-L, Banwell PE, Goodacre TE. Radiotherapy and wound healing. Int Wound J 2005; 2(2):112–27.
5. Payne WG, Naidu DK, Wheeler CK, et al. Wound healing in patients with cancer. Eplasty 2008;8:e9. Available at: http://www.ncbi.nlm.nih.gov/pubmed/18264518.
6. Gantwerker EA, Hom DB. Skin: Histology and Physiology of Wound Healing. Facial Plast Surg Clin North Am 2011;19(3):441–53.
7. Kwon D, Genden EM, de Bree R, et al. Overcoming wound complications in head and neck salvage surgery. Auris Nasus Larynx 2018;45(6):1135–42.
8. Hübner G, Brauchle M, Smola H, et al. Differential regulation of pro-inflammatory cytokines during wound healing in normal and glucocorticoid-treated mice. Cytokine 1996;8(7):548–56.
9. Beer H-D, Longaker MT, Werner S. Reduced Expression of PDGF and PDGF Receptors During Impaired Wound Healing. J Invest Dermatol 1997; 109(2):132–8.
10. Cronstein BN, Kimmel SC, Levin RI, et al. A mechanism for the antiinflammatory effects of corticosteroids: the glucocorticoid receptor regulates leukocyte adhesion to endothelial cells and expression of endothelial-leukocyte adhesion molecule 1 and intercellular adhesion molecule 1. Proc Natl Acad Sci 1992;89(21):9991–5.
11. Wang AS, Armstrong EJ, Armstrong AW. Corticosteroids and wound healing: clinical considerations in the perioperative period. Am J Surg 2013;206(3): 410–7.
12. Barcha CP, Ranzer MJ. Impact of Chronic Steroid Use on Plastic Surgery Outcomes. Plast Reconstr Surg 2018;142(5):770e–9e.
13. Zinder R, Cooley R, Vlad LG, et al. Vitamin A and Wound Healing. Nutr Clin Pract 2019;34(6):839–49.
14. Talas DU, Nayci A, Atis S, et al. The effects of corticosteroids and vitamin A on the healing of tracheal anastomoses. Int J Pediatr Otorhinolaryngol 2003; 67(2):109–16.
15. Phillips JD, Kim CS, Fonkalsrud EW, et al. Effects of chronic corticosteroids and vitamin a on the healing of intestinal anastomoses. Am J Surg 1992;163(1): 71–7.
16. Hunt TK, Ehrlich HP, Garcia JA, et al. Effect of Vitamin A on Reversing the Inhibitory Effect of Cortisone on Healing of Open Wounds in Animals and Man. Ann Surg 1969;170(4):633–41.
17. Mosely L, Finseth F. Cigarette smoking: impairment of digital blood flow and wound healing in the hand. Hand 1977;9(2):97–101.
18. Jensen JA. Cigarette Smoking Decreases Tissue Oxygen. Arch Surg 1991;126(9):1131.
19. Sørensen LT, Toft B, Rygaard J, et al. Smoking attenuates wound inflammation and proliferation while smoking cessation restores inflammation but not proliferation. Wound Repair Regen 2010;18(2): 186–92.
20. Sorensen LT, Karlsmark T, Gottrup F. Abstinence From Smoking Reduces Incisional Wound Infection. Ann Surg 2003;238(1):1–5.
21. Cetiner H, Cavusoglu I, Duzer S. The Effect of Smoking on Perforation Development and Healing after Septoplasty. Am J Rhinol Allergy 2017;31(1): 63–5.
22. Rees TD, Liverett DM, Guy CL. The Effect of Cigarette Smoking on Skin-Flap Survival in the Face Lift Patient. Plast Reconstr Surg 1984;73(6):911–5.
23. Parikh Sachin, Jacono A. Deep-Plane Face-life as an Alternative in the Smoking Patinet. Arch Facial Plast Surg 2011;13(4):283–5.
24. Rinker B. The Evils of Nicotine. Ann Plast Surg 2013; 70(5):599–605.
25. Jaleel Z, Blasberg E, Troiano C, et al. Association of vaping with decreased vascular endothelial growth factor expression and decreased microvessel density in cutaneous wound healing tissue in rats. Wound Repair Regen 2021;29(6):1024–34.
26. Troiano C, Jaleel Z, Spiegel JH. Association of Electronic Cigarette Vaping and Cigarette Smoking With

Decreased Random Flap Viability in Rats. JAMA Facial Plast Surg 2019;21(1):5–10.

27. Barchitta M, Maugeri A, Favara G, et al. Nutrition and Wound Healing: An Overview Focusing on the Beneficial Effects of Curcumin. Int J Mol Sci 2019; 20(5):1119.

28. Molnar JA, Underdown MJ, Clark WA. Nutrition and Chronic Wounds. Adv Wound Care 2014;3(11): 663–81.

29. Kirk SJ, Hurson M, Regan MC, et al. Arginine stimulates wound healing and immune function in elderly human beings. Surgery 1993;114(2):155–9. discussion 160. Available at: http://www.ncbi.nlm.nih.gov/pubmed/8342121.

30. ALVAREZ OM, GILBREATH RL. Effect of Dietary Thiamine on Intermolecular Collagen Cross-linking during Wound Repair. J Trauma Inj Infect Crit Care 1982;22(1):20–4.

31. Enoch S, Grey JE, Harding KG. Non-surgical and drug treatments. BMJ 2006;332(7546):900–3.

32. Lansdown ABG, Mirastschijski U, Stubbs N, et al. Zinc in wound healing: Theoretical, experimental, and clinical aspects. Wound Repair Regen 2007; 15(1):2–16.

33. WARNOLD I, LUNDHOLM K. Clinical Significance of Preoperative Nutritional Status in 215 Noncancer Patients. Ann Surg 1984;199(3):299–305.

34. Pierpont YN, Dinh TP, Salas RE, et al. Obesity and Surgical Wound Healing: A Current Review. ISRN Obes 2014;2014:1–13.

35. Nascimento AP, Costa AMA. Overweight induced by high-fat diet delays rat cutaneous wound healing. Br J Nutr 2006;96(6):1069–77.

36. Biondo-Simões M, Zammar GR, Fernandes RS, et al. Obesity and abdominal wound healing in rats. Acta Cir Bras 2010;25(1):86–92.

37. Baltzis D, Eleftheriadou I, Veves A. Pathogenesis and Treatment of Impaired Wound Healing in Diabetes Mellitus: New Insights. Adv Ther 2014;31(8): 817–36.

38. Cunningham DJ, Baumgartner RE, Federer AE, et al. Elevated Preoperative Hemoglobin A1c Associated with Increased Wound Complications in Diabetic Patients Undergoing Primary, Open Carpal Tunnel Release. Plast Reconstr Surg 2019;144(4):632e–8e.

39. Sgonc R, Gruber J. Age-Related Aspects of Cutaneous Wound Healing: A Mini-Review. Gerontology 2013;59(2):159–64.

40. Fenske NA, Lober CW. Structural and functional changes of normal aging skin. J Am Acad Dermatol 1986;15(4):571–85.

41. Gosain A, DiPietro LA. Aging and Wound Healing. World J Surg 2004;28(3):321–6.

42. Guo S, DiPietro LA. Factors Affecting Wound Healing. J Dent Res 2010;89(3):219–29.

43. Keylock KT, Vieira VJ, Wallig MA, et al. Exercise accelerates cutaneous wound healing and decreases wound inflammation in aged mice. Am J Physiol Integr Comp Physiol 2008;294(1):R179–84.

44. Emery CF, Kiecolt-Glaser JK, Glaser R, et al. Exercise Accelerates Wound Healing Among Healthy Older Adults: A Preliminary Investigation. Journals Gerontol Ser A Biol Sci Med Sci 2005;60(11): 1432–6.

45. O'Brien J, Finlayson K, Kerr G, et al. Evaluating the effectiveness of a self-management exercise intervention on wound healing, functional ability and health-related quality of life outcomes in adults with venous leg ulcers: a randomised controlled trial. Int Wound J 2017;14(1):130–7.

46. Seth AK, De la Garza M, Fang RC, et al. Excisional wound healing is delayed in a murine model of chronic kidney disease. PLoS One 2013;8(3): e59979. Sen U, ed.

47. Rijswijk L. Wound assessment and documentation. In: *Chronic wound care: a clinical source book for healthcare professionals*. Malvern, PA: HMP Communications; 2001. p. 101–15.

48. Hom DB, Dresner H. General approach to a poor healing wound- a practical overview. In: *Essential tissue healing of the face and neck*. Cary, NC: PMPH USA, Ltd; 2009. p. 317–29.

Reducing Risks for a Dissatisfied Patient in Facial Cosmetic Surgery

Donn R. Chatham, MD*

KEYWORDS

- Consultation • Patient selection • Expectations • Patient satisfaction • Patient dissatisfaction
- Management

KEY POINTS

- achieving satisfactory results from procedures administered by facial plastic surgeons is a combination of science, art and good fortune.
- Spending adequate time and effort (focused listening, candid discussion, explanation of reasonable pros and cons of treatment) before instituting treatment will pay huge dividends both for the patient and the surgeon.
- The surgeon needs to be attuned to types of patients who may possess either physical issues or emotional psychological issues which might pose additional risks of suffering a less-than-ideal procedural result.

Every procedure we perform and every patient encounter we experience aim to be a success, but sometimes we experience a less-than-ideal outcome.

And the only way to never have a less-than-ideal outcome and a dissatisfied patient is to never perform a procedure.

But short of this extreme and ungratifying strategy what can we do?

And why are some patients dissatisfied with the results of their experience? Did the result fall short of what they were expecting? Were there unpleasant or negative events they suffered through? Were there stressful surprises or traumas? Maybe their caregivers were rude, dismissive, or uncaring? Did they suffer a complication? Did they endure prolonged pain?

Did they feel cared for by their surgeon? Or not? Were they able to develop a rapport with their surgeon? Were they simply unpleaseable no matter what?

What might we physician surgeons do to reduce the risks of dealing with a dissatisfied patient in aesthetic procedures?

OUR GOAL SHOULD BE SATISFACTORY (BUT NOT NECESSARILY PERFECT) OUTCOMES, A SAFE PROCEDURE, AND A PLEASANT OVERALL EXPERIENCE

Very few things in life are perfect. Although we strive for perfection, it is rarely, if ever, obtained. It is impossible to make everyone happy with everything we do. Keep trying but understand the law of averages says no one "bats 1000."

It begins with the first encounter.

Selecting patients for elective procedures may at first glance seem simple, but it is indeed an art.[1]

The first consultation with a new physician can be stressful and uncertain. For the procedure naïve who may never have received aesthetic procedure care, this is a new territory. Some come armed with previous experiences, maybe from other practitioners, and even nonmedical spas. Others may feel ambivalent or wonder if they are being too vain or frivolous.

Helping reassure them that they have called the "right place" can be initiated by your office staff, who ideally possess not only accurate information

The author has no disclosures, nor conflicts of interest. All figures are mine and original.
Department Otolaryngology, University of Louisville Medical School
* 3015 Laura Drive, Floyds Knobs, IN 47119.
E-mail address: Donnchathammd@mindspring.com

Facial Plast Surg Clin N Am 31 (2023) 183–193
https://doi.org/10.1016/j.fsc.2023.01.004
1064-7406/23/© 2023 Elsevier Inc. All rights reserved.

but charming and even encouraging personalities. This time is crucial in deciding if this patient is a reasonable person with a reasonable view of the world. If not, the odds of satisfactory outcomes are low.

The office ambience and décor hopefully are welcoming, calm, and professional. No one wants to be kept waiting, and wait times greater than 13 minutes begin to produce negative feelings.[2] Longer wait times receive lower patient ratings.

Good questions include: what do you think this procedure might do for you?

Have you done something like this in the past? If so, how did it go? Is anyone else possibly affected by your decision?

In aesthetic surgery, the surgeon and patient agree to temporarily suspend the patient's good health in exchange for hopefully improved quality of life and self-esteem. Patients of their own volition agree to undergo a nonvital procedure, pay money, and experience pain and inconvenience while simultaneously believing this to be a wise decision; this illustrates "cognitive dissonance" at work, accepting 2 opposite positions at the same time.[3]

There is a significant difference between "usual surgery" and "aesthetic surgery." With "usual surgery," the patient hopes the surgery is not recommended. With aesthetic surgery, the patient hopes surgery is recommended. With trauma, tumors, or reconstruction, there is the expectation to proceed.

Are we perhaps "fortune tellers"? We predict that our skills combined with usual healing and a patient's expectations will result in a positive outcome.[4]

Every person has unique emotional strengths and weaknesses. Many have or are receiving counseling or other forms of psychiatric therapy and are prescribed psychotropic medicines. Others may self-medicate with alcohol or other mood-altering substances. Past history of psychiatric treatment is not an absolute contraindication for surgery, as this would disqualify many. Patients currently under psychiatric care should be asked if their current mental health professional is aware of their interest in plastic surgery.[5]

DO NOT RUSH THE INITIAL CONSULTATION. LISTEN CAREFULLY

A common patient complaint seeking medical care is that they were interrupted by the physician before completing their communications. Listening is an art and a discipline, and patients should be encouraged to tell their story without being rushed.

Consultation is a time of identification. Post-treatment is a time of management. The more carefully we learn during consultation, the less time we spend managing.

Not sure about a new patient? Make time for "courtship." Most people "court" before taking wedding vows. Begin with small minimal risk suggestions. Sometimes a second consultation on a different day is appropriate. And it is wise to listen to our staff's impression of new patients.

PEOPLE, WHO BUY DRILLS, DO NOT REALLY WANT DRILLS, THEY WANT HOLES

Those who "buy surgery" really do not want surgery. They want to "feel better about themselves" and appear reasonably attractive, to reduce stress and maximize their quality of life.

Are you and the patient compatible? Compatibility = skills + personality. We first need the skills to provide the procedure the patient seeks. But are we comfortable with that patient's personality? We could find them unlikable and even if well trained, this might suggest this would not be a good match.

EXPECTATIONS

"Blessed is the man who expects nothing, for he shall never be disappointed" said Alexander Pope, English poet, early 1700s.

Happiness is the elusive objective as the implied outcome of successful surgery.

Realistic expectations remain the cornerstone of a satisfying experience for every patient. Patients undergo aesthetic procedures to reduce stress and maximize quality of life.[6]

Will our procedure bring heightened self-esteem, enhanced social acceptance, feeling more attractive, and possibly other perks a more attractive person might garner?[7–9] It might even change their life for the better for the rest of their life.

Advertising in modern society is replete with enormous exaggerations as to how happy and full of life are those who are depicted having a light beer, driving a new vehicle, or cruising the Bahamas all while in perfect health.[10]

Likewise, the promotion of aesthetic results in the postprocedural world typically features smiling happy people who are likely popular, full of life, and possess something that the prospective patient does not have. So does advertising affect expectations? These heightened portrayals can sometimes set the prospective patient up for disappointment even before the initial visit with their doctor (**Fig. 1**).

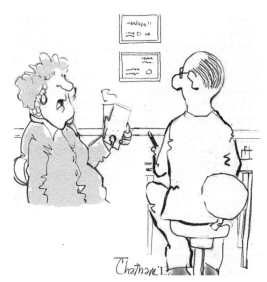

Fig. 1. "I want the "mini-procedures" but the "maxi-results"

Any marketing or advertising that creates unjustified expectations, promotes "world famous" personalities, and suggests a guarantee or that everyone is happy will only create problems (**Fig. 2**).

TEACH: PROCEDURE, EXPECTED OUTCOME, LIMITATIONS, ALTERNATIVES, AND RISKS INVOLVED

How well do patients truly understand what we tell them? All procedures carry a degree of risk. There are expected outcomes but not every outcome is

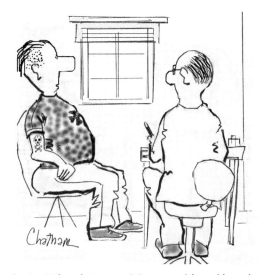

Fig. 2. "What do I expect? To meet girls and have lots of money."

the same. And we always have alternatives. (Sometimes the best alternative is to not proceed with a procedure.)

Patients need to know that in the days following a surgical procedure, they may experience a temporary "worsening" of the features we have addressed. Avoiding as many unanticipated surprises is good for all. Sometimes the postprocedure malaise, bruising, edema, and discomfort exceed what is customary and additional reassurance and sometimes early intervention to mitigate this is required. It is often asked *"when will the healing be done?"* and *"when will I see the final result?"*.

Although not every patient will correctly hear what they might be told, every caregiver needs to be clear and honest in describing the pros and cons of that procedure. For example, "minimal downtime" may mean maybe a day or so but not a week of swelling, bruising, or wound care. It seems wiser to help prepare our patients for a worsening experience rather than painting a Pollyanna picture.

WHAT IS INFORMED CONSENT?

Patients need enough reliable information on the pros and cons of the procedure they are entertaining but just how much detail? There are "expected results" and the most common possible "adverse events." But should every procedure come with the admonition that one possible outcome is a horrible death? Once our patients have access to data from verbal discussion, written material, and possibly on-line research, then they presumably are "well-informed enough" to make a decision. Our signed permits simply notarize their conscious decision. I sometimes tell my patients that "there is risk in everything we do: driving our cars, leaving our homes, eating in a restaurant...either you are me could get his by a cement truck driving home today....but we are playing the odds that bad things are unlikely. Such as it is with surgical procedures." And as the "small print" often states, results are not guaranteed and past performance is no guarantee of future performance.

Understand that information given preprocedure is "informed consent".

Information given postprocedure may be seen as "an excuse."

Patients often ask: "Doctor, do you think I am a good candidate for this procedure?" A reasonable verbal guidance may go something like: *"Sometimes there are problems that cannot be foreseen, but barring any unexpected problems I see no reason you should not do well. I will do everything I can to try to help you."*

And our "warranty" is one of service, not outcome.

BE CERTAIN OF YOUR OWN CAPABILITIES, SKILLS, AND LIMITATIONS

After adequate study, reasonable training, and development of confidence, there comes the first time we have actually performed a specific procedure, even though we may have scrubbed in or observed others. Our training is an ongoing experience, hopefully learning from each surgical case. But we are neither Gods nor superhuman and remain susceptible to the limitations of other humans. There is a fine line between performing "just enough" of a procedure versus pushing the boundaries into "careless experimentation." And proceeding with a procedure while our inner voice says "don't go there" is at best foolhardy. Avoiding an adverse outcome is much better for all rather than managing a damaging complication (**Fig. 3**).

TRUST YOUR INSTINCTS AS WELL AS YOUR RATIONAL MIND

Successful decisions are often based on objective data but listening to the inner voice that may whisper "pause," is part of a well-rounded approach. For example, if one feels pressured into scheduling a new patient for a procedure you do not 100% think is right, it might not be right.

You will never regret not performing surgery on a questionable patient. If you do not feel sure about a certain case or patient, but the rent is due, it will not be worth it (**Fig. 4**).

Some patients we simply do not like. We will know this within minutes of only meeting them. An unpleasant relationship will make dealing with an unanticipated result very difficult. An unhappy patient you never bonded with will consume an inordinate amount of our time and energy. Regrets will follow and consequences of an unfavorable outcome may be disproportionate to the result.

RAPPORT

The #1 reason for the dissatisfied patient is lack of rapport with the MD.

Communication is the *sine qua non* in building successful relationship and its by-product, rapport. And communication begins with listening.

Administering "awake procedures" is an excellent opportunity to build rapport and instill confidence and build trust. Often the first sensation of a minor procedure is a cold compress, the application of a peel, the heat of a laser, or the first needle prick. Perhaps these procedures should be preceded by a gentle touch on the shoulder, reassuring the patient that you are doing your best to minimize pain and achieve the best result in the safest manner possible. Letting each patient know in real time exactly what we are doing and what to expect helps alleviate anxiety and build trust. "Enhancing the Art of Care During Awake Procedures" is an excellent article articulating wise admonitions such as "be mindful", "creating

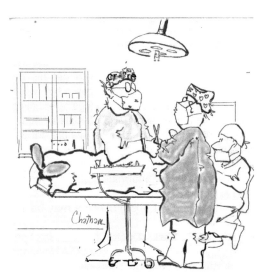

Fig. 3. "I don't know if this is a 'brilliant innovation' or a 'reckless experimentation,' but here goes."

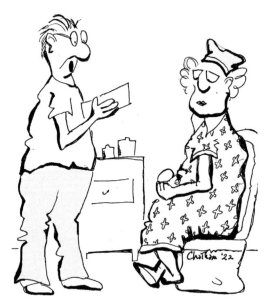

Fig. 4. "We are really not a good match, Mrs. Beanster, but you have the money so let's give it a try".

a peaceful environment," and knowing that "what we say matters."[11]

The doctor-patient relationship can be irreparably damaged by the surgeon's arrogance, hostility, coldness, or by rushing though the treatment seemingly not really caring.

YOU WILL ENCOUNTER DIFFICULT AND CHALLENGING PATIENTS. ACCEPT THIS REALITY

We all have the occasional challenging patient: perhaps an unattractive personality or we find them annoying or maybe with idiosyncrasies that we try to accept.

Difficult patients are ones who challenge the judgment of the doctor and puts unwanted stress on the staff.

Worse yet is the disruptive patient who interferes with the ability to deliver good care and whose behavior falls outside the limits of healthy.

Closely related is the manipulative patient who is not honest, seeking to control the situation, and is prone to act out, complain, and perhaps becomes sexually inappropriate.

There is the VIP patient who expects more and with whom we may unconsciously make exceptions with medical decisions that we may not make for others. Sometimes the VIP patient may even be another physician.

Patients who have been dissatisfied with previous adequately performed procedures seem more likely to become again dissatisfied with subsequent procedures.[12]

Not even the greatest surgeon in the world can please all of the people all of the time.

There inevitably will be those who will not be satisfied with what we have tried to do for them. And the memory of a dissatisfied patient will remain in the consciousness much longer than the most happy of patients.[13]

Difficult patients are more likely to become dissatisfied patients. So it is paramount to identify the truly difficult patient as early as possible to avoid scheduling them for a challenging surgery than having to manage a difficult and unhappy patient (**Fig. 5**).

Balancing a patient's perceived deformity and their level of concern cannot be overlooked. I remind patients that we humans tend to be harder on ourselves than most others. But when the "concern" is out of proportion to the "deformity" then red flags should go up[14] (**Fig. 6**).

Particularly difficult are those who suffer from body dysmorphic disorder (BDD). They seek cosmetic surgery but in reality may be dealing with an adverse childhood event, seeking healing

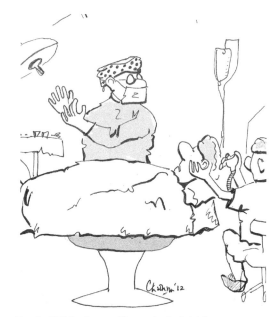

Fig. 5. "I'll be happy if you do it right."

from that. A minor physical trait may be described in language that is extreme, and this preoccupation can have extremely deleterious effects on their ability to function. Appropriate treatment is psychotherapy and not surgery.[15,16]

One study estimated that about 13% of patients seeking aesthetic surgery suffered from BDD as confirmed by the BDD severe combined immunodeficiency.[17]

Other maladies such as depression, anxiety, obsessive-compulsive disorder, personality disorders, narcissistic personalities, and others are prevalent in our society; it behooves us to discern when one of our patients brings this with them to our office (**Fig. 7**).

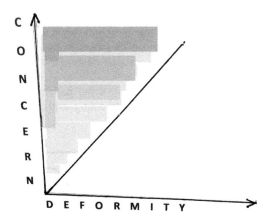

Fig. 6. Patient subjective deformity compared to patient concern. (As level of deformity rises, so should degree of concern)

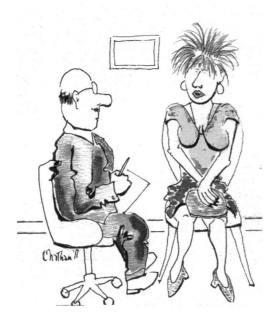

Fig. 7. "Why do you ask me if I know who Narcissus is?"

We must first strive to develop a reasonable set of psychological skills before becoming an excellent surgeon. Plastic surgery/psychiatrist John Goin and Maria Goin described the interplay of surgery and psychiatry.[18] This is a necessity, not a luxury.

It is wise to include a sampling of psychologically crafted questions in our initial patient questionnaires.[19] We include a smiley face emoji question asking "which of the following faces best represents how you see yourself on a day-to-day basis?" (**Fig. 8**).

Other more detailed personality testing has been proposed.[20]

We live in a world of gender fluidity and pronoun confusion. We once may have inhabited a world view with 2 genders, but present times in Western society reveal many more. The transgender patient deserves special care, a scope beyond this article but important nevertheless.[21]

On the other hand, many of the patients who consult with us are rather interesting, and a sense of humor is a value asset.[22]

Fig. 8. Which of the following faces describes how you feel most of the time?

ACCESS THE LEVEL OF DIFFICULTY

Choose the proper procedure for each unique patient.

Our treatment options usually cover a broad spectrum.........noninvasive low risk to very aggressive higher risk. Patient selection is easy with lower level aesthetic options but risk increases as difficulty of procedures increases. The higher the difficulty, the more the time/investment needed in consultation.[23]

Skills for successful injection of neurotoxins, although important, are not considered particularly difficult. Skills needed for a successful rhinoplasty may be among the most difficult. Revision rhinoplasty deserves a special note, as it is usually considered to be the most challenging of the facial aesthetic procedures. Understanding patient desires and concerns is paramount to achieving patient satisfaction.[23]

Gorney recommended avoiding rhinoplasty seekers who fit the "SIMON" criteria: single, immature, male, overexpectant, and narcissistic.[24]

Kridel devised a staging system to access the predicted difficulty in achieving patient satisfaction, which included number of prior surgeries, use of grafts, and patient expectations, graded "A" to "D." Clearly the "D" patient will likely never be satisfied and best avoided.[25]

A benefit when the surgeon personally performs lower risk procedures is the opportunity to evaluate patients for potential future more complicated procedures. One-on-one time spent will help determine the comfort level and compatibility between the patient and surgeon. One could even use a stepwise approach until the experience "maxes out."

DO EVERYTHING YOU CAN TO PREPARE INCLUDING ADEQUATE MENTAL PREPARATION AND REST

We may consider ourselves as nearly superhuman without need of the frivolous accoutrements of normal humans. Nevertheless, mortals do depend on food, rest, recovery, and other bodily care. As a medical student and resident, some of us could seemingly go for days without sleep fueled by coffee and candy bars. But more medical errors occur when doctors are sleep deprived and experiencing unhealthy stressors.

Just as we counsel our patients to prepare, thus should we also listen to our own words.

HAVE YOUR BEST TEAM AT THEIR BEST

Your surgical team also needs to perform at a high level and preparedness, having all necessary equipment and instruments readily available and maintain due concentration throughout the procedure and remain mindful and respectful of verbal communications where the patients may be listening to what is said. Background chatter from others in the room should be at the level comfortable to the surgeon.

EXECUTE THE PROCEDURE WITH YOUR BEST STRATEGY BUT BRING PLAN "B"

Unexpected factors require us to devise more than one strategy and possess alternative skills and options to adapt to changing circumstances. What, for example, do we do if the patient experiences excess bleeding or the anatomy is unusual or scar tissue is denser than expected? What if the cardiac monitor beeps out a new tachycardia or the oximeter numbers plummet or your favorite subcutaneous suture is missing or your favorite scrub assistant is not present? Expect the unexpected.

POSTPROCEDURE CARE

On leaving the operating room, a new phase of patient care begins. Communicating that surgery is finished and a report on how things went to the family is not only a simple etiquette but a necessary responsibility. Likely, this is a new experience and patients may have had little real knowledge of what to expect or do. Verbal and detailed written postoperative instructions may forestall them seeking random ill-conceived advice from others. Do not be hesitant to freely provide greater assurance to those who seem to need it.

Guiding our patients through this often-new experience for as many days as necessary helps reassure them that we know what we are doing, having seen this before. Healing is a "journey" rather than an "event."

Even when they return home, we remain responsible for their care. Simple things such as a phone call the next day to check on their well-being is smart and appreciated by the patient and their family; this conveys care and concern for them even though out of sight and helps continue rapport. It may at times prevent a minor issue from becoming a big problem and good business.[9]

If later there is some delayed issue with long-term healing, it is preferable they share this with you and not a potentially less-friendly practice.

DO WE KNOW HOW TO BEST EVALUATE RESULTS?

Postprocedural evaluation of results is subjective, sometimes needing just a glance to determine if our objectives were achieved. But this is not very scientific. Adding a bit more objectivity is the use of pretreatment and posttreatment photographs where even the patient can be expected to assume a bit of objectivity, and may offer an irrefutable documentation of change, hopefully for the better.

But sometimes the answer is less clear.[26]

Aside from the personal opinions of surgeon and patient, in recent years come psychometrically sound patient-reported outcome measures also known as P.R.O.Ms. Questionnaires measure items important to people such as general health, symptoms, and appearance and were first centered on general health outcomes and more recently applied to aesthetic surgery outcomes.

Attempts have been made to try to quantitate or score results with vehicles such as the FACE-Q test[27,28] and the Rosenberg self-esteem scales.[29]

These questionnaires survey appearance, adverse effects, experiences and quality of life, and self-esteem, which hopefully trend in a post-procedure positive direction, seeking to become "evidence-based."[30]

The 10-question SCHNOS survey for preprocedure and postprocedure analysis asks questions identified by patients as most relevant, such as on a 5-point scale "how much do I experience decreased mood and self-esteem due to my nose?"[31]

Being able, to some degree, to quantitating improvement would seem to be helpful in helping patients take on some bit of objectivity to their very subjective experience (**Fig. 9**).

INVITE HONEST COMMUNICATION

Honesty is the foundation of healthy doctor-patient relationships. Encouraging patients to

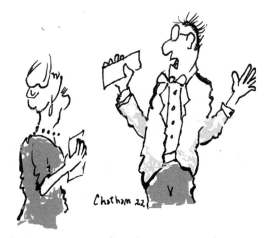

Fig. 9. "How can you be unhappy? Your early P.R.O.M scores were great!"

candidly share thoughts about their procedure does not entail questionnaires or statistical analysis. If pleased, this is reassuring. Perhaps they may share their experiences with others via online reviews. If less than pleased, they need a nonjudgmental avenue to speak. We offer empathy and perhaps solutions. Do not look for trouble but if it is there, do not ignore it. If body language or face expression is disconcerting we might ask: *"You don't seem too happy today. Is there something troubling you?"*

Management of a dissatisfied patient is less difficult if identified in the "dysplasia" stage rather than if discovered much later in the "malignant" stage (aka negative online review or letter from an attorney).

POSTPROCEDURE DISSATISFACTION

A technically perfectly executed surgery procedure is no guarantee of a satisfied patient. Outcomes do not always meet patient expectations.[32]

With a complaint, try not to take it personally: empathize, repeat what you are hearing, assure them you understand and want to do everything reasonable to help. They already feel disappointed, bewildered, confused, anxious, and possibly angry. Discuss your perspective in a straight-forward way, while reassuring them that their welfare is paramount.[33] Listen, empathize, identify the problem, and share your best strategy to find a remedial pathway.[34] Anger directed at a patient does no good but much harm.

A postoperative unhappy patient will consume an inordinate amount of our time and energy. Unhappiness can worsen in the face of ambiguity, so a treatment plan is reassuring even without a firm timetable. And frustration grows when asked to pay more for a second procedure.

Be candid: *"I know you are dissatisfied. I understand. But it's important that we work on this together. I need your support and I can assure you that you have mine."*

Not all "patients with a problem" need to become "problem patients." Early intervention may go a long way to helping ameliorate a smoldering bigger problem. Failure to identify and take action is tantamount to ignoring a fire.

Scenarios include the following:

1. Patient is unhappy and surgeon is unhappy
2. Patient is unhappy but surgeon is happy
3. Patient is unhappy and doctor is uncertain
   Is the problem anatomic? If so, can it be fixed? If contemplating another surgery, can you tolerate the patient? If the issue is likely improvable, discuss your plan with your patient. If another procedure is unlikely to change the outcome, do not proceed and explain why.

Do not see a problem? Then do not operate-...instead listen, reassure. There may be another yet unidentified issue driving the unhappiness.

Is the problem an overly expectant result? Is there criticism from an outside source such as a family member? Has there been an unexpected stress or loss in your patient's life that affected their mood?

Again, there are patients we cannot satisfy. It is disappointing not only for them but for us too. We may feel we have failed. Again, even though we practice in a highly demanding specialty, we must not gaze for too long in our own mirror of perfectionism.[35]

CAN YOU LEARN ANYTHING FROM THIS?

We learn from failures or shortcomings. But it is counterproductive to beat yourself up about it. It is ok to be human and not a god and we cannot control everything. Accept it. Sometimes healing lies distal, rather than proximal, to the scalpel.

ONLINE REVIEWS

Positive reviews from patients' experiences with us are desirable, whereas negative reviews rarely are a source of joy. The increasing prevalence of social media is a powerful force with tentacles extending into the daily lives of millions. Beyond platforms such as Facebook, Instagram, Tiktok, Twitter, and others, many are immersed in sharing, comparing, and seeking likes and affirmations, which have no end.

Patient consumers often study online reviews posted by others. Patients who had posted "5-star" reviews on behalf of their surgeon and asked "why" said "bedside manner" was the most important factor. The surgeon's knowledge and honesty was second, followed by results. The corollary was that for patients rating a doctor only 1 star, the chief complaint was lack of bedside manner. Less-than-ideal results are placed fourth[36] (**Fig. 10**).

What other factors best correlated with "likelihood to recommend practice"? Patients' confidence in the care provider and the provider's concern for questions were tops.[37]

Patients were asked to submit via phone a photograph to their surgeon in the first 48 to 72 hours, and 96% said this enhanced their total surgical experience.[38]

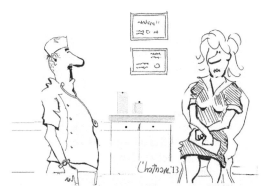

Fig. 10. "I want you to write a review, but only it it's 5-stars."

Social Media

Social media is both friend and foe. Surgical and procedural advice is easily obtained, and "Dr Google" is consulted for second opinions. Before and after photographs rarely show complications and exist in digital world free from discomfort, healing, and stress.

Comments made by others using online apps such as Instagram can have a profound effect especially when referring to the "appearance" of the poster and may lead to body dissatisfaction.

Regular exposure to social media posts focused on "fitspiration" (becoming more fit) and "thinspiration" (becoming thinner), leading to increased negative moods, also known as appearance comparison.

During the Covid pandemic, use of an image filter to change or enhance one's face also created anxiety when that person actually returned to work. Face-to-face encounters produced a "divergence" between the preferred "filtered face" and the actual "real face" and others likely noticed. "Snapchat dysmorphia," perhaps a form of BDD, refers to an obsessive preoccupation with one's looks using filters and imaging.[39]

"Zoom dysmorphia" is the condition of critiquing one's appearance after overuse of computer video conferencing and some seek changes in appearance. Patients may need reminding that the camera lens and distance may project a rounder face and broader nose that is not really accurate.[40]

Selfie face, also affected by camera optics, has been a factor in patients consulting surgeons[41] (Fig. 11).

In our society, women especially are "objectified" based on their appearance. Trying to comply with cultural standards of beauty and avoid judgments creates the stress of "body shaming." In addition, "appearance control" belief that humans are responsible for how they look and with

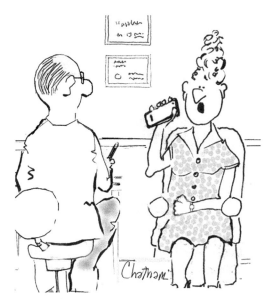

Fig. 11. "I thought my selfie face would look better!"

increased effort can control their appearance also leads to dissatisfaction.

BUT WHEN ALL ELSE FAILS...

There may be a time when we have exhausted all known personal resources with a patient who is dissatisfied or plain unhappy but demands something more. Sometimes it is best to terminate the relationship but we do not want to abandon a patient.

We might now determine whether another surgeon, hopefully a trusted one, might be helpful.

The conversation might become one of return of fees. Sometimes it may be easier to negotiate this as compared with ongoing headaches with a particular patient.[42] With candid communication with your medical liability insurance carrier, one can structure a document admitting to no deviation from the standard of care but documents a fee return for a more humanitarian reason and discourages an annoying legal experience.[43,44] This money can be money well spent.

Dismiss your patient only as a last resort, when no other recourse seems likely.

FINALLY

We seek to improve our clinical skills over our career, and thus should we learn to better our performance in the patient emotional and psychological realm. Skilled surgeons learn to meet the physical, emotional, and psychological needs of their various patients seeking advice from trusted colleagues, and learning from the experiences of others will benefit us and those whom we treat.[45]

Patient selection in aesthetic surgery is the ultimate inexact science, a mixture of surgical judgment, expertise, ego, gut feelings, personality interactions, and a spin of the roulette wheel. Using our procedural skills as well as our interpersonal skills will enhance our professional satisfaction and improve the quality of life for others as we try to reduce the likelihood of dissatisfaction, both for our patients and ourselves.

CLINICS CARE POINTS

- The evidence for pearls and pitfalls in this article are not traditional research-based studies or lab findings.
- Rather this is from actual patient experiences from a 37 year old private practice.
- Example: patient selection cannot be determined by specific answers to a questionnaire (objective) but rather by a combination of listening to a patient and using personal judgement skills (subjective).

REFERENCES

1. McCollough EG. The art of building a successful facial plastic surgery practice. Facial Plast Surg Clin North Am 2008;2(16):187–90. In: Chatham DR. ed. The difficult patient.
2. Patseavouras LL. The importance of staff in the facial plastic surgical practice: dynamic staff interface with the patients in support of the surgeons objectives. Facial Plast Surg Clin North Am 2008;16(2):191–4. In: Chatham DR. ed. The difficult patient.
3. Byrne P. The role of objective outcomes in surgery in overcoming cognitive dissonance. JAMA Facial Plast Surg 2016;18(3):163–4.
4. Hessler J, Moyer CA, Kim JC, et al. Predictors of satisfaction with facial plastic surgery: results of a prospective study. Arch Facial Plast Surg 2010;12:192–6.
5. Adamson PA, Strecker HD. Patient selection. Aesthetic Plast Surg 2002;26(Supp11):11.
6. Naraghi M, Atari M. Development and validation of the expectations of aesthetic rhinoplasty scale. Arch Plast Surg 2016;43(4):365–77.
7. VonSoest T, Kvalem IL, Roald HE, et al. The effects of cosmetic surgery on body image, self-esteem and psychological problems. J Plast Reconstruct Aesthet Surg 2009;62(10):1238–44.
8. Honigman TF, Phillips KA, Castle DJ. A review of psychosocial outcomes by patients seeking cosmetic surgery. Plast Reconstr Surg 2004;113(4):365–70, 1229 6;43(4).
9. Toni DP, Rossell SL, Tzimas N, et al. Assessing unrealistic expectations in clients undertaking minor cosmetic procedures: the development of the aesthetic procedure expectations scale. Facial Plast Surg Aesth Med 2021;23(4):263–9.
10. Kass LR. Ageless bodies, happy souls; biotechnology and the pursuit of perfection. Washington, D.C.: The New Atlantic; 2002. Spring.
11. Hom D. Enhancing the art of care during awake procedures, JAMA Facial Plast Verbal etiquette and practicing the art of giving comfort to those who seek our care will Pay huge rewards Surg. JAMA Facial Plast Surg 2015;12(1):5–6.
12. Gifford S. Cosmetic surgery and personality change: a review and some clinical observations. In: Goldwyn RM, editor. The unfavorable result in plastic surgery: avoidance and treatment. Boston: Little,Brown; 1972. p. 11–35.
13. Goin MK, Goin JM. Psychological effects of aesthetic facial surgery. Adv Psychosom Med 1986;15:84–108.
14. Gorney M. Mirror, mirror on the wall: the interface between illusion and reality in aesthetic surgery. Facial Plast Surg Clin North Am 2008;16(2):203–5. In: Chatham DR. ed. The difficult patient.
15. Ende KH, Lewis DL, Kabaker SS. Body dysmorphic disorder. Facial Plast Surg Clin North Am 2008;16(2):217–23. In: Chatham DR. ed. The difficult patient.
16. Constantian MB Childhood abuse, body shame, and addictive plastic surgery: the face of trauma. New York: Routledge; 2019.
17. Day J, Ishii M, Phillis M, et al. Body dysmorphic disorder in a facial plastic and reconstructive surgery clinic: measuring prevalence, assessing comorbidities, and validating a feasible screening. JAMA Facial Plast Surg 2015;17(2):137–43.
18. Goin J, Goin M. Changing the body: psychological effects of plastic surgery. Baltimore: Williams and Wilkins; 1981.
19. Anderson JP, Johnson C. A self-administered history questionnaire of cosmetic facial surgery candidates. Arch Otolaryngol 1978;104–89.
20. Terino E. Psychology of the aesthetic patient: the value of personality profile testing. Facial Plast Surg Clin North Am 2008;16(2):165–71. In: Chatham DR. ed. The difficult patient.
21. Spiegel JH. Challenges in care of the transgender patient seeking facial feminization surgery. Facial Plast Surg Clin North Am 2008;16(2):233–8. In: Chatham DR. ed. The difficult patient.
22. Chatham DR. It's a jungle out there survival guide for the facial plastic surgeon. Facial Plast Surg Clin North Am 2008;16(2):207–16. In: Chatham DR. ed. The difficult patient.
23. Tobin HA, Webster RC. The less-than-satisfactory rhinoplasty: comparison of patient and surgeon

satisfaction. Otolaryngol Head Neck Surg 1986;94: 86–95.

24. Gorney M, Martello J. Patient selection criteria: Medical legal issues in plastic surgery. Clin Plast Surg 1999;26:37–40.

25. Rodman R, Kridel R. A staging system for revision rhinoplasty A review. JAMA Facial Plast Surg 2016; 18(4):305–11. Available at: https://editorial.elsevier.com/app/login305-311.

26. Alasraff R, Larabee W, Anderson S, et al. Measuring facial plastic surgery outcomes: a pilot study. Arch Facial Plast Surg 2001;3(3):198–201.

27. Pusic A, Klassen AF, Scott AM, Cano SJ. Measuring outcomes that matter to facelift patients: development and validation of FACE-Q appearance appraisal : a new patient-reported outcome instrument for facial aesthetics patents. Clin Plast Surg 2013;40(2):249–60.

28. Klassen AF, Cano SJ, Eas CA, et al. Development and psychometric evaluation of the FACE-Q scales for patients undergoing rhinoplasty. JAMA Facial Plast Surg 2016;18(1):27–35.

29. Jacono A. Chastant RP. Dibelius G. Association of patient self-esteem with perceived outcome after face-lift surgery. published online October 29,29015. Facial Plast Surg. https://doi.org/10.1001/jamafaacial.2015.1460.

30. Stewart MG, Witsell DL, Smith TL, et al. Development and validation of the Nasal Obstruction Symptom Evaluation (NOSE) scale. Otolaryngol Head Neck Surg 2004;130(2):157–63.

31. Ioannidis JPA, Saltychev M, Most SP. The 10-Item Standardized Cosmesis and Health Nasal Outcomes Survey (SCHNOS) for Functional and Cosmetic Rhinoplasty. JAMA Facial Plast Surg 2018; 20(1):37–42. Moubayed Available at: https://pubmed.ncbi.nlm.nih.gov/28880988/SP.

32. Rohrich RJ. Mirror, mirror on the wall: when the postoperative reflection does not meet patients' expectations. Reconstr Surg 2001;108:507–9.

33. Sarwer DB. Psychological considerations in cosmetic surgery. In: Goldwyn DM, Cohen NN, editors. The unfavorable result in plastic surgery. Philadelphia: Lippincot Williamson & Williams; 2001. p. 14–23.

34. Wright MR. Management of patient dissatisfaction with results of cosmetic procedures. Arch Otolaryngo 1980;106:466–71.

35. Pfifferling JH. Healing he perfectionist surgeon. Facial Plast Surg Clin North Am 2008;16(2): 239–44. In: Chatham DR. Ed. The difficult patient.

36. Shemirani NL, Casrilliion J. Negative and positive online reviews of physicians-1 vs. 5 stars. JAMA Facial Plast Surg 2017;435–6.

37. Chen K, Congiusta S, Nash I, et al. Factors influencing patient satisfaction in plastic surgery: a nationwide analysis. Plast Reconstr Surg 2018; 142(3):820–5.

38. Dalla Pozza E, D'Souza G, DeLeonibus A, et al. Patient satisfaction with an early smartphone-based cosmetic surgery postoperative follow-up. Aesthe Surg J 2017;38(1):101–9.

39. Rajanalaa R, Maymone BC, Vashi NA. Selfies—living in the era of filtered photographs. JAMA Facial Plast Surg 2008;20(6):443–4.

40. Ric SM, Graber E, Kourish AS. A pandemic of dysmorphia: 'zooming' in the perception of our appearance. Facial Plast Surg Aesth Med 2020;22(6): 401–2.

41. 2019 survey from American Academy of Facial Plastic and Reconstructive Surgery. Available at: https://www.aafprs.org/Media/Press_Releases/Selfies%20Endure%20February%2027,%202020.aspx#:~:text=This%20year's%20results%20reveal%20that,%E2%80%93%20up%2015%25%20from%202018!.

42. Goode RL. The unhappy patient following facial plastic surgery: what to do? Facial Plast Surg Clin North Am 2008;16(2):183–6. In: Chatham DR. ed. The difficult patient.

43. Rhodes TW. Some legal thoughts on the unhappy patient. Facial Plast Surg Clin North Am 2008; 2(16):245–8. In: Chatham DR. ed. The difficult patient.

44. Gorney M. Claim's prevention for the aesthetic surgeon; preparing or the less-than-perfect outcome. Facial Plast Surg Clin North Am 2008;16(2): 2135–42. In: Chatham DR. Ed. The difficult patient.

45. Chatham DR. Essays on patient management and elective surgery. Facial Plast Surg Clin North Am 2008;16(2):259–65. In.Chatham DR, Ed.

Reducing Risks of Facial Scarring

David B. Hom, MD*, Jeffrey D. Bernstein, MD

KEYWORDS

- Facial scars • Prevention of scar • Scarring • Scar treatment • Facial plastics • Wound care • Face

KEY POINTS

- Many risk factors contribute to facial scarring which include wound healing status, surgical closure technique, evidence of infection, and post incisional care.
- Topical therapies for scar management such as silicone gel sheeting can be helpful adjuncts to mitigate the final appearance of the scar.
- Successful reduction in final scar appearance requires the proper surgical approach and medical treatment as determined by the individual patient and their scar.

INTRODUCTION

Tissue injury to the face carries a risk of scarring, which can have significant functional, social, and psychological implications for the patient.[1–3] Reducing facial scarring includes appropriate planning and care to reduce the risk of excessive scar formation. Management of facial scars involves a multifactorial approach with a host of preventive and treatment options. In this article, we outline the variety of scar types of the facial region. We discuss their etiology, describe the latest strategies for prevention, and highlight specific techniques to mitigate their final appearance.

Facial Scar Prevention: Identifying Risk Factors

Skin type

Skin type plays an important role in the formation an apparent scar.[4] Patients with Fitzpatrick types IV to VI (darker pigmentation) have a higher tendency for keloid scarring and hyperpigmentation. However, Fitzpatrick types I to III are more prone to hypopigmentation.[5] Certain ethnicities have a higher tendency of scarring: African Americans, Hispanics, Asians, and patients of Mediterranean origin have a higher risk of keloid formation.[5]

Facial scar location

Certain facial sites have a higher tendency to scar, often due to tension with facial expressions. The area of the jawline and the hair-bearing areas of the face have a higher tendency for hypertrophic scar and keloid formation.[6] In contrast, central sites on the face, nose, and upper lip have a lower tendency for keloid formation.[6]

Medical conditions

The propensity to form an excessive scar can be related to several medical conditions. Normal scar formation is contingent upon a delicate balance in wound healing. This balance exists between an initial controlled inflammatory response to combat infection and attenuation of this inflammatory process for the remaining wound healing cascade to continue. In some instances, excessive inflammation can be caused by a prolonged infection and foreign body reaction. Patients who are planned to have elective surgery should be screened for a tendency for scarring in their medical history.

Any medical condition that contributes to slower wound healing increases the risks of excessive scarring. These factors include older age, compromised immune status, collagen-vascular disease, chronic cardiopulmonary conditions, vascular,

Department of Otolaryngology–Head and Neck Surgery, University of California - San Diego, 200 West Arbor Drive, Mail Code 8895, San Diego, CA 92103, USA
* Corresponding author.
E-mail address: Dbhom@health.ucsd.edu

Facial Plast Surg Clin N Am 31 (2023) 195–207
https://doi.org/10.1016/j.fsc.2023.01.003
1064-7406/23/© 2023 Elsevier Inc. All rights reserved.

hepatic disease, diabetes, hypothyroidism, malnutrition, vitamin deficiency, tobacco and alcohol use, prior radiation treatments, a patient taking systemic steroids or chemotherapy, and the presence of psychiatric disease or other life stressors that may affect healing. Patients who have hyper-elastic joints are more prone to scarring due to increased elastin in the dermis.[7] This condition can be shown if the patient can bend their thumb to their forearm or touch their tongue to their nose (Gorlin's sign)[8] (Fig. 1). A patient's nutritional state affects wound healing, which influences scarring. A serum albumin of less than 2.5 can indicate a protein deficiency, which impairs wound healing and increases scar risk. Regarding radiation treatments, a threshold of >50 Gy has been associated with slower healing and greater complications.[9,10] A medication history should also be reviewed with consideration for chemotherapeutics, immunosuppressants, anticoagulants, antiplatelets, and steroids, as these all may delay wound healing and increase the risk of pathologic scar formation.

To optimize healing, a patient should stop using tobacco products for at least 4 weeks, aspirin, or aspirin-related products for at least 2 weeks. Nicotine decreases dermal perfusion, thus increasing the risk of skin breakdown due to its vasoconstrictive effects and damage to small vessels. For a patient taking isotretinoin (Accutane) for acne treatment, it is routinely advised that elective resurfacing procedures such as dermabrasion, deep chemical peels, and laser resurfacing should be postponed for at least 1 year after discontinuing this medication. This is based on the understanding that isotretinoin can delay re-epithelialization of a partial thickness dermal wound. However, this practice is now a topic of debate. A 2017 systemic review of 1485 cases found insufficient evidence to support delaying procedures in patients taking isotretinoin, with the exception of mechanical dermabrasion and ablative laser procedures.[11] Further research into how isotretinoin effects scarring is warranted.

Typically, a scar matures over a 6- to 12-month period after wounding. The strength of the scar will plateau to only 80% of the original strength of the skin. The remodeling phase of the scar is more prolonged in children with increased scar erythema and hypertrophy.

Pitfall: mistaken diagnosis
If a scar forms spontaneously, without a clear history of trauma, one should hold the suspicion that other pathologic conditions could be present. Malignant skin cancers can occur in facial scars (Fig. 2A–E). Clinically, when a scar has atypical features including, but not limited to ulceration, bleeding, fixation to underlying tissues, or a poor response to scar therapies, a biopsy should be performed to rule out malignancy.

Reducing Surgical Risks for Scarring

Surgical planning
Risk of scarring can be reduced by appropriate surgical planning. Use of the atraumatic and aseptic techniques is essential, along with diligent control of hemostasis without excess tissue thermal injury. It is important to titrate electrocautery settings to match the tissue sensitivity and thickness. Incisions should then be designed with the goal of having the least amount of tension possible on the final wound closure. In the face, this involves making incisions parallel with the relaxed skin tension lines (RSTLs). RSTLs are readily identified by pinching the skin perpendicular to the lines of tension. If the maximum tension vector on the incision approaches 90° to the incision, this can result in a wider scar. In addition, incisions may be more camouflaged when made within the boundaries of the facial subunits (Fig. 3). Incisions should be planned to lie within well-formed RSTLs or within the transition borders of esthetic facial subunits, such as the nasal ala or nasolabial fold.

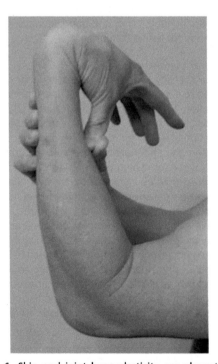

Fig. 1. Skin and joint hyperelasticity are phenotypic traits associated with an increased risk of scarring. This may be suspected if the patient can bend their thumb to their forearm or touch or touch their tongue to the nose (Gorlin's sign).

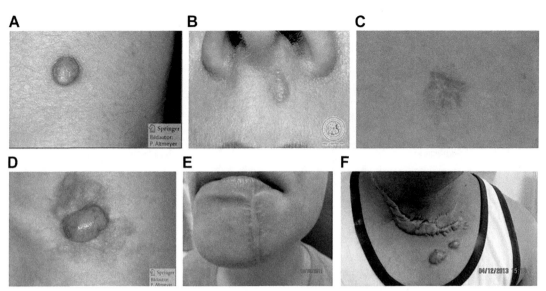

Fig. 2. Skin lesions can mimic scars. (*A*) Dermatofibroma. (*B*) Scar sarcoidosis. (*C*) Basal cell carcinoma. (*D*) Derma-tofibrosarcoma protuberans. (*E*) Hypertrophic scar. (*F*) Keloid scar. (*From* Hom DB. Pearls and Pitfalls in Scar Management. In: Thomas JR, Hom DB, editors. Facial Scars: Surgical Revision and Treatments. Shelton, CT: PMPH USA; 2019. p 222; with permission. (Figure 24-1 in original)).

Skin closure

When electively excising skin lesions using a fusiform shape, the apex angles should be 30° or less to minimize dog ear formation. Wide tissue undermining should be used to loosen the surrounding dermis to allow for more skin laxity for closure. This laxity will reduce tension on the wound and reduce scar widening. In addition, a layered closure with buried dermal anchor sutures in a halving technique will help relieve tension on the surface of a wound. In regard to cutaneous closure, running subcuticular sutures, fine running, or interrupted sutures can be used for surface skin closure. If the edges are very well apposed and aligned, one can consider applying a cyanoacrylate (skin tissue glue) to seal the incision instead of fine skin sutures. When closing skin, the epidermis should come together gently at the same level without step-offs and be free from tension. When making incisions or scar excisions in the scalp, incisions should be beveled and angled, such that hair follicles can later grow through the incision and disguise the scar (**Fig. 4**).

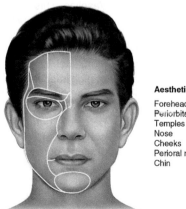

Aesthetic facial subunits

Forehead
Periorbital region
Temples
Nose
Cheeks
Perioral region
Chin

Fig. 3. The boundaries of the aesthetic facial subunits are useful locations to disguise scars to reduce their final appearance. (*From* Hom DB. Preoperative Scar Analysis and Planning. In: Thomas JR, Hom DB, editors. Facial Scars: Surgical Revision and Treatments. Shelton, CT: PMPH USA; 2019. p 94; with permission. (Figure 10-1 in original)).

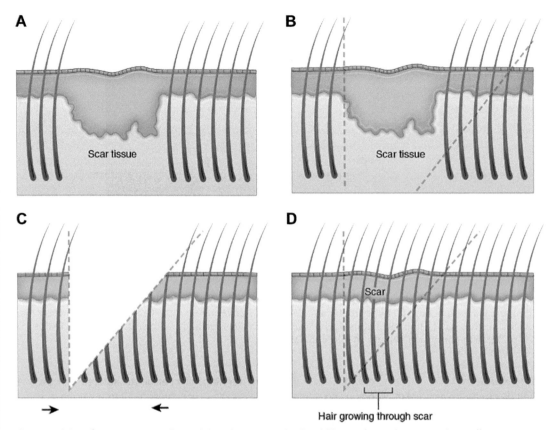

Fig. 4. Incisions for scar revision through hair-bearing scalp should be performed at an angle to allow for hair to grow through the scar and disguise its final appearance. (*A*) Scar tissue disrupts the hairline. (*B*) Planned angled incision through hair-bearing region. (*C*) Excised tissue with closure vectors to approximate hair-bearing regions. (*D*) Final closure with hair growing through the scar. (*From* Rousso DE, Kim Sw. Scar Revision in Hair-Bearing Areas. In: Thomas JR, Hom DB, editors. Facial Scars: Surgical Revision and Treatments. Shelton, CT: PMPH USA; 2019. p 151; with permission. (Figure 18-1 in original).)

Traumatic wounds

In a traumatic skin laceration, the risk of excessive scar formation is increased in a dirty wound environment, where excessive inflammation and delayed healing contribute to poor results. A contaminated wound with debris or bacteria will produce a prolonged inflammatory response and is more likely to produce an unsightly scar. This can be avoided with copious irrigation with sterile saline and/or dilute iodine solution, an important first step for the closure of nonsterile wounds. A wound with irregular edges can be conservatively freshened with a 15-blade scalpel. Attention to hemostasis and the placement of drains, when appropriate, can reduce the risk of hematoma and seroma formation, reducing subsequent infection risk.[12]

Wound care recommendations to reduce scarring

Keeping a wound clean and moist with ointments has been shown to promote re-epithelialization and enhance incision closure.[13] Following closure, wounds should be regularly cleansed with gentle soap and water, then dressed with non-antibacterial ointments, such as derivatives of Vaseline. This therapy should continue for weeks following the surgery or trauma. Antibiotics are routinely overprescribed and should be reserved only for cases in which the risk of infection is high, such as in dirty, traumatic wounds. In cases of high infection risk, a standard 7- to 10-day antibiotic course with close clinical follow-up is recommended. Skin cleansers such as hydrogen peroxide, betadine, Hibiclens (chlorhexidine gluconate 4%), or rubbing alcohol can be used acutely, but not chronically over an incision, as these increase the risk of cellular damage and increase inflammation. Applying a surgical dressing as needed to absorb exudate and reduce the risk of further trauma to the area can be helpful.

In the weeks following tissue injury, additional care recommendations should be followed. Wounds should be protected from excessive sun exposure with occlusive clothing or sunblock (>30 Sun Protection Factor with Ultraviolet A / B protection) starting 1 month after surgical incision closure for a 6-month duration to prevent scar hyperpigmentation.

If a scar seems to be indurated, manually massaging in a circular motion 3 to 4 times per day starting 1-month post-closure can help break up scar tissue. For immature or otherwise discolored scars in the postsurgical period, makeup can help camouflage their appearance. The principle of the color wheel can be followed: to disguise a shade, the opposite side of the wheel should be applied (**Fig. 5**). For example, a light green shade will hide erythema, whereas a yellow shade will hide ecchymoses.

Common Scar Types of the Head and Neck

Hypertrophic scar/widened scar

A hypertrophic scar is one which has proliferated to a size larger than expected for the wound, without extending beyond its original wound margins. These may be widened or raised in appearance, be darkened or reddened, and have an uncomfortable texture for the patient. Most often forming weeks following tissue injury, the incidence of hypertrophic scar is common, cited in as high as 39% to 68% of cases.[14] Hypertrophic scars may increase in size rapidly for 3 to 6 months,

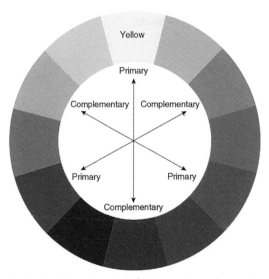

Fig. 5. Applying the color of makeup located opposite the color wheel from the undesired skin hue will best disguise the healing scar. (*From* Lam K, Sidle D: Cosmetics, Hairstyles and Facial Accessories for Scar Camouflage. In: Thomas JR, Hom DB, editors. Facial Scars: Surgical Revision and Treatments. Shelton, CT: PMPH USA; 2019. p 233; with permission. (Figure 25-1 in original).)

then begin to regress or fade as the scar matures. Complete maturation can take up to 2 years. The most common cause of hypertrophic scar is excessive tension placed upon a surgical wound. Common sites are convex areas of the face such as cheeks, forehead, chin, nasal tip, or sites of high tension and movement. These scars are not typically seen within RSTLs or at the intersection points between the facial subunits, such as the nasolabial fold. Unlike a Keloid scar, a hypertrophic scar may spontaneously regress (**Fig. 6**).

Keloid scar

Keloid scar is characterized by scar tissue overgrowth beyond the boundaries of the original wound. This aggressive, fibroproliferative scar is composed of whorls of thick, hyalinized collagen and a raised epidermis.[15] The most common sites of occurrence in the head and neck are the external ear, followed by the submental/submandibular region.[6,16] Risk of keloid scarring is greatest in areas of high tension and movement, whereas keloid risk in the central face is much less. Unlike hypertrophic scars, which typically appear within 1 month of injury, keloid scarring can appear up to 1 year after injury and frequently will not spontaneously regress. These scars tend to occur more frequently in patients with Fitzpatrick skin types IV to VI, patients who have a prior history of keloid scarring, and in patients of Asian, African, Mediterranean, and Hispanic descent.

Operative planning for a patient with a tendency to form keloid scars involves choosing the most conservative incision to limit scar formation and keeping all nonessential surgical incisions to a minimum. As always, a wound closure without tension and well-approximated edges are ideal to help reduce the risk of keloid scarring. During wound closure, prolonged inflammation should be minimized by selecting a monofilament synthetic suture. One month later, silicone gel or sheet can be considered.

Raised scar/trapdoor deformity

The trapdoor or "pincushion" scar has a characteristic raised appearance. This type of scar forms following a curved shaped incision, by which scar contracture and inadequate lymphatic drainage lead to a raised appearance of the skin. Like a hypertrophic scar, a trapdoor scar also has a propensity of developing on the convex areas of the face. Fortunately, this can be minimized by wide tissue undermining and proper incision planning. Use of straight-line or angulated planned incisions rather than curved incisions is helpful to minimize trapdoor deformity. If a rounded incision cannot be avoided, multiple Z-plasties can be used 6 months

Hypertrophic Scar   Keloid

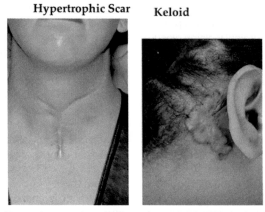

Fig. 6. Hypertrophic scar (*left*) may be mistaken for keloid scar (*right*); these can be differentiated clinically by their growth pattern and by histology. (*From* Hom DB. Preoperative Scar Analysis and Planning. In: Thomas JR, Hom DB, editors. Facial Scars: Surgical Revision and Treatments. Shelton, CT: PMPH USA; 2019. p 95; with permission. (Figure 10-3 in original)).

later to redistribute the scar contracture and minimize the trap door deformity (**Fig. 7**).

Discolored scar/hypo- and hyperpigmented scar

In normal scarring, scars usually fade to a slightly lighter shade than the patient's skin tone. Hypo- or hyperpigmentation is hypothesized to occur because of damage to the basal dermal layer. With the disruption of the tissue, migration of melanocytes into scar tissue is reduced, and melanin precursors within migratory melanocytes may be up- or downregulated, producing the characteristic appearance.[17] Hyperpigmented scars may be significantly darker or reddened, standing out and contributing to poor cosmesis, whereas hypopigmented scars will be pale, and more noticeable on patients with naturally darker skin. Hypopigmented scars will be most noticeable in heavily sun-exposed areas. This type of scar may be reduced by instructing patients to avoid excessive direct sun exposure of the scar for up to 6 months after surgery, apply daily sun protection cream (SPF 30+), and use protective clothing or an occlusive dressing. This advice is especially important in Fitzpatrick IV-VI patients.

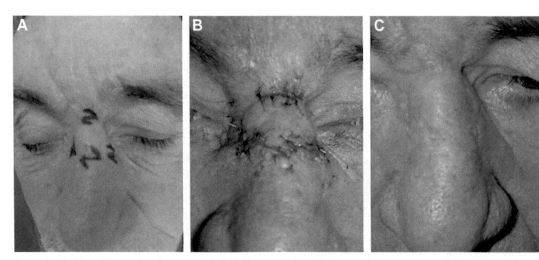

Fig. 7. Multiple Z-plasties for flattening trapdoor scar. Z-plasty design with concentric Z-plasties on a patient's nose to smooth out a trap door deformity from a paramedian forehead island ski flap. (*A*) Preoperative photo with planned Z-plasty markings. (*B*) Immediate postoperative photo with four Z-plasties performed. (*C*) 6-month postoperative visit. (*From* Hom DB. Preoperative Scar Analysis and Planning. In: Thomas JR, Hom DB, editors. Facial Scars: Surgical Revision and Treatments. Shelton, CT: PMPH USA; 2019. p 101; with permission. (Figure 10-12 in original).)

General Principles for Management of Facial Scars

Setting expectations for scar revision
In evaluating the patient with scarring, it is important to first determine which parameters of the scar are most bothersome (eg, color, contour, shape, tightness, and raised appearance). The patient may have different priorities from the surgeon about what bothers them most. Determining what the patient desires from scar revision (eg, improving appearance, maximizing function, and/ or relieving pruritis or pain) is important to make sure their goals are realistic and obtainable. The patient should be counseled that the goal of scar revision is not to erase the scar but to make it less noticeable. There are advantages and disadvantages to every approach; the goals of the patient and the goals of the surgeon should correlate as closely as possible to achieve the best-desired result (**Table 1**).

Classifying the severity of the scar can help both patient and provider establish realistic expectations for the outcome. The authors prefer using a 5-step severity scale (**Box 1**). A more severe scar deformity will have more difficulty attaining improved levels of scar appearance. Often, scar revision procedures can improve the degree of appearance by one to two steps on this scale. An additional step can be obtained with the use of camouflage makeup.

Approaches to scar management are outlined in **Fig. 8**.

Medical Therapy

Steroid injection
Injections of corticosteroids are a popular first-line adjunct to surgical scar revision. Serial steroid injections help to treat raised or contracted scars by reducing the proliferation of fibroblasts, reducing collagen formation, and softening or loosening the tension surrounding a scar.[18] Steroids are often more effective for treating early scars rather than mature scars, but can be used in any setting. For prevention in cases of recurrent hypertrophic or keloid scar, treatment may be offered in the weeks following surgery with an intralesional injection of triamcinolone acetonide (Kenalog; Bristol–Myers Squibb; 10 to 40 mg/mL) within the scar without going beyond its borders. Injections typically occur at 3- to 4-week intervals, with a duration of therapy dependent on observed response. Although easily administered and cost-effective, steroid injections require multiple treatments and may not entirely resolve the scar. Other potential side effects include telangiectasia, hypopigmentation, ulceration, or skin thinning.[19]

Topical treatments
Topical treatment of scar reduction is a widely used approach due to its high accessibility, ease of use, and relatively low cost compared with more invasive treatment. Scar massage, with or without the use of ointments such as Vaseline, silicone gel, Vitamin E, or a combination thereof has been the subject of limited studies showing varying efficacy.[20,21] Due to the lack of high-quality data, no single widely-accepted treatment paradigm has been consistently recommended, however, silicone gel/sheeting has the most evidence-based support to reduce scarring by, topical treatment.

For treating a hyperpigmented or reddened scar, topical hydroquinone may be used to lighten tissue. Common side effects include contact dermatitis and inflammatory reactions causing worsened pigment changes.

Silicone sheeting and gel
Silicone sheeting or gel is a simple and effective treatment for treating a scar. An occlusive silicone gel sheet is applied directly to the wound after re-epithelialization has occurred and then worn for 12 to 18 h per day for several months. Silicone topical treatment has been hypothesized to work in various ways: by reducing tissue water loss and increasing tissue hydration, by modulating the fibroblast and cytokine milieu, and by reducing keratinocyte activity.[19] For keloid scar, silicone gel sheeting can reduce scar thickness, improve discoloration, and reduce pain and pruritis.[22–25] In addition, silicone gel sheeting may reduce the incidence of keloid and hypertrophic scar formation in patients who are prone to pathologic scarring.[25] Silicone gel ointments can be used postoperatively if sheeting is not feasible.

Common adverse effects of silicone sheeting and silicone gel are temporary and include skin irritation and skin breakdown from prolonged occlusion. Drawbacks of this therapy include the inconvenience of wearing a daily dressing. Compliance with therapy may prove challenging, especially in sensitive areas of the face where a daily dressing may not be practical, such as the lips or eyelids.

Wound taping
The use of surgical nonstretch tape to aid in wound healing is an inexpensive adjunct to surgery and medical therapy. Nonstretch tape, such as flesh-colored Micropore, is applied by the patient perpendicular to the wound daily. Taping works to counteract the mechanical forces which may stretch or widen the wound and cause a hypertrophic scar. A recent review reported that taping could reduce scar height, reduce the incidence of abnormal scar color, improve pruritis, and significantly reduce

Table 1
Measures to prevent and reduce scars

Therapy	Advantages	Disadvantages
Surgical excision	Excess scar removed	High recurrence without adjuvant therapy, cost
Surgical lengthening (Z-plasty and W-plasty)	Increased mobility and range of motion	Some excess scar persists, occasionally worse cosmesis
Steroid intralesional Injection	Cost, ease	Multiple treatments; telangiectasia hypopigmentation
Silicone gel sheeting	Cost, ease of use, noninvasive	Difficulty application on the head, neck across joints
Pressure therapy	Noninvasive, some proven efficacy	Cumbersome facial garments, cost high if custom-made, and constant use for months to years. Perception in public
Radiation after surgery	Some proven efficacy	Risk of carcinogenesis, cost
Laser	Pulsed dye 585 nm laser best for decreasing red color; Carbon dioxide, Nd:YAG, pulsed Erb: YAG lasers have some reported efficacy	Cost, multiple treatments, emerging technology
Cryotherapy	Some proven efficacy in keloid reduction	Hypopigmentations, pain, skin atrophy
Microporous tape	Ease, low cost	Keeping tape on the skin
Popular over-the-counter topical treatments: (vitamin E, onion extract, and other plant creams)	Ease, low cost	No proven benefits
Physical therapy treatments: ultrasound, pulsed electrical stimulation, Hydrotherapy, massage	Patient participation-increase joint range of motion; can decrease scar pain, pruritus	No quantitative proven efficacy, cost
Anti-inflammatory/proliferative medication injections(interferons,5-fluorouracil,bleomycin, mitomycin)	Early controlled studies report success	Emerging therapy, indications are still being determined
Dermabrasion	Lower costs	Operator-dependent, aerosolization of blood

From Hom DB. Preoperative Scar Analysis and Planning. In: Thomas JR, Hom DB, editors. Facial Scars: Surgical Revision and Treatments. Shelton, CT: PMPH USA; 2019. p 97; with permission. (Table 10-5 in original).

median scar width.[26] This treatment approach is favorable for its low cost, minimal side effects, and potential for improving outcomes. The greatest potential drawback of tape therapy is the need for daily compliance. Placing tape on highly visible regions of the face may make some patients uncomfortable and less compliant with this approach. Other potential side effects include local reactions to adhesives.

Pressure therapy

Similar to silicone sheeting, pressure therapy works by compressing tissue for many months to reduce the final scar appearance. It has been shown to be successful in the management of keloid scars.[27] Consistent pressure on the skin leads to dermal thinning, reduction of blood flow and oxygen, and a hypoxic environment with less edema. Compression reduces fibroblast activity as well as levels of scar-inducing cytokines.[28] Downsides of compression therapy are patient discomfort, patient appearance, and the cost associated with more elaborate compression devices.

Dermabrasion

Dermabrasion is a mechanical skin-resurfacing technique used to blend and topically smooth

---

Box 1
Five-step rating for appearance of facial scars

Excellent

Good

Average

Deformity

Gross disfigurement

---

out existing scars with the surrounding skin. This could be best used on uneven surfaces, such as hypertrophic, discolored, or raised scars. Importantly, this technique is not suited for keloid scar, as it may cause severe recurrence. For dermabrasion, wire brushes, sandpaper, or diamond fraise brushes are used to smooth the upper layers of the skin, removing the epidermis and papillary dermis to a depth no deeper than the superficial reticular layer (when collagen stranding is visible). The local tissue injury creates a fresh wound which then produces new collagen and epithelium with a more favorable appearance.[29,30] Optimal re-epithelialization occurs over the partial thickness wound by keeping the wound continuously moist. Light dermabrasion can be considered 6 weeks after the incision.

Complications include acute facial reddening, worsened scars (if the plane of dissection is too deep), or delayed hyperpigmentation. This can be mitigated by regular use of sun protection (>SPF 30) after full re-epithelialization. Risk of complications may be higher in females taking birth control pills or hormonal medications due to associated pigmentary changes. In addition, patients of Asian ethnicity, among others, may be at increased risk for pigmentary changes with dermabrasion. In patients with Fitzpatrick IV to VI skin, one could consider doing a test dermabrasion treatment in an inconspicuous region (eg, behind the ear) to ensure pigmentary changes would not likely occur.

Cryotherapy

Cryotherapy involves freezing the lesion to stimulate a favorable healing response. Although topical cryotherapy has been less successful for scar management, multiple small studies have had promising results in treating hypertrophic and keloid scars with intralesional cryotherapy.[31] Performed under local anesthetic, intralesional cryotherapy uses a microneedle cooled with liquid nitrogen to freeze the lesion from the inside. It is best performed on pedunculated lesions with a narrow base, to minimize trauma to surrounding tissues. Side effects include pain, recurrence, slow healing, and temporary hypopigmentation of nearby tissues.

Radiation

For the treatment of severe, recalcitrant keloid scarring, radiation therapy is the most aggressive adjunctive option. Under the direction of a trained practitioner, external beams of high-energy particles are aimed at the affected area with 1 cm margins and a depth of 0.5 to 1 cm. Recommended dosages range from 12 to 20 Gy delivered in 1 to 3 fractions over 5 to 7 days. Local tissue inflammation may occur, causing irritation, reddening, desquamation, edema, and necrosis. Delayed complications include dermatitis, fibrosis, impaired wound healing, pigment change, and a theoretic risk of delayed carcinogenesis of the tissues, including the salivary glands. Rates of recurrence after surgical excision plus radiation therapy, or after radiation alone have been reported to be 22% to 37%, respectively, with rates of recurrence as low as 12% for keloids of the ear.[32] Although effective, the risk and cost profile of radiation therapy reserve this modality for only the most severe or refractory cases of keloid scarring.

Surgical scar revision

After allotting 6 to 12 months to allow the scar to fully mature, surgical scar revision may be considered. In some instances, scar revision may be performed as early as 3 months; however, this is typically reserved for cases of functional compromise, such as ectropion, lip retraction, or nasal alar contraction. Revision techniques will differ depending on the goals for treatment. Before the revision, the diagnosis of keloid scarring should be ruled out for risk of negative outcome. Simple scar excision can be performed by either fusiform excision of the mature scar, by lengthening and redirecting the mature scar to improve tension on the wound, or by breaking up an elongated scar.

Management of Common Scar Types

Hypertrophic scar

For simple hypertrophic scars, a fusiform excision with wide tissue undermining and a layered closure can be used. This technique may also be used for scars that are too wide, scars with misaligned edges, and scars lying within RSTLs. As stated above, the apices of the fusiform incision should be 30° or less to prevent a dog ear.

If scar reorientation, scar lengthening, or effacement of scar webbing is required, Z-plasty techniques can be very helpful to redirect tension vectors to lie within the RSTLs. This technique creates two triangular flaps, which are transposed to rotate and lengthen the scar, placing it more favorably within the RSTL. This serves the dual purpose of reducing wound tension and risk of hypertrophic scar while also camouflaging the scar by disrupting its linear configuration (**Fig. 9**A–C). Repositioning the scar allows for the scar to fall more within the normal skin creases, behind the hair-bearing areas, or within the boundaries of the facial subunits, making it less apparent.

If revising an elongated scar, one can consider multiple Z-plasties, a W-plasty, or a geometric closure. The W-plasty and geometric closure can flatten and break up a long scar into multiple smaller patterns. This makes the scar look more irregular and less apparent (**Figs. 10** and **11**).

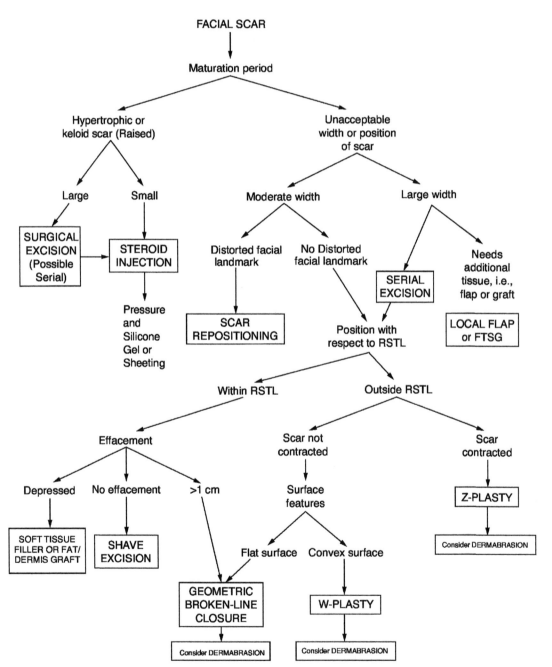

Fig. 8. Algorithm for the systematic approach to scar revision. (*Adapted from* Thomas JR: Dermabrasion and Scar Treatment. In: Thomas JR, Hom DB, editors. Facial Scars: Surgical Revision and Treatments. Shelton, CT: PMPH USA; 2019. p 104; with permission. (Figure 11-1 in original).)

A

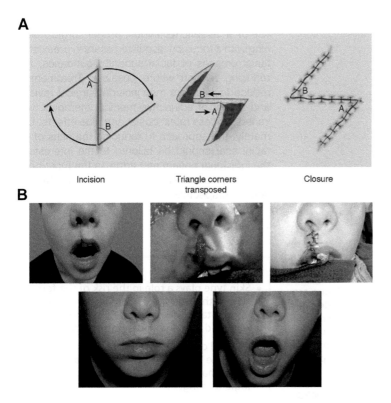

Incision   Triangle corners   Closure
                  transposed

B

Fig. 9. (*A*) Z-plasty principle for linear scar reorientation by triangular flap transposition. The scar being excised is the vertical central limb of the Z. The angles of the lateral limbs can be 30°, 45°, and 60°, thus lengthening the vertical axis by 25%, 50%, and 75%, respectively. (*B*) Example of a patient with a retracted upper lip scar who underwent two serial Z-plasties to excise and lengthen scar, with postoperative results 1 year. (*From* [*A*] Thomas JR, Hom DB: Z-plasty. In: Thomas JR, Hom DB, editors. Facial Scars: Surgical Revision and Treatments. Shelton, CT: PMPH USA; 2019. p 113; with permission. (Figure 13-1 in original); [*B*] Thomas JR, Hom DB: Z-plasty. In: Thomas JR, Hom DB, editors. Facial Scars: Surgical Revision and Treatments. Shelton, CT: PMPH USA; 2019. p 118; with permission. (Figure 13-15 in original)).

Keloid scar

Owing to the high rate of recurrence and the need for prolonged treatments, the management of keloid scar presents a significant challenge. Typical scar revision techniques do not apply to keloids as they could make the keloid worsen in its growth pattern. In treating patients with keloids, one should prioritize addressing both symptoms (pain, pruritis) and appearance. Because rates of recurrence are so high, patients should be counseled that the goals of treatment are to control rather than cure. Historically, successfully treated cases have used a multimodality strategy to address this type of scar.

If surgical excision of a keloid is planned, priority should be made in reducing skin tension and mitigating the inflammatory tissue response, and consider placing incisions within the keloid border. Care must be taken to properly align wound edges, reduce wound dead space, and use

A   **B**   **C**

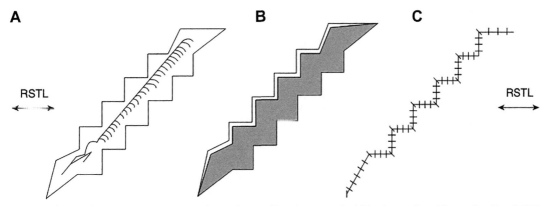

RSTL   RSTL

Fig. 10. (*A*) A W-plasty zig-zag incision is planned to realign the wound within the resting skin tension line (RSTL). (*B*) The defect after excision. (*C*) The closure creates a zig-zag pattern to modify the skin contractile forces and break up the linear scar into smaller scars. (*From* Thomas JR, Hom DB: W-plasty. In: Thomas JR, Hom DB, editors. Facial Scars: Surgical Revision and Treatments. Shelton, CT: PMPH USA; 2019. p 126; with permission. (Figure 14-1 in original)).

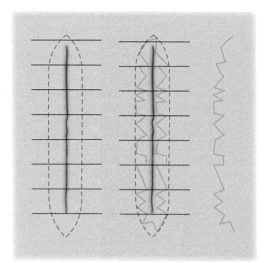

Fig. 11. Geometric broken line closure. Irregular, matching geometric edges measuring 5 to 7 mm are excised to make the scar irregular and to provide camouflage. (*From* Thomas JR: Geometric Broken Line Closure (GLBC) and Scar Revision. In: Thomas JR, Hom DB, editors. Facial Scars: Surgical Revision and Treatments. Shelton, CT: PMPH USA; 2019. p 132; with permission. (Figure 15-1 in original).)

monofilament sutures such as prolene, polydioxanone (PDS), or monocryl. Any area with excised tissue is prone to form a keloid, potentially compounding, rather than alleviating the issue. As such, the best strategy is for the most conservative excision possible. Adjuvant therapy, such as steroid injection, should be considered along with surgical excision, as rates of recurrence of keloid with surgery alone have been reported ranging from 45% to 100%.[33] If adjuvant therapy is planned, a steroid injection can be done at the time of excision or after waiting 1 month until the wound is further healed to decrease the risk of wound dehiscence. Postoperatively, silicone sheeting or gel for 6 months should be considered to reduce regrowth, along with serial steroid injections every 4 to 6 weeks over several months.

Discolored scar
Hypo- or hyperpigmented scars may be surgically excised to allow for more favorable healing. Patients should be thoroughly counseled on the risks of developing a pigmented scar with exposure to UV light. Hypopigmented scars will often be amenable to conservative concealment with makeup; however, more permanent solutions, such as tattooing may be used.

SUMMARY

The consequences of facial scarring should be considered during any surgical treatment of the

head or neck. Primary prevention includes the use of an aseptic technique, proper surgical planning with a focus on disguising scars in preexisting facial creases or facial subunit boundaries, and reducing tension where possible. Treatment to reduce facial scars may include surgical revision and a host of adjunctive medical therapies, with varied success rates, costs, and side effects. Ultimately, the approach to reducing the risks of the facial scar should be tailored to the interests of the individual patient and address the most bothersome characteristics of the scar from the patient's perspective.

CLINICS CARE POINTS

- Skin type plays a role in the risk of the formation of the scar; lighter skin is prone to hypopigmentation, whereas darker skin is prone to keloid scar and hyperpigmentation.

- Medical conditions that delay wound healing decrease collagen formation or cause excess inflammation to increase the risk of pathologic scarring.

- The risk of scar can be mitigated with proper surgical planning including designing incisions within the resting skin tension lines or boundaries of facial subunits.

- Surgical scar revision uses a variety of techniques including Z-plasty, W-plasty, and Geometric Closure to camouflage existing scars.

- Some nonsurgical treatments for scar revision include steroid injection, wound taping, dermabrasion, and silicone gel sheeting.

DISCLOSURE

The authors have nothing to disclose.

REFERENCES

1. Chu EA, Farrag TY, Ishii LE, et al. Threshold of Visual Perception of Facial Asymmetry in a Facial Paralysis Model. Arch Facial Plast Surg 2011;13(1):14–9.
2. Wang TT, Wessels L, Hussain G, et al. Discriminative Thresholds in Facial Asymmetry: A Review of the Literature. Aesthetic Surg J 2017;37(4):375–85.
3. Price P, Tebble N. Psychological Consequences of Facial Scarring. In: Téot L, Banwell PE, Ziegler UE, editors. Surgery in wounds. Berlin Heidelberg: Springer; 2004. p. 519–26.
4. Visscher MO, Bailey JK, Hom DB. Scar Treatment Variations by Skin Type. Facial Plastic Surgery Clinics of North America 2014;22(3):453–62.

5. Girardeau-Hubert S, Pageon H, Asselineau D. In vivo and in vitro approaches in understanding the differences between Caucasian and African skin types: specific involvement of the papillary dermis. Int J Dermatol 2012;51:1–4.

6. Wang JC, Fort CL, Hom DB. Location Propensity for Keloids in the Head and Neck. Facial Plast Surg Aesthet Med 2021;23(1):59–64. https://doi.org/10.1089/fpsam.2020.0106.

7. Thomas JR, Hom DB. Facial scars: surgical revision and treatment. May 2019.

8. Scar revision and local flap refinement. Local Flaps in Facial. In: Leake D, Baker S, editors. Reconstruction 2007;723–60.

9. Payne WG, Naidu DK, Wheeler CK, et al. Wound healing in patients with cancer. Eplasty 2008;8:e9.

10. Hom DB, Odland RM. Prognosis for facial scarring. Surgical techniques for cutaneous scar revision. Boca Raton, FL, USA: CRC Press; 2000. p. 47–60.

11. Spring LK, Krakowski AC, Alam M, et al. Isotretinoin and Timing of Procedural Interventions: A Systematic Review With Consensus Recommendations. JAMA Dermatology 2017;153(8):802–9.

12. Welshhans JL, Hom DB. Soft tissue principles to minimize scarring: an overview. Facial Plast Surg Clin 2017;25(1):1–13.

13. Junker JPE, Kamel RA, Caterson EJ, et al. Clinical Impact Upon Wound Healing and Inflammation in Moist, Wet, and Dry Environments. Adv Wound Care 2013;2(7):348–56.

14. Niessen FB, Spauwen PH, Schalkwijk J, et al. On the nature of hypertrophic scars and keloids: a review. Plast Reconstr Surg 1999;104(5):1435–58.

15. Berman B, Bieley HC. Adjunct Therapies to Surgical Management of Keloids. Dermatol Surg 1996;22(2):126–30.

16. Lindsey WH, Davis PT. Facial Keloids: A 15-Year Experience. Arch Otolaryngol Head Neck Surg 1997;123(4):397–400.

17. Carney BC, Chen JH, Luker JN, et al. Pigmentation Diathesis of Hypertrophic Scar: An Examination of Known Signaling Pathways to Elucidate the Molecular Pathophysiology of Injury-Related Dyschromia. J Burn Care Res 2018;40(1):58–71.

18. Jalali M, Bayat A. Current use of steroids in management of abnormal raised skin scars. Surgeon 2007;5(3):175–80.

19. Thomas JR, Somenek M. Scar Revision Review. Arch Facial Plast Surg 2012;14(3):162–74.

20. Grigoryan KV, Kampp JT. Summary and evidence grading of over-the-counter scar treatments. nternational Journal of Dermatology 2020;59(9):1136–43.

21. Hom DB, Hom KA. Do topical products reduce post-incision scars? Laryngoscope 2015;125(2):282–3.

22. Berman B, Perez OA, Konda S, et al. A review of the biologic effects, clinical efficacy, and safety of silicone elastomer sheeting for hypertrophic and keloid scar treatment and management. Dermatol Surg 2007;33(11):1291–303.

23. Katz BE. Silicone gel sheeting in scar therapy. Cutis 1995;56(1):65–7.

24. O'Brien L, Jones DJ. Silicone gel sheeting for preventing and treating hypertrophic and keloid scars. Cochrane Database Syst Rev 2013;2013(9):CD003826.

25. Stavrou D, Weissman O, Winkler E, et al. Silicone-Based Scar Therapy: A Review of the Literature. Aesthetic Plast Surg 2010;34(5):646–51.

26. O'Reilly S, Crofton E, Brown J, et al. Use of tape for the management of hypertrophic scar development: A comprehensive review. Scars, Burns & Healing 2021;7. https://doi.org/10.1177/20595131211029206. 20595131211029206.

27. Juckett G, Hartman-Adams H. Management of keloids and hypertrophic scars. Am Fam Physician 2009;80(3):253–60.

28. Chang L-W, Deng W-P, Yeong E-K, et al. Pressure Effects on the Growth of Human Scar Fibroblasts. J Burn Care Res 2008;29(5):835–41.

29. Harmon CB, Skinner DP. Dermabrasion. Cosmet Dermatol 2022;547–54.

30. Lee Peng G, Kerolus JL. Management of Surgical Scars. Facial Plast Surg Clin North Am 2019;27(4):513–7.

31. O'Boyle CP, Shayan-Arani H, Hamada MW. Intralesional cryotherapy for hypertrophic scars and keloids: a review. Scars, Burns & Healing 2017;3. https://doi.org/10.1177/2059513117702162. 2059513117702162.

32. Mankowski P, Kanevsky J, Tomlinson J, et al. Optimizing Radiotherapy for Keloids: A Meta-Analysis Systematic Review Comparing Recurrence Rates Between Different Radiation Modalities. Ann Plast Surg 2017;78(4):403–11.

33. Mustoe TA, Cooter RD, Gold MH, et al. International clinical recommendations on scar management. Plast Reconstr Surg 2002;110(2):560–71.

Risks for Specific Procedures

Reducing Surgical Risks in the Rhinoplasty Patient

Deborah Watson, MD*, Kayva L. Crawford, MD

KEYWORDS

- Rhinoplasty • Complications • Prevention • Risk reduction

KEY POINTS

- Optimization of patient outcomes begins in the preoperative period with thorough informed consent, setting of realistic expectations, pausing all anticoagulating medications and supplements as tolerated, and administration of perioperative steroids.
- The risk of nasal deformities can be minimized by avoiding overresection of the nasal bones or any components of the cartilaginous framework.
- Maintaining tip and dorsal-septal support is a critical element of open septorhinoplasty.

INTRODUCTION

Although rhinoplasty is one of the most frequently performed surgeries within facial plastic surgery, the reported overall complication rate remains relatively low at 0.7% (**Table 1**).[1] Despite the rare occurrence of major complications, studies have shown that litigation rates after rhinoplasty are among the highest in facial plastic surgery, with litigation more common in cases of a perceived poor cosmetic outcome.[2,3]

Reducing complications in the rhinoplasty patient is essential to ensuring optimal functional, aesthetic, and patient satisfaction outcomes. This process begins with thorough informed consent to review the full spectrum of risks, benefits, and alternatives. Many of the complications of rhinoplasty are technical in nature and are preventable with meticulous attention to surgical technique and postoperative care. This article aims to review preoperative, intraoperative, and postoperative considerations to reduce surgical risks in the rhinoplasty patient.

PREOPERATIVE CONSIDERATIONS
Preoperative Planning

Adequate preoperative planning is instrumental in establishing reasonable expectations and ensuring that patients are adequately equipped for postoperative recovery. Beginning with a thorough informed consent process, patients should be advised of the approximate duration of surgery, expected postoperative pain level, and length of anticipated recovery. Risks including bleeding, infection, numbness, scar, damage to surrounding structures including the eyes, poor cosmetic or functional outcome, and need for revision surgery should be explained in detail with time set aside to address patient questions. In a recent meta-analysis of rhinoplasty consent forms, Heilbronn and colleagues found that only 83% of consents included the possibility of an unsatisfactory result, and only 75% mentioned need for revision surgery. The authors advocate for a thorough discussion of these possibilities, especially given that the typical revision rate for rhinoplasty falls between 5% and 15%.[4–6] The investigators also recommend a detailed review of preoperative patient photos between the patient and surgeon to review a tentative surgical plan and discuss expected outcomes.

In patients who can tolerate a pause in their anticoagulation regimen, all blood thinning medications, supplements, and foods should ideally be discontinued 7 to 10 days before the procedure. It is also advisable that patients fill their prescriptions in advance of surgery to streamline the postoperative experience. These prescriptions often

Department of Otolaryngology–Head & Neck Surgery, University of California San Diego, 9350 Campus Point Drive, La Jolla, CA 92037, USA
* Corresponding author. 3350 La Jolla Village Drive, 112-C, San Diego, CA 92161.
E-mail address: dewatson@health.ucsd.edu

Facial Plast Surg Clin N Am 31 (2023) 209–220
https://doi.org/10.1016/j.fsc.2023.01.005
1064-7406/23/Published by Elsevier Inc.

Table 1
Preventative measures against common rhinoplasty complications

Anatomic Region	Complication	Preventative Measures
Upper vault	Open roof deformity	• Conservative bony dorsal hump reduction • After performing dorsal hump reduction, use lateral osteotomies to realign nasal bones
	Rocker deformity	• Avoid extending osteotomies too far into the frontal bone
	Stair step deformity	• Precise alignment of lateral osteotomies at the junction of the nasal bones with the ascending process of the maxilla
Middle vault	Asymmetry	• Spreader graft placement with variable widths • Clocking sutures
	Pollybeak deformity	• Ensure adequate take-down of cartilaginous dorsal septum with removal of anterior septal angle • Ensure adequate columellar support with columellar strut graft or caudal septal extension graft if patient has short medial crura • Judicious use of dorsal resection in thick-skinned patients • Postoperative Kenalog injections to minimize scar tissue
	Inverted V deformity	• Avoid aggressive dorsal hump removal • Spreader or autospreader graft placement • Reattachment of upper lateral cartilages to spreader grafts (if applicable) and dorsal septum
	Saddle nose deformity	• Preserve a minimum 1.0–1.5 cm dorsal cartilaginous strut during septoplasty • Cartilaginous onlay grafts
Nasal tip	Asymmetry	• Stabilize columella with columellar strut graft, medial crural setback, or caudal septal extension graft • Ensure transdomal sutures are symmetric • Avoid catching edge of alar cartilage during closure of marginal incision
	Skin necrosis	• Avoid excessive thinning of skin soft tissue envelope • Avoid excessive compression if using supra-alar basting sutures
	Bossae	• Adequate undermining of vestibular skin from asymmetric lower lateral cartilages • Maintain 5–8 mm of lower lateral cartilage during cephalic trim to prevent buckling
	Visible cartilage grafts	• Avoid use of cartilage grafts in thin-skinned patients if possible • Soft tissue and fascial camouflage onlay grafts
	Columellar deformity	• Avoid overaggressive tightening of marginal sutures during skin soft tissue envelope closure • Avoid overresection of caudal septum • Avoid excessive medial crural setback • Ensure appropriate length of caudal septal extension graft
Septum	Septal hematoma	• Quilting/basting sutures • Doyle or silastic splint placement
	Septal perforation	• Careful elevation of submucoperichondrial flaps • Close large rents with chromic suture • Crushed cartilage, fascia, and perichondrium can be placed between opposing rents to reduce risk of perforation

include opioid analgesics, nonopioid analgesics such as celecoxib, and an option for antibiotics depending on the patient's comorbid factors. Factors affecting the decision to prescribe postoperative antibiotics are discussed in greater detail later in this article.

INTRAOPERATIVE CONSIDERATIONS
Anesthesia Considerations

On the day of surgery, the authors recommend initiating a conversation with the anesthesiologist or anesthesia practitioner about measures that can be taken to reduce intraoperative bleeding, postoperative pain, and postoperative edema.

Studies have shown that a regimen of perioperative steroids, which may include Decadron, Solu-Medrol, or other intravenous (IV)-administered steroids, can significantly reduce both intraoperative and postoperative edema. Steroids have also been shown to reduce postoperative ecchymosis in the first 7 days by more than 30%.[7] A recent analysis by Gurlek and colleagues[8] investigated whether results varied between different steroid regimens and found no statistically significant difference.

Local anesthetic injections are also an important component of preoperative vasoconstrictive effect on the nasal tissues several minutes before the initial incision is made. The investigators advocate a local anesthetic such as lidocaine with 1:100,000 epinephrine placed into the columella, nasal tip, site of planned marginal incisions, extraperiosteal planes lateral and medial to the ascending processes of the maxilla, and in the submucoperichondrial plane of the nasal septum on both sides to facilitate hydrodissection. After intubation, many institutions implement routine bilateral infraorbital nerve blocks as an adjunctive method for postoperative pain control. In a recent randomized, double-blind, placebo-controlled study, patients who underwent bilateral infraorbital and infratrochlear nerve blocks with 0.25% Marcaine had lower perioperative morphine equivalents and shorter postanesthesia care unit recovery times compared with controls.[9]

Finally, numerous methods of reducing intraoperative blood loss have been described in recent literature. Controlled hypotension with a goal mean arterial pressure between 60 and 70 mm Hg has been shown to significantly reduce intraoperative bleeding, the duration of surgery, postoperative bleeding, and ecchymosis.[10] Oral or IV tranexamic acid administration has also been described as an effective method of reducing intraoperative blood loss. In a recent meta-analysis, patients who received preoperative tranexamic acid lost an average 50 mL less of blood compared with controls.[11] Another systematic review and meta-analysis showed a mean difference of −42.3 mL of blood loss with oral administration and −23.9 mL with IV administration of tranexamic acid. This study also found no reported cases of thromboembolic events.[12] Tranexamic acid should be used with caution in patients with genetic predisposition to hypercoagulability, and any discussion of its administration should involve the patient's anesthesia provider.[12]

Preventing Common Surgical Complications in Rhinoplasty

The upper vault

Dorsal reduction is a common component of rhinoplasty that involves resection and smoothing of the dorsal aspect of the nasal bones and lowering the dorsal septal height, often in the case of a "dorsal hump." Without attention to detail, dorsal reduction can result in well-described deformities such as pollybeak, inverted-V, and open roof deformities. Prevention is key, as correcting overreduction is much more difficult than addressing residual convexity.[13] An inappropriately concave nasal dorsum with overreduction of the dorsal hump is also the hallmark of an obvious rhinoplasty, far from the natural results that most patients seek.[13] The key to preventing these complications is to avoid overresection of the dorsal nasal bones and to close the gap created by dorsal resection with osteotomies, as described later.

Open roof deformity The open roof deformity, defined as a trapezoidal, wide-appearing nasal bridge with a "flat top," is caused by dorsal hump reduction without realignment of the nasal bones with osteotomies (**Fig. 1**).[14] This deformity is easily prevented with judicious, conservative use of bony dorsal hump reduction or by performing lateral osteotomies with medialization of the nasal bones in the event of more extensive dorsal hump removal.[13] A persistent open roof deformity may also require the addition of tissue to restore dorsal volume; this can be achieved with dermal fillers or preferably autologous tissue sources such as temporalis fascia, fat, postauricular fascia, and cartilage.[13]

Rocker deformity The ideal technique for medial and lateral osteotomies results in discrete cuts, 2 along each nasal bone, that terminate at the junction of the nasal and frontal bones. Rocker deformities occur when osteotomies extend too far into the frontal bone, destabilizing the nasal bones so that once they are medialized, the superior portion cantilevers laterally.[14] These deformities

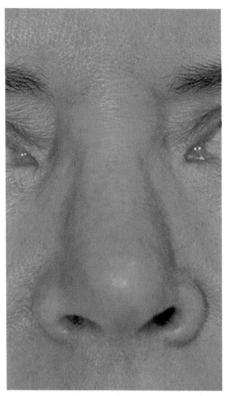

Fig. 1. Patient photo after prior septorhinoplasty demonstrating an open roof deformity caused by dorsal reduction without sufficient medialization of the nasal bones.

can be prevented with attentive planning of osteotomies, as well as through auditory and haptic feedback while creating the bony cuts. Using a conventional osteotome, you may notice a "dull" sound as the osteotome reaches the thicker frontal bone; this can be used as auditory confirmation that the osteotomy is complete. If a rocker deformity is inadvertently created, Surowitz and colleagues[14] advocate for transverse percutaneous osteotomies with a controlled back fracture to correct it.

Stair step deformity The stair step deformity, often identified by patients as a palpable ridge over the lateral aspect of the nasal bone near the medial canthus, occurs when lateral osteotomies are performed too far anterior to the ascending process of the maxilla[15]; this creates an unsightly "stair step" between the nasal bone and the ascending process of the maxilla that is both visible and palpable once postoperative edema resolves. Thankfully, the stair step deformity can be avoided by careful palpation and alignment of the lateral osteotomy at the junction between these 2

bones and avoiding excessive infracturing of the nasal bones.[15]

The middle vault

The middle vault, also known as the cartilaginous vault, comprises the dorsal surface of the quadrangular cartilage and bilateral upper lateral cartilages. This area is of utmost importance during rhinoplasty, as it influences the overall appearance of nasal width and symmetry and contributes to the overall brow-tip aesthetic line. Middle vault irregularities such as general asymmetry, the pollybeak deformity, the inverted V deformity, and the saddle nose deformity can have disastrous consequences on overall aesthetic appearance. Similar to the previously discussed upper vault deformities, these can be avoided with meticulous attention to detail and frequent reassessment for fine-tuning.

Middle vault asymmetry Middle vault asymmetry can be the result of congenital deformity, nasal trauma, or iatrogenic injury after prior surgery. See **Fig. 2** for a representative photo of middle vault asymmetry. Often, the middle vault can be corrected with spreader graft placement between the dorsal nasal septum and upper lateral cartilages. Spreader grafts can also be an essential component in restoring the brow-tip aesthetic line and augmenting the patency of the internal nasal valve to improve nasal obstruction (**Fig. 3**).[14] It is imperative to conduct an independent assessment of the required spreader graft thickness for each side of the nose; in some circumstances, asymmetric thickness is necessary to correct middle vault narrowing on one side.[16,17] Toriumi[16] also advocate for spreader graft usage in patients with short nasal bones, narrow noses, long weak upper lateral cartilages, and thin skin, as these patients are at increased risk of upper lateral cartilage collapse, especially after dorsal hump removal. Clocking sutures can also be used to correct mild middle vault asymmetries.

Pollybeak deformity The pollybeak deformity is defined as cartilaginous convexity of the supratip, most commonly arising from overresection of the nasal bones, leading to a disproportionately full-appearing middle vault and supratip regions (**Fig. 4**).[13] It is best detected on the lateral profile view. This deformity can also be caused by loss of support of the columella support; for example, patients with short medial crura and a widened columella require additional tip support during open septorhinoplasty to prevent loss of projection during healing.[13] Because of the variety and complexity of technical errors that can cause this frequently encountered deformity, some case

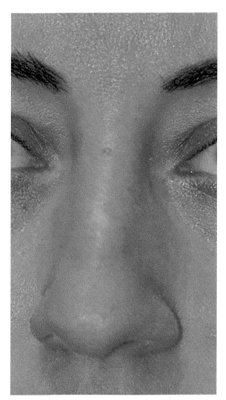

Fig. 2. Patient photo demonstrating middle vault asymmetry and tip deviation.

series report the pollybeak deformity as the underlying reason for revision rhinoplasty in up to 64% of cases.[18–21]

To prevent a pollybeak deformity, it is important to ensure that you take down a proportionate amount of cartilaginous dorsal septum when performing dorsal reduction, including removing a portion of the anterior septal angle.[13,22] The competent rhinoplasty surgeon can also compensate for short medial crura with the use of a columellar strut graft or a caudal septal extension graft to ensure adequate tip support (**Figs. 5** and **6**). Additional preventative measures include avoiding tip over-rotation in thick-skinned patients and repositioning the lateral crura with or without lateral crural strut grafts in the case of cephalic malpositioning.[13] The pollybeak deformity can also arise from supratip scar formation; this can be avoided by performing dorsal resection in thick-skinned patients who are prone to scar tissue formation and with early postoperative mitigation with Kenalog injections.

Inverted V deformity The inverted V deformity refers to a narrowing of the middle vault due to collapse of the upper lateral cartilages against the nasal septum, resulting in disruption of the desired brow-tip aesthetic line (**Fig. 7**). This deformity is most common in patients who have undergone prior rhinoplasty or who have short nasal bones relative to the length of their upper lateral cartilages. The inverted V deformity is also often related to aggressive dorsal hump removal and can cause significant nasal obstruction due to nasal airway stenosis.[23] This error can be easily avoided or corrected with spreader or autospreader graft placement and reattachment of the

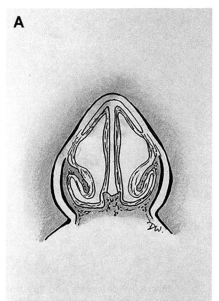
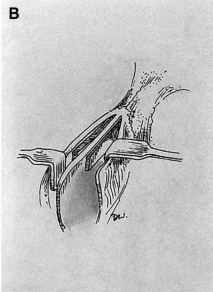

Fig. 3. (A) the internal nasal valve. (B) Spreader graft placement, commonly used for correction of middle vault asymmetry and augmentation of internal nasal valve patency.

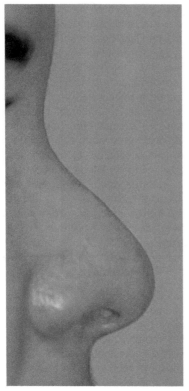

Fig. 4. Pollybeak deformity on lateral profile view resulting from prior septorhinoplasty with characteristic supratip fullness and loss of tip projection.

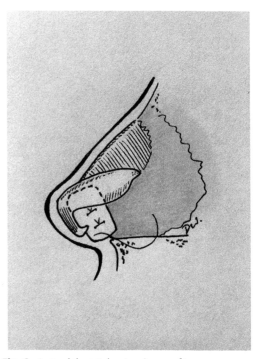

Fig. 6. A caudal septal extension graft.

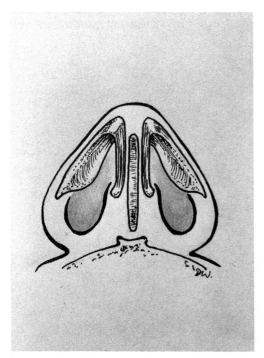

Fig. 5. A columellar strut graft.

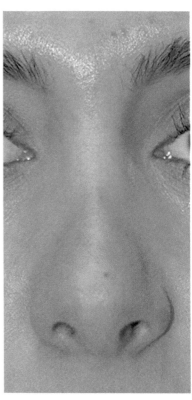

Fig. 7. Inverted V deformity resulting from prior septorhinoplasty with characteristic collapse of the upper lateral cartilages against the nasal septum and loss of the brow-tip aesthetic line.

upper lateral cartilages to the dorsal septum, which will restore nasal width and patency of the internal nasal valve.[23–25] A study by Yoo and Most[23] found that performing autospreader grafts after dorsal reduction was especially helpful in reducing postoperative NOSE and VAS scores in patients with preoperative nasal obstruction who were undergoing combined cosmetic and functional rhinoplasty.

Saddle nose deformity Saddle nose deformity, one of the most devastating complications of rhinoplasty and septoplasty, is used to describe collapse of the middle vault after excessive removal of cartilaginous support from the quadrangular cartilage (**Fig. 8**). It can also be caused by disarticulation of the superior fusion of the quadrangular cartilage with the perpendicular plate of the ethmoid, otherwise known as the keystone area.[14] This deformity can be avoided by preserving a minimum 1.0 to 1.5 cm dorsal cartilaginous strut during septoplasty.[13] Depending on severity, the saddle nose deformity can be corrected by placement of camouflage onlay grafts such as crushed cartilage or the "Turkish delight," autologous rib cartilage reconstruction with or without the use of a caudal septal

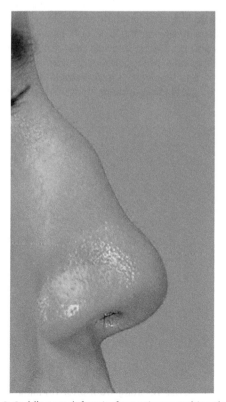

Fig. 8. Saddle nose deformity from prior septorhinoplasty.

extension graft for caudal support, or a cantilevered calvarial bone graft anchored to the nasal dorsum.[13]

The lower third and nasal tip

Tip and nostril asymmetry Although asymmetry can be congenital, tip and nostril asymmetry are common complications of rhinoplasty that may not be apparent until late in the postoperative period once nasal edema decreases and skin envelope begins to shrink and contract. With careful attention to the size, relative position, and contour of the lower lateral cartilages, tip and nostril asymmetry can often be avoided.

First, to ensure proper contour of the nasal tip, many rhinoplasty cases require stabilization of the columella with a columellar strut graft, caudal septal extension graft, or medial crural setback before any work on the lower lateral cartilages or domes (see **Figs. 5** and **6**; **Fig. 9**).[26] Without these guardrails, one risks an unpredictable loss of tip projection after the first several postoperative months due to a failure of tip support; this tends to occur more frequently in noses with short medial crura that do not reach the posterior nasal spine.[26]

Meticulous attention should be paid to transdomal sutures, as irregularities or asymmetries in suture placement may be magnified as gross tip asymmetries when nasal edema begins to subside.[27] Toriumi advocates the use of 2 separate dome sutures to prevent alteration of the columellar lobular angle and avoid creating a pinched appearance of the nasal tip with alar notching.[26] Extended spreader grafts can also be used when placing cap, peck, or shield grafts. The size, orientation, and placement of these grafts must be carefully considered because they can dramatically alter overall tip appearance and nasal projection.[26] Tip grafts should be cephalically curved to preserve the natural columellar-lobular double break. Alar deformity can also be prevented by avoiding aggressive suture tightening when closing marginal incisions. Nostril asymmetry can be prevented and corrected with conservative wedge or alar base skin resection.[28]

In the postoperative period, tip asymmetry and deviation can also be influenced by cartilage memory or intrinsic asymmetry of the strength and shape of the lower lateral cartilages. In mild cases of residual asymmetry, the patient can be instructed to apply regular compression to their nasal tip or can be encouraged to perform directional taping during the healing process.

Skin necrosis Skin necrosis is a rare complication seen in less than 2% of open septorhinoplasty

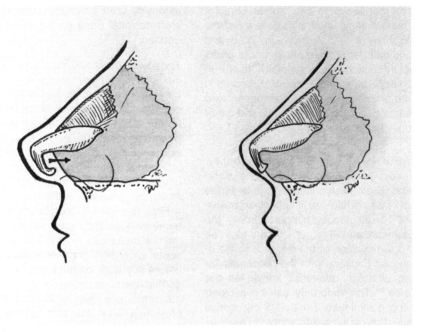

Fig. 9. The medial crural setback technique.

cases that occurs due to excessive thinning of the skin-soft tissue envelope during the elevation process with compromise of the blood supply found in the adipose layer above the nasal superficial musculoaponeurotic system.[29] During soft tissue elevation, care must be taken to elevate the skin, superficial areolar tissue, fibromuscular layer, deep areolar tissue, perichondrium, and periosteum in order to preserve maximal blood supply. The investigators advocate for the supplemental use of cotton-tip blunt dissection to ensure that all soft tissue is elevated off the nasal cartilage during this process. In addition, avoiding excessive external compression and metal splints can help reduce the risk of skin necrosis.[30,31]

Bossae The term "bossae" stems from the Latin word for "bump" and is used to encompass a wide range of protuberances of nasal tip cartilage that are caused by scar contracture and a weak cartilage framework.[32] According to Kridel and colleagues,[32] factors that contribute to bossa formation include intralobular bifidity, thin skin, strong alar cartilages, failure to undermine vestibular skin from asymmetric cartilages, splayed medial crura, and improper dome suturing. A classic example of bossae can be found in **Fig. 10.** This deformity can be prevented by maintaining a minimum of 5 to 8 mm of lateral crus intact during cephalic trim to prevent buckling in the postoperative period.[32,33] Bossa formation

may also be more common after rhinoplasty via an endonasal approach.[32]

Visible cartilage grafts Patients with thin skin are prone to the development of visible or palpable cartilage grafts as the skin soft tissue envelope thins and contracts, and this may not be obvious until the late postoperative period once nasal edema has resolved. It is preferable to avoid the use of cartilage grafts in thin-skinned patients

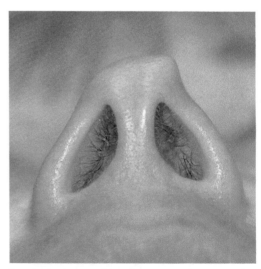

Fig. 10. Bossae resulting from prior rhinoplasty in a thin-skinned patient.

entirely due to the high probability of visibility late in the postoperative period.[14] However, if grafting is necessary, one can prevent visibility by placing soft tissue and fascial camouflage grafts over the cartilage grafts to soften the contour.[34]

Columellar deformity Columellar deformity, as a complication of rhinoplasty, can result from alar retraction, columellar retraction, or hanging columella. Alar retraction can be prevented by avoiding overaggressive tightening of marginal sutures during skin soft tissue envelope closure and by avoiding aggressive cephalic trimming. Overresection of the caudal septum or excessive medial crural setback should be avoided to reduce the likelihood of a retracted columella. One can also prevent a hanging columella by ensuring that the use of columellar and caudal septal extension grafts is not too long.[14]

The nasal septum
Septal hematoma Septal hematoma is the accumulation of blood in the dead space between mucoperichondrial flaps after resection of cartilage and can happen during any surgery involving the septum. Quilting sutures have been described as the best method of preventing septal hematoma formation.[34] In a study by Ahmed and colleagues,[34] in patients who presented with a septal hematoma, drainage and placement of quilting sutures prevented recurrence in 100% of cases. Other methods, such as Doyle splints and flat silastic splints, have not been shown to decrease rates of hematoma formation, although they have remained a popular option due to their ability to prevent intranasal synechiae by ensuring that inferior turbinate mucosa is not in direct contact with a septal mucosal tear.[35]

Septal perforation Iatrogenic septal perforation can occur at sites of opposing rents in the bilateral mucoperichondrial flaps; this can be avoided with careful elevation of the submucoperichondrial flaps and by making sure that all mucosa has been lifted off all surrounding portions of the deviated septum to be excised. Some investigators favor closing large rents with chromic suture. There is also some evidence to support crushed cartilage, fascia, or perichondrium placement between opposing rents to serve as a barrier to through-and-through perforation.[36–38]

POSTOPERATIVE CONSIDERATIONS

In the early postoperative period after rhinoplasty, the focus should be on reducing postoperative epistaxis, edema, ecchymosis, pain, and infection.

Reducing Epistaxis

After any nasal surgery, a small amount of postoperative nasal bleeding is expected. The quantity of bleeding can be minimized by restricting exertional activity, avoiding blood thinning agents for 3 to 5 days after surgery if tolerated by medical comorbidities, keeping the head elevated, and avoiding environmental heat. If submucous resection is performed during inferior turbinate reduction, ensuring that mucosal edges have adequate hemostasis is a helpful preventative measure.

Reducing Postoperative Edema and Ecchymosis

Multiple studies have shown that the degree of postoperative edema and ecchymosis correlates directly with patient satisfaction and perception of functional result.[39,40] As such, patients may benefit psychologically from measures that minimize postoperative edema and ecchymosis. These measures can include taping, a restricted salt diet, elevation of the head of the bed, and low exertional activity.[40] In thick-skinned patients who may be more prone to increased swelling, extended taping to compress the skin and postoperative Kenalog injections can help mitigate prolonged edema.

Recent studies have also shown that avoiding subperiosteal tunneling during osteotomy can reduce the severity of postoperative edema and ecchymosis.[41,42] In a prospective study of 18 patients who underwent lateral osteotomies with subperiosteal tunneling performed only on one side, postoperative edema was found to be significantly increased on the side with tunneling when reviewed by a second independent observer.[41] A meta-analysis of 6 randomized control in which patients were randomized to undergo either subperiosteal tunneling before lateral osteotomy or supraperiosteal osteotomies, subperiosteal tunneling was associated with significantly increased edema and ecchymosis.[42]

Preventing Infection

Postoperative antibiotic prophylaxis is highly surgeon dependent, with a great deal of variability existing between individual surgeon practices. Currently, the American Academy of Otolaryngology does not recommend the routine use of prophylactic antibiotics for greater than 24 hours after rhinoplasty, except in cases of revision or complicated surgery, nasal packing, cartilage grafting, patients with known methicillin-resistant *Staphylococcus aureus* colonization, immunocompromise, and medical comorbidities requiring antibiotics.[29] Studies examining the role of prophylactic antibiotics in the setting of nasal packing have not clearly demonstrated benefit. A meta-analysis of 990 by Lange and colleagues[43] published in 2017 found no significant difference in infection rates among patients with epistaxis in whom nasal packing was placed whether or not they were treated with antibiotics.

SUMMARY POINTS

- An in-depth knowledge of nasal anatomic relationships, the tissue planes, and the 3-dimensional structure is critical to reducing risks in a rhinoplasty patient and can prevent many of the common complications.
- Upper vault complications can be reduced by paying attention to the placement of medial and lateral osteotomies, proper repositioning of the nasal bones, and ensuring overresection of the dorsum is avoided.
- Middle vault risks include asymmetry, pollybeak deformity, inverted V deformity, and saddle nose deformity. These risks can be prevented with awareness to the amount of bony and cartilaginous septum that is resected, avoiding overresection of the nasal bones, placing spreader grafts of appropriate widths, and preserving adequate dorsal and caudal septal strut support.
- Lower vault complications include tip and nostril asymmetry, bossa, visible or palpable cartilage grafts over the tip, alar deformities, and columellar deformities. These can be avoided with meticulous attention to detail during surgical dissection.

CLINICS CARE POINTS

- Upper vault deformities can largely be prevented by avoiding overresection of the nasal bones and medializing the nasal bones with osteotomies in cases where significant dorsal resection is necessary.
- The pollybeak deformity is among the most common rhinoplasty complication, with some studies estimating it as the underlying reason for revision in up to 64% of cases.
- Columellar strut grafts, caudal septal extension grafts, avoiding tip over-rotation and over-deprojection in thick-skinned patients, and lateral crural repositioning can all be used to avoid creating a pollybeak deformity.
- During cephalic trim, maintaining a minimum of 5 to 8 mm of intact lateral crus can prevent buckling and minimize bossae formation.

- Postoperative epistaxis can be reduced by restricting exertional activity, avoiding blood thinning agents for 3 to 5 days after surgery if tolerated by medical comorbidities, keeping the head elevated, and avoiding environmental heat.

DISCLOSURE

No funding was received for this publication.

REFERENCES

1. Layliev J, Gupta V, Kaoutzanis C, et al. Incidence and preoperative risk factors for major complications in aesthetic rhinoplasty: analysis of 4978 patients. Aesthet Surg J 2017;37(7). https://doi.org/10.1093/asj/sjx023.
2. Svider PF, Keeley BR, Zumba O, et al. From the operating room to the courtroom: a comprehensive characterization of litigation related to facial plastic surgery procedures. Laryngoscope 2013;123(8). https://doi.org/10.1002/lary.23905.
3. Razmpa E, Saedi B, Safavi A, et al. Litigation after nasal plastic surgery. Iran J Otorhinolaryngol 2011; 23(65):119–26.
4. Heilbronn C, Cragun D, Wong BJF. Complications in rhinoplasty: a literature review and comparison with a survey of consent forms. Facial Plast Surg Aesthet Med 2020;22(1). https://doi.org/10.1089/fpsam.2019.29007.won.
5. Crawford KL, Lee JH, Panuganti BA, et al. Change in surgeon for revision rhinoplasty: the impact of patient demographics and surgical technique on patient retention. Laryngoscope Investig Otolaryngol 2020;5(6). https://doi.org/10.1002/lio2.496.
6. Rettinger G. Risks and complications of rhinoplasty. Laryngorhinootologie 2007;86(Suppl 1):S40–54.
7. Valente DS, Steffen N, Carvalho LA, et al. Preoperative use of dexamethasone in rhinoplasty a randomized, double-blind, placebo-controlled clinical trial. JAMA Facial Plast Surg 2015;17(3). https://doi.org/10.1001/jamafacial.2014.1574.
8. Gurlek A, Fariz A, Aydogan H, et al. Effects of different corticosteroids on edema and ecchymosis in open rhinoplasty. Aesthetic Plast Surg 2006; 30(2). https://doi.org/10.1007/s00266-005-0158-1.
9. Boselli E, Bouvet L, Augris-Mathieu C, et al. Infraorbital and infratrochlear nerve blocks combined with general anaesthesia for outpatient rhinoseptoplasty: a prospective randomised, double-blind, placebo-controlled study. Anaesth Crit Care Pain Med 2016; 35(1). https://doi.org/10.1016/j.accpm.2015.09.002.
10. Rokhtabnak F, Motlagh SD, Ghodraty M, et al. Controlled hypotension during rhinoplasty: a comparison of dexmedetomidine with magnesium

sulfate. Anesth Pain Med 2017;7(6). https://doi.org/10.5812/aapm.64032.

11. McGuire C, Nurmsoo S, Samargandi OA, et al. Role of tranexamic acid in reducing intraoperative blood loss and postoperative edema and ecchymosis in primary elective rhinoplasty: a systematic review and meta-analysis. JAMA Facial Plast Surg 2019;21(3). https://doi.org/10.1001/jamafacial.2018.1737.

12. de Vasconcellos SJDA, do Nascimento-Júnior EM, de Aguiar Menezes MV, et al. Preoperative tranexamic acid for treatment of bleeding, edema, and ecchymosis in patients undergoing rhinoplasty a systematic review and meta-analysis. JAMA Otolaryngol 2018;144(9). https://doi.org/10.1001/jamaoto.2018.1381.

13. Hamilton GS. Dorsal failures: from saddle deformity to pollybeak. Facial Plast Surg 2018;34(3). https://doi.org/10.1055/s-0038-1653990.

14. Surowitz JB, Most SP. Complications of rhinoplasty. Facial Plast Surg Clin North Am 2013;21(4). https://doi.org/10.1016/j.fsc.2013.07.003.

15. Acartürk S, Gencel E. The spreader-splay graft combination: a treatment approach for the osseocartilaginous vault deformities following rhinoplasty. Aesthetic Plast Surg 2003;27(4). https://doi.org/10.1007/s00266-003-3030-1.

16. Toriumi DM. Management of the middle nasal vault in rhinoplasty. Oper Tech Plast Reconstr Surg 1995;2(1). https://doi.org/10.1016/S1071-0949(05)80013-7.

17. Kim L, Papel ID. Spreader grafts in functional rhinoplasty. Facial Plast Surg 2016;32(1). https://doi.org/10.1055/s-0035-1570127.

18. Foda HMT. Challenging problems in rhinoplasty. Facial Plast Surg 2016;32(4). https://doi.org/10.1055/s-0036-1585574.

19. Hussein WKA, Foda HMT. Pollybeak deformity in middle eastern rhinoplasty: prevention and treatment. Facial Plast Surg 2016;32(4). https://doi.org/10.1055/s-0036-1585571.

20. Kamer FM, McQuown SA. Revision rhinoplasty: analysis and treatment. Arch Otolaryngol 1988;114(3). https://doi.org/10.1001/archotol.1988.01860150039014.

21. Vuyk HD, Watts SJ, Vindayak B. Revision rhinoplasty: review of deformities, aetiology and treatment strategies. Clin Otolaryngol Allied Sci 2000;25(6). https://doi.org/10.1046/j.1365-2273.2000.00353.x.

22. Tardy ME, Kron T, Younger R, et al. The cartilaginous pollybeak: etiology, prevention, and treatment. Facial Plast Surg 1989;6. https://doi.org/10.1055/s-2008-1064718.

23. Yoo S, Most SP. Nasal airway preservation using the autospreader technique: analysis of outcomes using a disease-specific quality-of-life instrument. Arch Facial Plast Surg 2011;13(4). https://doi.org/10.1001/archfacial.2011.7.

24. Rohrich RJ, Hollier LH. Use of spreader grafts in the external approach to rhinoplasty. Clin Plast Surg 1996;23(2). https://doi.org/10.1097/00006534-199801000-00062.

25. Sheen JH. Spreader graft: a method of reconstructing the roof of the middle nasal vault following rhinoplasty. Plast Reconstr Surg 1984;73(2). https://doi.org/10.1097/00006534-198402000-00013.

26. Toriumi DM, Checcone MA. New concepts in nasal tip contouring. Facial Plast Surg Clin North Am 2009;17(1). https://doi.org/10.1016/j.fsc.2008.10.001.

27. Baker SR. Suture contouring of the nasal tip. Arch Facial Plast Surg 2000;2(1). https://doi.org/10.1001/archfaci.2.1.34.

28. Kridel RWH, Chiu RJ. The management of alar columellar disproportion in revision rhinoplasty. Facial Plast Surg Clin North Am 2006;14(4). https://doi.org/10.1016/j.fsc.2006.06.015.

29. Eytan DF, Wang TD. Complications in rhinoplasty. Clin Plast Surg 2022;49(1). https://doi.org/10.1016/j.cps.2021.07.009.

30. Mrad MA, Almarghoub MA. Skin necrosis following rhinoplasty. Plast Reconstr Surg Glob Open 2019;7(2). https://doi.org/10.1097/GOX.0000000000002077.

31. Bilgen F, Ince B, Ural A, et al. Disastrous complications following rhinoplasty: soft tissue defects. J Craniofac Surg 2020;31(3). https://doi.org/10.1097/SCS.0000000000006185.

32. Kridel RWH, Yoon PJ, Koch RJ. Prevention and correction of nasal tip bossae in rhinoplasty. Arch Facial Plast Surg 2003;5(5). https://doi.org/10.1001/archfaci.5.5.416.

33. Gillman GS, Simons RL, Lee DJ. Nasal tip bossae in rhinoplasty. Etiology, predisposing factors, and management techniques. Arch Facial Plast Surg 1999;1(2). https://doi.org/10.1001/archfaci.1.2.83.

34. Ahmed S, Ashfaq M, Shabbir A. Modified quilting sutures: a new technique for hematoma and abscess of nasal septum. J Coll Physicians Surg Pak 2016;26(6):531–2.

35. Kim SJ, Chang DS, Choi MS, et al. Efficacy of nasal septal splints for preventing complications after septoplasty: a meta-analysis. Am J Otolaryngol 2021;42(3). https://doi.org/10.1016/j.amjoto.2020.102389.

36. Fairbanks DNF. Nasal septal perforation repair: 25-year experience with the flap and graft technique. Am J Cosmet Surg 1994;11(3). https://doi.org/10.1177/074880689401100308.

37. Kridel RWH, Delaney SW. Approach to correction of septal perforation. Facial Plast Surg Clin North Am 2019;27(4). https://doi.org/10.1016/j.fsc.2019.07.002.

38. Kridel RWH. Considerations in the etiology, treatment, and repair of septal perforations. Facial Plast Surg Clin North Am 2004;12(4). https://doi.org/10.1016/j.fsc.2004.04.014.

39. Gadkaree SK, Shaye DA, Occhiogrosso J, et al. Association between pain and patient satisfaction after rhinoplasty. JAMA Facial Plast Surg 2019;21(6). https://doi.org/10.1001/jamafacial.2019.0808.

40. Farahvash MR, Khorasani G, Mahdiani Y, et al. The effect of steri-strip dressing on patients' satisfaction and reduction of ecchymosis in lower eyelid, malar and cheek following rhinoplasty. World J Plast Surg 2016;5(1):51–7.

41. Kara CO, Kara IG, Topuz B. Does creating a subperiosteal tunnel influence the periorbital edema and ecchymosis in rhinoplasty? J Oral Maxillofac Surg 2005;63(8). https://doi.org/10.1016/j.joms.2005.04.008.

42. Kim JS, Kim SH, Lee H, et al. Effects of periosteal elevation before lateral osteotomy in rhinoplasty: a meta-analysis of randomized controlled trials. Clin Exp Otorhinolaryngol 2020;13(3). https://doi.org/10.21053/ceo.2019.01599.

43. Lange JL, Peeden EH, Stringer SP. Are prophylactic systemic antibiotics necessary with nasal packing? a systematic review. Am J Rhinol Allergy 2017;31. https://doi.org/10.2500/ajra.2017.31.4454.

Reducing Surgical Risks for Septal and Turbinate Surgery

Sapideh Gilani, MD, FACS

KEYWORDS

- Nasal septum • Nasal obstruction • Septoplasty • Obstructive sleep apnea • Trauma • Surgery
- Fracture • Reconstruction

KEY POINTS

- Review complications of septoplasty and turbinate surgery with preventive measures.

PREOPERATIVE CONSIDERATIONS

Indications for septoplasty include the relief of nasal obstruction caused by the deviation, improved access for endoscopic sinus surgery, and skull base surgery;[1] choanal atresia correction; nasal obstruction requiring a concomitant rhinoplasty; and first-line treatment of obstructive sleep apnea.

Preoperative Workup

Age of the patient

Deviated septum in neonate is typically a result of nasal trauma during vaginal delivery. Although these injuries were often overlooked in the past, increasingly pediatricians check for this neonatal injury in the newborn nursery. With gentle manual pressure, the deviation can easily be corrected in the neonate. This injury is less often encountered in surgeon offices as pediatricians are increasingly reducing deviated or injured neonatal noses in the newborn nursery.

In toddlers, deviations are often due to birth trauma or secondary to trauma later in life. Traumatic deviations can be corrected acutely. Long-standing deviations may be deferred until midface growth is complete in order to prevent midface hypoplasia.[2,3]

In children and teenagers who have completed midface growth, a conservative septoplasty can be performed with care taken not to resect or

damage cartilage and bone areas that are essential to growth.[4,5]

History

Inquiries into history include the assessment of nasal obstruction, sense of smell, discolored nasal discharge, and facial pain.[6] Clinical practice guidelines recommend assessment to rule out chronic sinusitis in patients who have had nasal obstruction for more than 3 months. If patients have one out of the three symptoms of decrease sense of smell, discolored nasal discharge. or facial pain in addition to nasal obstruction from septal deviation, then endoscopy is recommended to check for purulence or polyps in the nose. If the examination is negative for findings consistent with chronic sinusitis, then a computed tomography scan without contrast is indicated to assess the patient for chronic sinusitis.[7,8]

In addition, preoperative inquiry should include an assessment of witnessed apneas, previous sleep studies, continuous positive airway pressure (CPAP) or bi-level positive airway pressure use, snoring and sleep concerns, previous nasal surgery, or previous nasal trauma. The previous use of nasal dilator strips *and/or nasal breathing cones* and the patient perceived efficacy should be assessed.

Medication

Medication inquiry should include assessment for the use of alpha-adrenergic agonists such as

Department of Otolaryngology, University of California San Diego, 200 West Arbor Drive, MC 8654, San Diego, CA 92103, USA
E-mail address: sapideh.research@gmail.com

Facial Plast Surg Clin N Am 31 (2023) 221–226
https://doi.org/10.1016/j.fsc.2023.01.010
1064-7406/23/© 2023 Elsevier Inc. All rights reserved.

facialplastic.theclinics.com

oxymetazoline and phenylephrine as well as nasal steroid use and 0.09% normal saline irrigations.

Allergy

Allergy evaluation should include inquiry of allergy symptoms such as runny nose, itchy eyes, or skin pruritus as well as non steroidal anti inflammatory (NSAID) allergy and previous immunotherapy or allergy evaluation.

Social history

Social history should include smoking and history of drug use as well as housing situation and support after discharge and patient occupation and hobbies that will affect post-op recovery.

Review of systems

An assessment of bleeding and coagulopathic disorders, air hunger at rest, and autoimmune disorders such as granulomatous polyangiitis or relapsing polychondritis should be made.

Physical examination

Anterior rhinoscopy and nasal endoscopy are performed in the office, and the degree of obstruction is assessed based on patient symptoms and well as physical examination. The examination should include visualization as well as careful palpation of the exterior of the nose to assess for corresponding septal deviation associated with external deformities of the nose that will need to be corrected. Palpation of the anterior septum to assess the position in relation to the anterior nasal spine is performed. Nasal endoscopy is performed to check for findings that cannot be seen with anterior rhinoscopy such as adenoid hypertrophy, posterior septal spurs, posterior perforations in patients who have had previous nasal surgery, choanal narrowing, and nasal polyps in the frontal recess, middle meatus, or posterior airway. Unusually enlarged middle turbinates suggesting concha bullosa may later be assessed with computed tomography. Nasal endoscopy is also necessary to check for discolored nasal discharge. Support of the nasal ala and the upper lateral cartilages and the degree of collapse on deep inspiration and the effect of deep inspiration on the internal and external nasal valve are assessed.

Surgery Considerations

Posterior deviations

These may be addressed under endoscopic guidance or with a speculum for exposure. The incision may be placed posteriorly and vertically. After elevation of the mucoperichondrial or mucoperiosteal layer, the incision can be carried through bone or cartilage to the opposite side. After elevation of the mucosa in a subperichondrial or subperiosteal layer, deviated areas of bone and cartilage may be removed. If the septoplasty is being done in conjunction with skull base surgery, often the posterior aspect of the septum is entirely removed. Often drilling is required to correct posterior deviations that are associated with choanal narrowing or atresia.

Mid-septal deviations

Mid-deviations are addressed through mid-septal mucosal incisions or through a hemitransfixion or Killian incision. Care is taken to leave both an anterior strut as well as a dorsal strut of at least 10 to 15 mm.

Superior septal deviations

Often these are associated with external deformities that are corrected with concomitant rhinoplasty. The septum must be dissected free from the upper lateral cartilages bilaterally. Often this relieves much of the deviation. However, often medial and lateral osteotomies and a dorsal strut graft of cartilage *or spreader grafts may be* needed to maintain a straight dorsum.

Deviations of the maxillary crest

This is dissected free through either a Killian or more commonly through a hemitransfixion incision. The decussating fibers must be freed, and this dissection cannot be easily performed with an endoscope. The use of the nasal speculum allows for isolation of the bony maxillary crest and the subsequent removal with an osteotome.

Caudal deviations

These are the most challenging and require a number of techniques to achieve long-term results. If the septum is to the left or the right of the anterior nasal spine, then it is dissected free from the nasal spine and must be secured in place in the midline periosteum of the anterior nasal spine using an anchor suture. Alternatively, the septum may be secured using a tongue in groove technique between the medial crura and the anterior nasal spine that can be split sagittally with an osteotome.

If the septum is deviated sagittally or horizontally, then that may also be corrected by scoring the concave side, morselizing the cartilage, batten grafts to the concave side or extracorporeal resection and replacement of the whole septum and use of polylactic acid sheets, costal cartilage graft, organ donor costal cartilage, conchal bowl cartilage graft, or hydroxyapatite sheets. A modified extracorporeal resection or anterior septal reconstruction may also be performed with less impact on the dorsum of the nose. This is performed by preserving the dorsal strut of the nose especially at the junction of the quadrangular cartilage, perpendicular plate of the ethmoid, and nasal bones.[9]

Choice of Anesthesia

Although some have advocated for the use of laryngeal mask airway with septoplasty,[10–13] many surgeons and anesthesiologists can do monitored or general endotracheal anesthesia for nasal surgery.

Complications

Complications include septal hematoma, septal perforation, persistent septal deviation, synechia, atrophic rhinitis, rhinitis sicca, epistaxis, cosmetic changes, and change in smell, litigation, and failure to consent properly.

Septal Hematoma

When blood collects between the septal cartilage and the mucoperichondrial layer, this collection interferes with appropriate blood supply to the septum. Coagulative necrosis ensues with subsequent absorption of the tissue when severe. These hematomas are prevented with quilting absorbable suture which allows for thorough coaptation of the mucoperichondrial layer to the underlying septum. Silastic splints with or without magnets may also be used to coapt the mucoperichondrial layer to the underlying septal cartilage. If not diagnosed, a septal hematoma can develop into a septal abscess which can later lead to a severe embolic infection to the cavernous sinus.

Septal Perforation

A failure to raise the mucoperichondrial flaps in the correct plane is the most common cause of this complication. Splitting and damaging the mucosa during the dissection leave the septum vulnerable to necrosis. This complication is more common in patients with previous intranasal drug use with substances that cause severe vasoconstriction of the mucosal vasculature. Often previous damage to the nasal lining creates scar between the mucosa and the septal cartilage. The dissection of the damaged mucoperichondrial layer from the underlying septum is then fraught with less certainty.

Persistent Septal Deviation

Persistent septal deviation after surgery has many causes. Often failure to recognize a posterior spur of the perpendicular plate of the ethmoid or a deviation of the maxillary crest will leave the nasal airway obstructed if not addressed with septoplasty. Often the need for a concurrent rhinoplasty may be overlooked. Common causes are when a dorsal deviation of the septum or a caudal deviation is overlooked preoperatively. Without a concurrent rhinoplasty, the septal deviation will be persistent, and if not addressed, it will result in unfavorable outcomes. Revision surgery is often the solution.

Synechia

Scarring between the septum and the lateral nasal wall can be the result of previous trauma, previous surgery, or intranasal drug use. If not addressed at the time of septoplasty, this may contribute to persistent nasal obstruction. When this complication is found after a septoplasty, it is often due to approximation of the septum to the lateral nasal wall during the healing process. Using saline nasal spray to keep blood from collecting between the septum and lateral nasal wall is helpful. Using Silastic sheeting to prevent adhesions in the first week of postoperative healing is another method to avoid this complication. Meticulous dissection and placement of quilting sutures to coapt the mucosa to the septum helps keep the septum a safe distance from the lateral nasal wall and helps to prevent this complication. Some advocate the use of Silastic sheeting or splints for 2 weeks after revision nasal surgery when the patient's previous surgery was complicated by formation of synechia. Although uncomfortable for the patient, this practice reduces the chance of repeat formation of synechia in a revision case.

Litigation

Although complications are rare, one review found that septoplasty was of the top 12 procedures in otolaryngology involved in litigation and ranks six out of twelve following endoscopic sinus surgery, mastoid, tonsil, thyroid, and septorhinoplasty.[14] Another study found that septoplasty followed by functional endoscopic sinus surgery and septorhinoplasty was the three most common procedures involved with claims in rhinology.[15] Failure to consent and manage patient outcomes was the most common complaints.[15] Other complaints involved cosmetic changes, change in vision, septal perforation, retained splints, and or packs and failure to improve symptoms.[15] In both Italy and England, complaints and malpractice payouts have increased in the last decade.[15,16] In the United States, 34.1% of otolaryngology claims are related to the nose and sinuses.[17]

Expectations

Snoring
Septoplasty is not a treatment of snoring and outcomes for snoring are variable. Patients who

present with nasal obstruction and snoring should be advised beforehand that appropriate workup of a patient with snoring and nasal obstruction includes evaluation with polysomnography. Snoring with sleep apnea is treated with positive airway pressure. Snoring without sleep apnea may be addressed with radiofrequency reduction of the palate. Rarely snoring is from vibration of the epiglottis. If this is suspected diagnostic sleep endoscopy may be performed to assess for snoring sound originating from the epiglottis.[18,19]

Sleep apnea

Nasal surgery including septoplasty improves compliance with the use of CPAP devices and significantly helps with the comfort of using CPAP.[20–22] Apnea hypopnea index also reduces after nasal surgery.[22] The quality of life also improves after nasal surgery in patient with obstructive sleep apnea.[23]

Hyposmia or smell disorders

Patients presenting with deficient sense of smell and nasal obstruction as part of the chief complaint should be advised that a workup for chronic sinusitis is indicted. If nasal endoscopy shows no abnormality to account for the loss of sense of smell and no blockage of the olfactory cleft is visualized, then computed tomography without contrast of the sinuses is recommended as part of clinical practice guidelines for chronic sinusitis. If there is evidence for sinusitis, the patient is advised that sinusitis will need to be managed medically or surgically if indicated.[24–26]

Facial pain

Patients presenting with this chief complaint in addition to septal deviation causing nasal obstruction should be advised of the work up for facial pain in this setting. Although pain can be caused by contact between a spur and the lateral nasal wall (*Sluder syndrome*) or pressure changes and the presence of concha bullosa, often pain requires further work up. The patient is advised that workup recommended by clinical practice guidelines include nasal endoscopy to check for source of pain and computed tomography without contrast of the sinuses. Often severe pain should be addressed by neurology before surgery to relieve nasal obstruction is recommended. The patient should be advised that pain outcomes after nasal surgery are variable. Pain may worsen if there is an underlying neuralgia.[8]

Air hunger at rest

Often patients feel short of breath at rest. Opening of the mouth does not resolve this feeling those patients often attribute to nasal obstruction from septal deviation. Patients presenting with this complaint must be advised that air hunger will not resolve with septoplasty.[27]

Nasal obstruction in a previously operated nose

Often residual deviations of the septum are noted. However, correction may not necessarily resolve the feeling of nasal obstruction as previously operated nasal lining is often rendered insensate and therefore not able to detect the feeling of airflow and the evaporation of nasal secretions necessary for the feeling of airflow through the nose. The patient should be advised that this will not be corrected with septal surgery.

Dry nose

Aggressive removal of nasal turbinate mucosa or damaging of the nasal turbinate mucosa may lead to the sensation of dry nose. Using current techniques of submucosal work of the inferior turbinates, this complication is rarely encountered. Patients who have the sensation of dry nose preoperatively should be cautioned against repeat surgery.

Septal perforation

Often an underreported complication of previous nasal surgery, septal perforations are often asymptomatic. Examination with endoscopy is often needed to detect septal perforations. If present before surgery, the outcome expectations for breathing improvement given a previously visible septal perforation should be discussed. Subcentimeter perforations can easily be repaired; however, larger ones would require more extensive surgery to close the perforation. Because the covering of the perforation is often insensate, breathing expectations for septoplasty with repair of larger perforations should be discussed beforehand. Because of the insensate lining, often repair of the perforation of the septum with septoplasty does not improve breathing but can help with reducing crusting and rhinitis in the nose.[28] The placement of a septal button may be a conservative option to reduce nasal whistling.

Allergic rhinitis

Patients should be advised that septoplasty does not resolve allergy symptoms.[29]

SUMMARY

Septoplasty is a safe and effective procedure to address nasal airway obstruction when patients are carefully selected, post-op expectations are discussed thoroughly with the patient, and shared decision-making is practiced.

CLINICS CARE POINTS

- Consent for septoplasty must include expectations for the following complaints: snoring, sleep apnea, smell disorders, facial pain, air hunger at rest, continued nasal obstruction in secondary septoplasty, dry nose, and allergic rhinitis.

- Complications of septoplasty include the following: septal hematoma, perforation, persistent septal deviation, synechiae, litigation, and continued feeling of obstruction in addition to the risks typically associated with general anesthesia.

FINANCIAL DISCLOSURES, CONFLICTS OF INTEREST

None.

REFERENCES

1. Tatreau JR, Patel MR, Shah RN, et al. Anatomical considerations for endoscopic endonasal skull base surgery in pediatric patients. Laryngoscope 2010;120(9):1730–7.
2. Verwoerd CD, Verwoerd-Verhoef HL. Developmental aspects of the deviated nose. Facial Plast Surg 1989;6(2):95–100.
3. Huizing EH. Septum surgery in children; indications, surgical technique and long-term results. Rhinology 1979;17(2):91–100.
4. Shandilya M, Den Herder C, Dennis SC, et al. Pediatric rhinoplasty in an academic setting. Facial Plast Surg 2007;23(4):245–57.
5. Justicz N, Choi S. When should pediatric septoplasty be performed for nasal airway obstruction? Laryngoscope 2019;129(7):1489–90.
6. Kohli P, Naik AN, Harruff EE, et al. The prevalence of olfactory dysfunction in chronic rhinosinusitis. Laryngoscope 2017;127(2):309–20.
7. Fokkens WJ, Lund VJ, Mullol J, et al. European Position Paper on Rhinosinusitis and Nasal Polyps 2012. Rhinol Suppl 2012;3(23):1–298. p preceding table of contents.
8. Fokkens WJ, Lund VJ, Hopkins C, et al. European Position Paper on Rhinosinusitis and Nasal Polyps 2020. Rhinology 2020;58(Suppl S29):1–464.
9. Most SP, Rudy SF. Septoplasty: Basic and Advanced Techniques. Facial Plast Surg Clin North Am 2017;25(2):161–9.
10. Karaaslan E, Akbas S, Ozkan AS, et al. A comparison of laryngeal mask airway-supreme and endotracheal tube use with respect to airway protection in patients undergoing septoplasty: a randomized, single-blind, controlled clinical trial. BMC Anesthesiol 2021;21(1):5.
11. Swamy RS, Most SP. Preoperative, anesthetic, and postoperative care for rhinoplasty patients. Facial Plast Surg Clin North Am 2009;17:7–13. United States. v.
12. Ahmed MZ, Vohra A. The reinforced laryngeal mask airway (RLMA) protects the airway in patients undergoing nasal surgery–an observational study of 200 patients. Can J Anaesth 2002;49(8):863–6.
13. Kantas I, Balatsouras DG, Papadakis CE, et al. Aesthetic reconstruction of a crooked nose via extracorporeal septoplasty. J Otolaryngol Head Neck Surg 2008;37(2):154–9.
14. Navaratnam AV, Hariri A, Ho C, et al. Otorhinolaryngology litigation in England: 727 clinical negligence cases against the National Health Service. Clin Otolaryngol 2021;46(1):9–15.
15. Harris AS, Edwards SJ, Pope L. Litigation in English rhinology. J Laryngol Otol 2015;129(3):244–9.
16. Motta S, Nappi S. Current trends for medico-legal disputes related to functional nasal surgery in Italy. Acta Otorhinolaryngol Ital 2014;34(3):210–4.
17. Dawson DE, Kraus EM. Medical malpractice and rhinology. Am J Rhinol 2007;21(5):584–90.
18. Lurie A. Obstructive sleep apnea in adults: epidemiology, clinical presentation, and treatment options. Adv Cardiol 2011;46:1–42.
19. De Vito A, Carrasco Llatas M, Ravesloot MJ, et al. European position paper on drug-induced sleep endoscopy: 2017 Update. Clin Otolaryngol 2018;43(6):1541–52.
20. Camacho M, Riaz M, Capasso R, et al. The effect of nasal surgery on continuous positive airway pressure device use and therapeutic treatment pressures: a systematic review and meta-analysis. Sleep 2015;38(2):279–86.
21. Ishii L, Roxbury C, Godoy A, et al. Does Nasal Surgery Improve OSA in Patients with Nasal Obstruction and OSA? A Meta-analysis. Otolaryngol Head Neck Surg 2015;153(3):326–33.
22. Wu J, Zhao G, Li Y, et al. Apnea-hypopnea index decreased significantly after nasal surgery for obstructive sleep apnea: a meta-analysis. Medicine 2017;96(5):e6008.
23. Li HY, Lin Y, Chen NH, et al. Improvement in quality of life after nasal surgery alone for patients with obstructive sleep apnea and nasal obstruction. Arch Otolaryngol Head Neck Surg 2008;134(4):429–33.
24. Rosenfeld RM, Piccirillo JF, Chandrasekhar SS, et al. Clinical practice guideline (update): adult sinusitis. Otolaryngol Head Neck Surg 2015;152(2 Suppl):S1–139.
25. Desrosiers M, Evans GA, Keith PK, et al. Canadian clinical practice guidelines for acute and chronic

rhinosinusitis. J Otolaryngol Head Neck Surg 2011;
40(Suppl 2):S99–193.

26. Hummel T, Whitcroft KL, Andrews P, et al. Position
paper on olfactory dysfunction. Rhinology 2017.

27. Bhattacharyya N. Does chronic rhinosinusitis relate
to systemic hypoxemia? Laryngoscope investigative
otolaryngology 2020;5(5):809–12.

28. Daudia A, Alkhaddour U, Sithole J, et al.
A prospective objective study of the cosmetic
sequelae of nasal septal surgery. Acta Otolaryngol
2006;126(11):1201–5.

29. Wise SK, Lin SY, Toskala E, et al. International
consensus statement on allergy and rhinology:
allergic rhinitis. Int Forum Allergy Rhinol 2018;8(2):
108–352.

Reducing Surgical Risks in a Blepharoplasty

Bobby S. Korn, MD, PhD[a,b,*], Michelle Ting, MA (Cantab), MBBS, FRCOphth[a,c]

KEYWORDS

- Blepharoplasty • Cosmetic surgery • Eyelid • Complications

KEY POINTS

- Thorough preoperative assessment and counseling of expectations is essential to reduce the risk of complications and maximize patient satisfaction after blepharoplasty surgery.
- Upper eyelid blepharoplasty markings should consider the patient's natural eyelid crease, desired crease placement, and ethnic background. Judicious and conservative removal of skin prevents postoperative lagophthalmos and corneal exposure.
- Be cautious about the possible worsening of dry eye symptoms following blepharoplasty in patients with known dry eye syndrome or previous history of laser in situ keratomileusis surgery.
- Blepharoplasty revisions are expected. Avoid the temptation to intervene too early after surgery when unexpected results occur. Wait until healing is completed and stability has been achieved.
- Be able to recognize the symptoms and signs of vision-threatening retrobulbar hemorrhage and know how to manage it promptly.

INTRODUCTION

The term *dermatochalasis* describes the presence of loose and redundant eyelid skin. It is a common sign of periocular aging. Although usually more pronounced in the upper lid, it can also affect the lower lids. Upper lid dermatochalasis can create a hooding effect, which blocks peripheral vision. Furthermore, the presence of a prolapsed nasal fat pad can contribute to a dissatisfactory cosmetic appearance. In the lower lid, additional involutional changes create the appearance of "eye bags": the tethering effect of the orbitomalar ligament contributes to the tear trough deformity, which is accentuated by inferior orbital fat prolapse due to septal weakening.[1] A sound understanding of these aetiologic factors is essential before undertaking blepharoplasty surgery.

The aims of upper lid blepharoplasty are functional and cosmetic improvement,[2,3] whereas usually the sole goal of lower lid blepharoplasty is cosmetic improvement. The potential complications of upper and lower lid blepharoplasty are numerous and can occur at any stage. In the preoperative stage, important steps to take include the following.

- A careful examination of the patient's periocular anatomy
- A review of medications
- Clinical photographs
- Detailed consent and counseling of patient expectations
- An explanation of postoperative care.

Addressing each of these steps minimizes the risk of complications or patient dissatisfaction.

Intraoperatively, safe technique and a sound anatomical understanding are paramount to avoid complications. Upper lid blepharoplasty involves

[a] Division of Oculofacial Plastic and Reconstructive Surgery, Viterbi Family Department of Ophthalmology, UC San Diego Shiley Eye Institute, 9415 Campus Point Drive, La Jolla, CA 92093-0946, USA; [b] Division of Plastic Surgery, UC San Diego Department of Surgery, La Jolla, CA, USA; [c] Royal Free London NHS Foundation Trust, Pond Street, London, NW3 2QG, UK
* Corresponding author. Division of Oculofacial Plastic and Reconstructive Surgery, Viterbi Family Department of Ophthalmology, UC San Diego Shiley Eye Institute, 9415 Campus Point Drive, La Jolla, CA 92093-0946.
E-mail address: bkorn@health.ucsd.edu

Facial Plast Surg Clin N Am 31 (2023) 227–238
https://doi.org/10.1016/j.fsc.2023.01.012
1064-7406/23/© 2023 Published by Elsevier Inc.

excision of redundant upper lid skin and in some cases also a corresponding portion of orbicularis oculi muscle and prolapsed upper lid fat. The approach to lower lid blepharoplasty depends on the individual patient's anatomical factors. Broadly, the techniques can include either a trans-conjunctival or transcutaneous approach, orbital fat resection and/or fat redraping, conservative skin excision, orbicularis pexy, suborbicularis oculi fat (SOOF) or midface lift, and horizontal lid tightening. In this article the authors discuss safe intra-operative technique in more detail.

Postoperative follow-up is essential, and patients must be educated on appropriate activity restrictions and wound care. It is important to be able to distinguish which complications require prompt treatment and which are best suited to observation with possible revision later. In the next section the authors describe the major common complications of blepharoplasty and discuss keys ways in which to prevent them.

DISCUSSION
Lid Malpositions and Poor Aesthetic Outcomes

Lagophthalmos
The term *lagophthalmos* refers to incomplete eyelid closure. It is common to encounter mild lagophthalmos (<2 mm) in the immediate postoperative period due to orbicularis paresis from local anesthesia, traumatic myopathy from the surgical incision, or patient discomfort resulting in poor lid closure effort. Long-term lagophthalmos is more problematic, as it can cause dry eye and exposure keratopathy. Signs include an "incomplete blink" and a gap between the upper and lower lid margin on gentle eyelid closure (Fig. 1). In mild to moderate cases, the resultant dryness of the ocular surface can be seen as punctate epithelial erosions of the inferior cornea, highlighted with topical fluorescein dye under a cobalt blue light. In severe cases a frank corneal epithelial defect can develop, which if left untreated may lead to microbial keratitis and in the worst cases corneal perforation.[4]

The first step in preventing lagophthalmos is appropriate preoperative assessment of eyelid closure and orbicularis function. Look for preexisting lagophthalmos by asking the patient to gently close their eyes. Test orbicularis strength by asking the patient to squeeze their eyes shut and resist manual opening. Bells phenomenon is reflexive upward movement of the globe on lid closure and provides a protection against corneal exposure. Document the presence or absence of Bells reflex as well as corneal sensation, which is tested by gently touching the cornea with the end of a tissue and

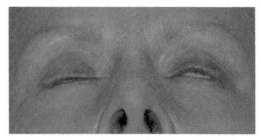

Fig. 1. Bilateral lagophthalmos, worse on the left side. Note the incomplete lid closure and exposure of the inferior cornea bilaterally.

observing the patient blink reflex. Be particularly alert to the patient with a history of refractive laser in situ keratomileusis, as they are at higher risk of developing postoperative dry eye syndrome.[5]

Once the patient is on the operating table, accurate preoperative marking before the injection of local anesthetic is critical to achieve a pleasing cosmetic result and avoid excessive skin excision. The inferior incision line should be made along the patient's natural eyelid crease, taking care to respect ethnic variations in anatomy. Once the skin crease is marked, a pair of nontoothed forceps is placed with one tip at the skin crease and with the other tip used to grasp the redundant skin superiorly. The grasped skin is folded over, and care is taken to check that this does not induce lagophthalmos. The position of the upper tip is marked with a pen, and this is repeated centrally, medially, and laterally along the lid. The 3 points are then joined together and connected to the inferior incision line (Fig. 2). Another tip to avoid excising excessive skin is to recognize the demarcation between thin upper lid skin and thicker brow skin and avoid going beyond this transition zone. There should remain a minimum of 21 mm of skin between the lid margin and inferior brow. Fig. 3 demonstrates a patient with lagophthalmos due to excessive skin excision beyond the transition zone.

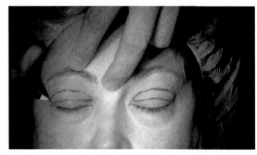

Fig. 2. Bilateral upper lid blepharoplasty markings. The skin within the purple markings is to be excised.

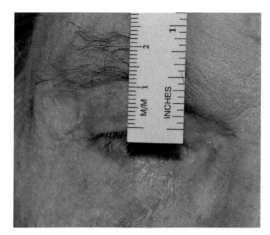

Fig. 3. Right upper lid lagophthalmos. Note there is only 12 mm of residual skin between the inferior brow and lid margin. Also note the stark interface between the thicker brow skin superiorly and the thin lid skin inferiorly, due to surgical incision beyond the transition zone.

Intraoperatively, once the premarked skin has been excised, a small strip or orbicularis can also be removed. However, avoid excessive orbicularis excision, as this can weaken lid closure.

Despite the aforementioned measures, if lagophthalmos is encountered postoperatively, it should be managed with frequent topical lubrication, asking the patient to instill artificial tears at least 4 to 6 times a day. Mild cases tend to resolve. If persistent for longer than 3 months or there is a risk to corneal integrity, the patient may require further treatment, such as a lateral canthopexy to aid lid closure, or in severe cases a skin graft.

Lid crease malposition and asymmetry

Preoperative discussion regarding the patient's desired lid crease height is important particularly in cases where there is already skin crease asymmetry or in patients of Asian ethnicity who have significant skin crease variability.[6] Preoperative clinical photographs enable documentation of preexisting asymmetry, which can be specifically pointed out to patients.

When performing lid crease marking, note that in Caucasians and African Americans the natural skin crease lies at around 7 to 8 mm above the lid margin in men and 8 to 11 mm in women.[7] In East Asians the crease is lower at 4 to 6 mm or may be completely absent, in which case it must be created.[6,8] The use of calipers aids accuracy in marking and helps to avoid asymmetry. Fig. 4 shows an example of postoperative skin crease asymmetry.

In cases of lid crease malposition, steps may be taken to reposition the lid crease. However, wait at least 3 months for healing to be complete before considering revision surgery. One possible approach to raise a low skin crease is to perform a secondary open blepharoplasty, marking the new skin crease superior to the old and then excising redundant skin and orbicularis superior to this.[9] To lower a high skin crease, a nonsurgical option includes the injection of filler superior to the skin crease, which effectively displaces the skin fold inferiorly (Fig. 5).

A surgical approach to lower a skin crease involves secondary open blepharoplasty in which the upper incision is along the fold that is to be revised, and the lower margin marks the new crease height. If the skin lacks redundancy and lagophthalmos is expected, skin is not resected. Rather, a lower incision can be used to undermine the upper flap and release the high fold. The flap should then be fixed at the lower height.[9-11]

Excess residual skin

The persistence of excess residual upper lid skin usually occurs laterally and sometimes medially. In patients who complain of residual lateral dermatochalasis, first assess the brow height—a ptotic brow may be the cause of residual lateral skin redundancy. In this case, it may be better to reposition the brow than to remove more upper lid skin, which could result in skin deficiency and further brow descent. Again, it is advisable to wait a minimum of 3 months before reassessing the need for revision surgery. Always reassess for ocular exposure and dry eye before excising more skin.

Periocular hollowing and superior sulcus deformity

Fat prolapse in the upper and lower lids occurs with age and should be corrected but excessive excision will result in a hollow appearance that will contribute to an aged appearance (Fig. 6).

In the upper lid, fat resection can be limited to the nasal fat pad in most cases, leaving the preaponeurotic fat pad untouched (Fig. 7).[12] Avoiding excessive orbicularis removal also prevents hollowing.

If postoperative hollowing does occur, again it is recommended to wait at least 3 months until healing is complete. At this point, if the patient is still dissatisfied, consider revolumizing with filler injectables.

Eyelid retraction

Lower eyelid retraction is a common and dreaded complication of lower lid blepharoplasty. It is defined as the inferior malposition of the lid margin without lid eversion. Patients with lid retraction will

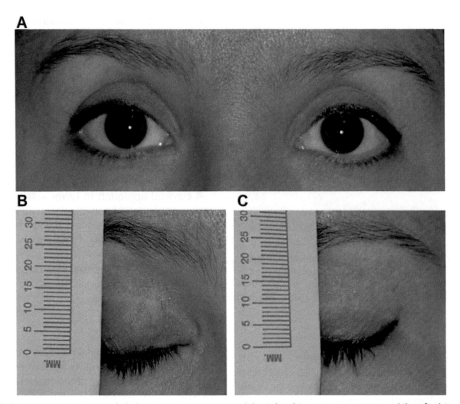

Fig. 4. (A) Postoperative upper lid skin crease asymmetry. (B) Right skin crease at 14 mm. (C) Left skin crease at 10 mm.

complain of dry eyes with foreign body sensation and tearing and an unsatisfactory cosmetic appearance. On examination, the lid margin will be situated below the inferior corneal limbus, resulting in inferior scleral show (**Fig. 8**).

The causes of lower lid retraction after blepharoplasty are multifactorial[13] and can include the following:

- Excessive skin excision resulting in anterior lamellar deficiency
- Lateral canthal laxity or disinsertion

- Scarring and contraction of the orbital septum
- Negative vector orbit configuration, resulting in the lower lid "slipping" under the globe when it is tightened

To minimize the risk of lower lid retraction, a careful preoperative anatomical assessment is imperative to inform the surgeon of the most appropriate choice of surgical technique. Identify the presence of lateral canthal laxity by distracting the lid medially away from the lateral canthus. If laxity is present, then plan to perform lateral

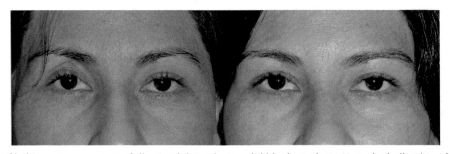

Fig. 5. (*Left*) Skin crease asymmetry following bilateral upper lid blepharoplasty. Note the hollowing of the right superior sulcus and right skin crease higher than left. (*Right*) Following injection of hyaluronic acid filler to the right superior sulcus.

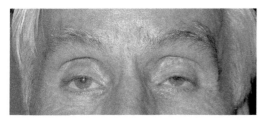

Fig. 6. An example of excess fat excision resulting in bilateral superior sulcus hollowing.

canthal tightening during lower lid blepharoplasty. If the patient exhibits a significant amount of redundant lower lid skin, then conservative skin excision can be considered. In cases of mild lower lid dermatochalasis, the authors prefer to perform a transconjunctival lower lid blepharoplasty paired with a subciliary skin pinch. Limited to approximately 2 mm of skin excision, this is a very safe approach with a minimal risk of resultant anterior lamellar deficiency. In cases of moderate to severe lower lid dermatochalasis, a transcutaneous approach can be taken, with conservative excision of the lateral wedge portion of the skin flap, excising no more than 4 to 5 mm. However, because the risk of lower lid retraction is higher in transcutaneous lower lid blepharoplasty, simultaneous orbitomalar ligament resuspension is required.[14]

In patients who present with postoperative lower lid retraction, the treatment depends on the severity of retraction and the patient-specific anatomical factors. Allow sufficient time for healing, ideally at least 6 months, before performing further surgery. In cases of mild lid retraction, tightening the lateral canthal tendon may be sufficient to correct lid position.[15] More moderate cases with septal scarring require a middle lamellar spacer graft such as acellular dermal

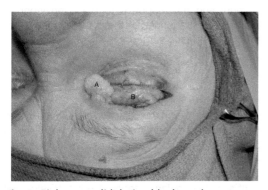

Fig. 7. Right upper lid during blepharoplasty surgery. Note the pale-yellow nasal fat pad (A) and the dark yellow preaponeurotic fat pad (B). Only the nasal fat pad should be resected.

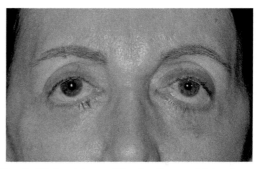

Fig. 8. Bilateral lower lid retraction and lateral canthal dystopia following lower lid blepharoplasty. In this case there had been excessive excision of lower lid skin. Note the inferior scleral show on both eyes.

matrix[16] or hard palate graft in conjunction with SOOF suspension and horizontal lid tightening. Severe lid retraction requires midface lifting in addition to a spacer graft and lateral canthal tightening. Several techniques have been described[17,18]; the authors prefer to take a transconjunctival approach with subperiosteal dissection to access the midface. Midface lifting provides inferior support to the lower lid and aids in the recruitment of anterior lamella. Consider placing a temporary Frost suture to reduce the chance of early postoperative recurrence (Fig. 9).

The management of postblepharoplasty lower lid retraction is complex and results are highly dependent on surgeon experience. Therefore, for patients with lower lid retraction following blepharoplasty, referral to an oculoplastic surgeon is recommended.

Ectropion
Lower lid ectropion can occur in isolation but is commonly seen in conjunction with lower lid retraction following blepharoplasty. Ectropion is defined as when the eyelid turns away from the globe. In the immediate postoperative setting, paralytic ectropion may be present due to orbicularis paresis from local anesthetic or surgical trauma. In such cases, observation and reassurance are sufficient. However, persistent or late ectropion may be due to involutional lower lid laxity not addressed intraoperatively (Fig. 10) or excessive skin excision resulting in cicatricial ectropion (Fig. 11). Sometimes there is a combination of the two.

In cases of purely involutional ectropion, correction can be achieved by horizontal lid tightening. Many surgeons will employ a lateral tarsal strip procedure. The authors prefer to perform a modified Bick "quick strip" procedure, in which a triangular portion of the lateral lower eyelid is excised

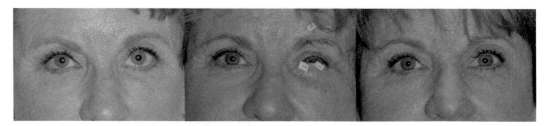

Fig. 9. (*Left*) Patient presenting after lower lid blepharoplasty done elsewhere, complicated by left lower lid retraction and inferior scleral show; (*center*) week 1 status after left lower lid retraction repair by SOOF lift, collagen implant graft, lateral canthoplasty, and Frost suture; (*right*) at month 3 status after retraction repair.

without disruption of the lateral canthal tendon.[19] Lateral canthal tightening alone may also be sufficient to correct lid position in cases of mild cicatricial ectropion. However, in more moderate cases of cicatricial ectropion, lifting of the SOOF or midface will also be required to recruit deficient anterior lamella. Severe cases of cicatricial ectropion require skin grafting,[20,21] although this is often cosmetically unsatisfactory to the aesthetically minded patient and should only be used as a last resort (see **Fig. 11**).[22]

Canthal webbing

Webbing of the canthus can occur medially or laterally. Medially, webbing results from misplacement of the incision line (**Figs. 12** and **13**). To avoid webbing, the medial portion of the incision should not be angled down too close to the lid margin, nor extended too far nasally. Lateral canthal webbing occurs when upper and lower lid blepharoplasty incisions meet or the upper lid blepharoplasty incision is angled downward toward the canthus.[23]

Canthal webs are difficult to efface, and their correction can lead to scarring and a worsened cosmetic appearance.[24] Allow 6 months to 1 year before proceeding with revision and only proceed after detailed explanation of possible outcomes with the patient.

Ptosis

The presence of ptosis should be identified preoperatively. Dermatochalasis with skin obscuring the upper eyelid margin may give the false impression of ptosis (pseudoptosis) but elevating the excess skin gently allows measurement of the true margin-to-reflex distance (the distance of the corneal light reflex to the lid margin in primary gaze). Ptosis is defined by a margin-to-reflex distance of 2.5 mm or less. If true ptosis is present, then correction is required at the same time as blepharoplasty.

The development of new ptosis following blepharoplasty may be due to lid edema in the early postoperative period. However, if ptosis remains after resolution of swelling, it is possible that the levator muscle or aponeurosis was stretched, damaged, or inadvertently disinserted during surgery.[25] If levator function is reduced after surgery, muscle damage should be suspected. Damage to the levator structures usually occurs during fat removal. If fat removal is to be performed, it should be done conservatively and with a sound knowledge of eyelid anatomy. Avoid excision of the preaponeurotic fat pad, which is intimately related to the levator aponeurosis.[26]

If ptosis correction is required after blepharoplasty, wait until at least 3 months postoperatively before reassessing lid position and levator function. Repair may be performed by an internal or external levator advancement, depending on the severity and the response to the phenylephrine test.[27] If inexperienced in these techniques, refer to an oculoplastic surgeon.

Postoperative Wound Complications

Hemorrhage

The lids have a rich vascular supply. Bleeding and hematoma formation may occur in a preseptal plane or posterior to the septum, which can result in a vision-threatening retrobulbar hematoma.[28] To minimize the risk of bleeding, check the patient's anticoagulant status preoperatively and stop the relevant medications 7 to 10 days before surgery if systemically safe to do so. Consult the patient's prescribing physician if needed.

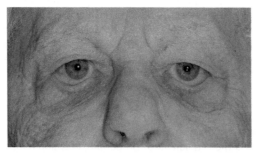

Fig. 10. Bilateral lower lid involutional ectropion.

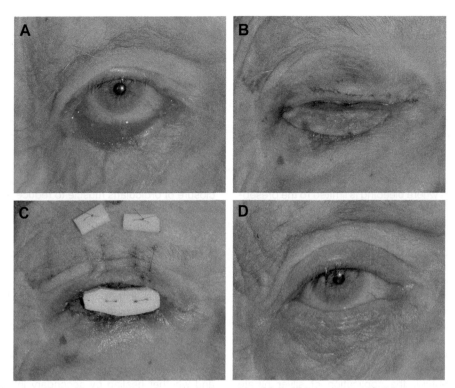

Fig. 11. (*A*) Cicatricial right lower lid ectropion. (*B*) Placement of full-thickness skin graft. (*C*) Frost suture retained until 2 weeks postoperatively. (*D*) At postoperative month 1.

During surgery, inject local anesthesia slowly—this prevents the sudden painful distension of soft tissues, which causes eye squeezing, resulting in hematoma formation. If sedation is being used, wait until the patient is adequately sedated before injecting. Using local anesthetic mixed with 1:100,000 or 1:200,000 epinephrine helps with vasoconstriction. Apply pressure to the eyelid for 30 seconds after local injection to minimize

hematoma formation. Intraoperatively, adequate diathermy should be performed. Postoperatively the patient should be told to avoid eye rubbing, physical straining, and heavy lifting (avoid lifting >15Lb) for 2 weeks; this helps to prevent dislodging of microclots and minimizes the risk of postoperatively bleeding.

If the patient presents with postoperative bleeding, it is critical to be able to distinguish between preseptal and postseptal bleeding. The latter can result in a retrobulbar hematoma, which places the patient at acute risk of compressive optic neuropathy and vision loss.[29] Signs of

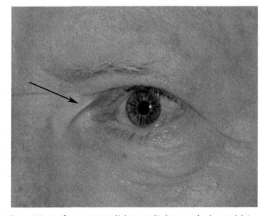

Fig. 12. Left upper lid medial canthal webbing (*arrow*).

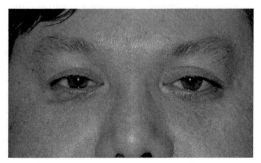

Fig. 13. Significant bilateral lower lid scars along asymmetrically placed subciliary incisions.

retrobulbar hemorrhage include a painful tense orbit with significantly reduced vision, reduced extraocular movements, high intraocular pressure, and signs of optic neuropathy, including an afferent pupil defect and reduced color vision. Immediate decompression by way of lateral canthotomy and cantholysis is imperative to prevent permanent visual loss, which can occur within less than an hour. If there is still no improvement in signs of orbital compartment syndrome following canthotomy and cantholysis then urgent evacuation of the hematoma should be performed.

In cases where bleeding is limited to the preseptal plane, there will be an absence of the aforementioned symptoms and signs. Advise the patient to apply ice and pressure to the lid and sit with the head elevated. In most cases, the bleeding resolves, and the only treatment required is observation and reassurance. However, in the occasional instance where bleeding persists despite conservative measure, the incision should be reopened and repeat diathermy performed to actively bleeding vessels. Consider at this point withholding the patient's anticoagulants if not already done so. In extreme cases resistant to repeat cautery, the application of silver nitrate may be required.

Infection
Steps taken to prevent infection include adequate skin preparation with iodine solution, operating within a sterile field, and the application of topical antibiotic ointment to incisions for 2 weeks postoperatively. Prophylactic oral antibiotics are usually not required. Use of a monofilament suture such as nylon (Ethilon) or polypropylene (Prolene) carries lower risk of infection than braided sutures. Patients should be advised to keep incisions free of dirt and contamination.

Postoperative infection is uncommon and is usually limited to the preseptal soft tissues (preseptal cellulitis) but occasionally can involve structures posterior to the septum (orbital cellulitis). The latter poses higher risk to vision and requires more aggressive treatment.[30] Common causative pathogens are staphylococcus, streptococcus, and pseudomonas.[31] Patients present with skin erythema, swelling, warmth, and tenderness. In the case of abscess formation there may be fluctuance. Signs to look for that indicate involvement of the posterior orbit include limitation of eye movements, reduced visual acuity, a relative afferent pupil defect, reduced color vision, and high intraocular pressure. The patient may also be febrile. In cases of preseptal cellulitis, treatment is with broad spectrum oral antibiotics with close outpatient follow-up. In the rare instance of orbital cellulitis, the patient requires inpatient admission, intravenous antibiotics, and computed tomography of the head and orbit to identify drainable collections and cavernous sinus involvement.

Wound dehiscence
The risk of wound dehiscence is highest in the first 2 weeks postoperatively. Smoking increases the risk, and cessation should be counseled preoperatively.[32] Intraoperative techniques to reduce the risk of subsequent wound dehiscence include avoiding excessive cauterization of wound edges, closure of orbicularis muscle to reduce tension on the skin wound, unrolling skin wound edges before suture placement to avoid apposition of epithelialized edges, and tying suture knots securely. Use of a fast-absorbing suture may be associated with increased risk of dehiscence.[33] Therefore, if using an absorbable suture, select one that takes at least 7 days to dissolve or use nonabsorbable sutures and remove these after 1 week. Advise the patient to avoid bending, heavy lifting, or sleeping face down in the 2 weeks postoperatively.

If wound dehiscence does occur, the management depends on the extent of skin separation and whether healing by secondary intention has started to take place. In cases of complete wound dehiscence along much of the incision, the wound edges require repeat deepithelialization with a blade or Westcott scissors, then reclosure. In cases where only a small area of slight dehiscence has occurred, observation may be the best option, allowing the wound to heal by secondary intention.

Wound scarring and hypertrophy
Hypertrophy of the incision line is related to suture choice and skin type. It is more common in patients of East Asian, Latino, and African descent (Fig. 13). Preoperatively, ascertain from the patient if there is a history of keloid scarring. The suture of choice should ideally be a monofilament such as nylon or polypropylene, which are minimally tissue reactive. Avoid skin closure with inflammatory sutures such as silk or polyglactin 910 (Vicryl), which are associated with suture granuloma formation.[34] Postoperative use of a steroid-containing ointment can also help to reduce scar formation.[35] Note, however, that steroid ointment should not be continued beyond a month postoperatively due to the risk of ocular complications including high intraocular pressure and the development of cataract. Some patients will enquire about the use of arnica gel to aid wound healing. The authors do not routinely recommend this, given the lack of evidence for its efficacy.[36]

If wound hypertrophy seems to be developing, consider injecting steroid or 5-fluorouracil (5-FU) along the incision, starting approximately 4 to 6 weeks postoperatively.[37,38] In the case of 5-FU, a total of 3 or 4 injections may be required, spaced at least a week apart. In milder cases of wound hypertrophy, consider the use of a topical silicone gel twice a day for up to 3 months.[39] In cases of discrete suture granulomas, observation is usually all that is required, as many resolve with time. If the granuloma persists beyond the 3-month period, consider surgical excision.

Inadvertent Intraoperative Damage of Surrounding Structures

Globe perforation
Ocular globe perforation during blepharoplasty is extremely rare but can be visually devastating.[40] Upmost care must be taken to avoid this complication. During local anesthetic injection, an assistant should help to steady the patient's head to avoid sudden movements. If performing the case under sedation, consider discussing with anesthesiologist whether it is appropriate to use fentanyl in addition to propofol to reduce the risk of patient sneezing.[41] When injecting, direct the needle away from the globe and apply gentle traction to the lid to distract soft tissues away from globe. Furthermore, manually guiding the soft tissues onto a stationary needle tip can be safer than forcefully directing the tip into tissue. Consider using corneal protector intraoperatively to minimize the risk of inadvertent globe perforation. If globe perforation is suspected, consult an ophthalmologist *immediately*, as delaying treatment can result in permanent visual loss.

Corneal abrasion
Corneal abrasions can occur either due to direct trauma from surgical instruments[42] or due to lagophthalmos with resultant corneal exposure and epithelial breakdown. In addition to taking the preventative measures described for globe perforation, be sure to liberally apply ointment to the ocular surface at the end of the case. Patients should continue to apply ointment to the eye at least twice a day for 2 weeks.

Symptoms of corneal abrasion include pain, foreign body sensation, photophobia, tearing, and a red eye. If the patient complains of any of these, urgent postoperative evaluation is required. The corneal epithelial defect can be visualized easily with topical fluorescein staining under a cobalt blue light. Treatment includes regular antibiotic and lubricant eye drops with close follow-up.

Diplopia
Binocular diplopia or "double vision" occurs due to misalignment of the 2 eyes. Following

blepharoplasty surgery, this is usually due to paresis or injury of one or more of the extraocular muscles.[43] In lower lid blepharoplasty, the most likely culprit is the inferior oblique muscle, which is situated between the medial and central inferior orbital fat pads (**Fig. 14**); this can be temporarily paralyzed due to local anesthetic, or it can inadvertently be damaged during fat pad resection. Following upper lid blepharoplasty, the trochlea of the superior oblique may be affected, as it lies in close relation to the nasal fat pad (see **Fig. 14**; **Fig. 15**). Injury to the superior rectus has also been reported.[44] It is important to have an understanding of the extraocular muscle anatomy in relation to the upper and lower lids before embarking on blepharoplasty surgery. Intraoperatively, look out for the pinkish color of the inferior oblique while handling the medial and central lower lid fat pads. During upper lid blepharoplasty, when performing nasal fat pad resection, avoid tissue manipulation too close to the superomedial bony orbit where the trochlea resides.[45]

In patients who complain of double vision immediately following blepharoplasty surgery, determine whether the diplopia occurs only with both eyes open (binocular diplopia) or is still present with just one eye open (monocular diplopia). The latter is usually due to refractive error or an intraocular problem and requires referral to an ophthalmologist. In cases of binocular diplopia, observation for 24 to 48 hours will determine if there is any improvement once the local anesthetic wears off. If symptoms persist, referral to a strabismus surgeon for ocular motility assessment is required.

Lacrimal gland injury
The lacrimal gland can be inadvertently damaged during upper lid blepharoplasty, resulting in postoperative symptoms of dry eye and in severe cases filamentary keratitis and vision loss. The lacrimal gland is located in the lacrimal gland fossa, just posterior to the superolateral orbital rim (see **Fig. 14**). Lacrimal gland prolapse may be present, placing the gland at higher risk of injury (**Fig. 16**). The lacrimal gland may be mistaken for a third fat pad in the upper lid and subsequently resected.[46] It is critical to understand that there is not a third fat pad in the upper lid and to be familiar with the appearance of a prolapse lacrimal gland. It is possible to reposition the lacrimal gland into its correct position by placing a 5-0 polypropylene (Prolene) suture through the lacrimal gland capsule and resuspending the gland in the lacrimal gland fossa.

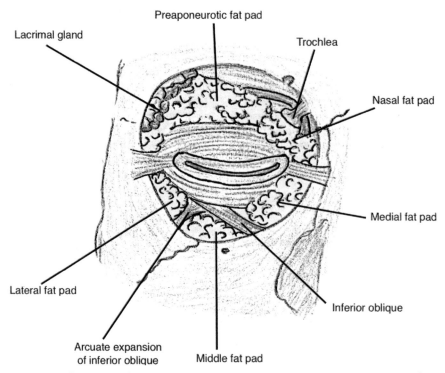

Fig. 14. Diagrammatic illustration of the relationship between the trochlea and upper lid nasal fat pad and the inferior oblique and lower lid medial and central fat pads. Also note the position of the lacrimal gland in relation to the upper lid central fat pad.

Tissue burns

Surgery can pose a fire risk due to the combination of intranasal oxygen delivery, heat from the diathermy, and fuel in the form of drapes and soft tissues. Singed lashes are the commonest result of flame ignition but more serious burns to the lids and ocular surface may also occur.[47] To reduce the risk of fire, avoid placing the oxygen nasal cannulae underneath the drape, as this results in the creation of an oxygen reservoir pool. When performing fat resection, use saline to wash away highly flammable fat globules before performing diathermy. If possible, avoid the use of monopolar cautery or high temperature cautery to achieve hemostasis; opt instead for bipolar diathermy, which has a lower fire risk. If monopolar cautery must be used then avoid using the machine in fulguration mode, as this leads to spark creation.

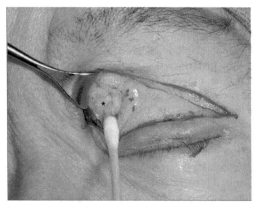

Fig. 15. Identification of the trochlea (*asterisk*) in relation to the nasal fat pad during left upper lid blepharoplasty.

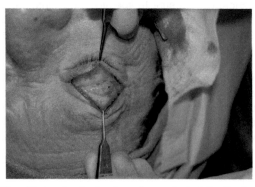

Fig. 16. Lacrimal gland prolapse (*asterisk*) situated lateral to the preaponeurotic fat pad, noted during right upper lid blepharoplasty.

SUMMARY

- Blepharoplasty is a commonly sought-after surgery with many potential pitfalls. However, if performed well, it can lead to high levels of patient satisfaction.
- Care taken at each step—preoperatively, intraoperatively, and postoperatively—can significantly reduce the risk of complications. However, even experienced surgeons experience complications and should have a knowledge of how to mitigate these.
- Complications can be aesthetic or related to visual function. Know how to recognize sight-threatening complications and act quickly.
- Aesthetic complications should only be addressed once postoperative swelling gone and stability has been achieved. Careful discussion with the patient is required.

CLINICS CARE POINTS

- Preoperative evaluation is key for suitable patient selection, planning the surgical approach, identifying the risk of potential complications, managing patient expectations, and taking photographs for documentation.
- Sound intraoperative technique includes careful marking with respect for patient's natural anatomy and full understanding of vital anatomical structures to avoid intraoperative damage. Avoid overzealous removal of soft tissues. Meticulous hemostasis and wound closure with appropriate choice of suture minimizes complications.
- Postoperative wound care plays an important role in wound healing and requires patient cooperation and appropriate follow-up.
- Vision threatening complications include corneal abrasions, exposure keratopathy, infection, and retrobulbar hemorrhage. Know how to recognize and manage these complications appropriately in an acute setting. Do not hesitate to consult an ophthalmologist for specialist management.
- Revision surgery should only be contemplating after wound healing is complete and stability has been achieved.

DISCLOSURE

The authors have nothing to disclose.

REFERENCES

1. Kikkawa DO, Lemke BN, Dortzbach RK. Relations of the superficial musculoaponeurotic system to the orbit and characterization of the orbitomalar ligament. Ophthalmic Plast Reconstr Surg 1996;12(2): 77–88.
2. Akidan M, Turgut Coban D, Erol MK, et al. Evaluation of visual field and balance function alterations in patients who underwent dermatochalasis surgery. J Ophthalmol 2020;2020:1310947.
3. Cahill KV, Bradley EA, Meyer DR, et al. Functional indications for upper eyelid ptosis and blepharoplasty surgery: a report by the American Academy of Ophthalmology. Ophthalmology 2011;118(12):2510–7.
4. Baek JS, Kim KH, Lee JH, et al. Ophthalmologic complications associated with oculofacial plastic and esthetic surgeries. J Craniofac Surg 2018; 29(5):1208–11.
5. Korn BS, Kikkawa DO, Schanzlin DJ. Blepharoplasty in the post-laser in situ keratomileusis patient: preoperative considerations to avoid dry eye syndrome. Plast Reconstr Surg 2007;119(7):2232–9.
6. Song HM, Tran KN. Incisional Blepharoplasty for the Asian Eye. Facial Plast Surg Clin North Am 2021; 29(4):511–22.
7. Price KM, Gupta PK, Woodward JA, et al. Eyebrow and eyelid dimensions: an anthropometric analysis of African Americans and Caucasians. Plast Reconstr Surg 2009;124(2):615–23.
8. Saonanon P. Update on Asian eyelid anatomy and clinical relevance. Curr Opin Ophthalmol 2014; 25(5):436–42.
9. Cho IC. Revision upper blepharoplasty. Semin Plast Surg 2015;29(3):201–8.
10. Mendelson BC, Luo D. Secondary upper lid blepharoplasty: a clinical series using the tarsal fixation technique. Plast Reconstr Surg 2015;135(3):508e–16e.
11. McKinney P, Camirand A, H Carraway J, et al. Secondary upper eyelid blepharoplasty. Aesthet Surg J 2004;24(1):51–9.
12. Korn BS, Kikkawa DO, Hicok KC. Identification and characterization of adult stem cells from human orbital adipose tissue. Ophthalmic Plast Reconstr Surg 2009;25(1):27–32.
13. Patipa M. The evaluation and management of lower eyelid retraction following cosmetic surgery. Plast Reconstr Surg 2000;106(2):438–53 [discussion: 454–9].
14. Korn BS, Kikkawa DO, Cohen SR. Transcutaneous lower eyelid blepharoplasty with orbitomalar suspension: retrospective review of 212 consecutive cases. Plast Reconstr Surg 2010;125(1):315–23.
15. Kim JW, Ellis DS, Stewart WB. Correction of lower eyelid retraction by transconjunctival retractor excision and lateral eyelid suspension. Ophthalmic Plast Reconstr Surg 1999;15(5):341–8.

16. McGrath LA, Hardy TG, McNab AA. Efficacy of porcine acellular dermal matrix in the management of lower eyelid retraction: case series and review of the literature. Graefes Arch Clin Exp Ophthalmol 2020;258(9):1999–2006.

17. Patel A, Wang Y, Massry GG. Management of post-blepharoplasty lower eyelid retraction. Facial Plast Surg Clin North Am 2019;27(4):425–34.

18. Le Louarn C. Concentric malar lift in the management of lower eyelid rejuvenation or retraction: a clinical retrospective study on 342 cases, 13 years after the first publication. Aesthetic Plast Surg 2018;42(3):725–42.

19. Vahdani K, Ford R, Garrott H, et al. Lateral tarsal strip versus Bick's procedure in correction of eyelid malposition. Eye (Lond) 2018;32(6):1117–22.

20. Vahdani K, Thaller VT. Anterior lamellar deficit ectropion management. Eye (Lond) 2021;35(3):929–35.

21. Medina A. Management of severe multifactorial eyelid ectropion with lateral tarsal strip procedure and full-thickness skin graft. Cureus 2022;14(3):e23462.

22. Liebau J, Schulz A, Arens A, et al. Management of lower lid ectropion. Dermatol Surg 2006;32(8):1050–6 [discussion: 1056–7].

23. Lee HBH, Bradley EA. Surgical repair of lateral canthal web. Am J Ophthalmol 2006;142(2):339–40.

24. Massry GG. Cicatricial canthal webs. Ophthalmic Plast Reconstr Surg 2011;27(6):426–30.

25. Wolfort FG, Poblete JV. Ptosis after blepharoplasty. Ann Plast Surg 1995;34(3):264–6 [discussion: 266–7].

26. Steinsapir KD, Kim YD. Pathology of "Post-Upper Blepharoplasty Syndrome": implications for upper eyelid reconstruction. Clin Ophthalmol 2019;13:2035–42.

27. Nacaroglu SA, Karabulut GO, Fazil K, et al. Comparing the outcome of Muller's muscle conjunctival resection for mild/moderate versus severe involutional aponeurotic ptosis. Eur J Ophthalmol 2021;31(6):3436–41.

28. Hass AN, Penne RB, Stefanyszyn MA, et al. Incidence of postblepharoplasty orbital hemorrhage and associated visual loss. Ophthalmic Plast Reconstr Surg 2004;20(6):426–32.

29. Teng CC, Reddy S, Wong JJ, et al. Retrobulbar hemorrhage nine days after cosmetic blepharoplasty resulting in permanent visual loss. Ophthalmic Plast Reconstr Surg 2006;22(5):388–9.

30. Chiu ES, Capell BC, Capel B, et al. Successful management of orbital cellulitis and temporary visual loss after blepharoplasty. Plast Reconstr Surg 2006;118(3):67e–72e.

31. Shih EJ, Chen JK, Tsai PJ, et al. Differences in characteristics, aetiologies, isolated pathogens, and the efficacy of antibiotics in adult patients with preseptal cellulitis and orbital cellulitis between 2000-2009 and 2010-2019. Br J Ophthalmol 2021. https://doi.org/10.1136/bjophthalmol-2021-318986.

32. Liu D, Zhu L, Yang C. The effect of preoperative smoking and smoke cessation on wound healing and infection in post-surgery subjects: a meta-analysis. Int Wound J 2022;19(8):2101–6.

33. Homer NA, Zhou S, Watson AH, et al. Wound dehiscence following upper blepharoplasty: a review of 2,376 cases. Ophthalmic Plast Reconstr Surg 2021;37(3S):S66–9.

34. Cartmill BT, Parham DM, Strike PW, et al. How do absorbable sutures absorb? A prospective double-blind randomized clinical study of tissue reaction to polyglactin 910 sutures in human skin. Orbit 2014;33(6):437–43.

35. Ogawa R. Keloid and hypertrophic scars are the result of chronic inflammation in the reticular dermis. Int J Mol Sci 2017;18(3):E606.

36. van Exsel DCE, Pool SMW, van Uchelen JH, et al. Arnica ointment 10% does not improve upper blepharoplasty outcome: a randomized, placebo-controlled trial. Plast Reconstr Surg 2016;138(1):66–73.

37. Fitzpatrick RE. Treatment of inflamed hypertrophic scars using intralesional 5-FU. Dermatol Surg 1999;25(3):224–32.

38. Gold MH, McGuire M, Mustoe TA, et al. Updated international clinical recommendations on scar management: part 2–algorithms for scar prevention and treatment. Dermatol Surg 2014;40(8):825–31.

39. De Decker I, Hoeksema H, Verbelen J, et al. The use of fluid silicone gels in the prevention and treatment of hypertrophic scars: a systematic review and meta-analysis. Burns 2022;48(3):491–509.

40. Parikh M, Kwon YH. Vision loss after inadvertent corneal perforation during lid anesthesia. Ophthalmic Plast Reconstr Surg 2011;27(5):e141–2.

41. Tao J, Nunery W, Kresovsky S, et al. Efficacy of fentanyl or alfentanil in suppressing reflex sneezing after propofol sedation and periocular injection. Ophthalmic Plast Reconstr Surg 2008;24(6):465–7.

42. Shoji MK, Tran AQ, Nikpoor N, et al. Corneal laceration associated with upper eyelid blepharoplasty. Ophthalmic Plast Reconstr Surg 2020;36(1):e21–3.

43. Galli M. Diplopia following cosmetic surgery. Am Orthopt J 2012;62:19–21.

44. Lee JY, Cho K, Choi DD, et al. Superior rectus muscle insertion injury following cosmetic upper lid blepharoplasty: a case report. BMC Ophthalmol 2018;18(1):187.

45. Wilhelmi BJ, Mowlavi A, Neumeister MW. Upper blepharoplasty with bony anatomical landmarks to avoid injury to trochlea and superior oblique muscle tendon with fat resection. Plast Reconstr Surg 2001;108(7):2137–40 [discussion: 2141–2].

46. Smith B, Lisman RD. Dacryoadenopexy as a recognized factor in upper lid blepharoplasty. Plast Reconstr Surg 1983;71(5):629–32.

47. Maamari RN, Custer PL. Operating room fires in oculoplastic surgery. Ophthalmic Plast Reconstr Surg 2018;34(2):114–22.

Reducing Surgical Risks in a Rhytidectomy

William H. Truswell IV, MD[a],*, Albert J. Fox, MD[b]

KEYWORDS

• Facelift • Complications • Hematoma • Infection • Nerve injury • Scarring

KEY POINTS

- Establishing good rapport, along with supportive staff, can help create a positive relationship with your patient that will aid both the surgeon and patient should a complication arise.
- The consultation process should include a thorough discussion of expectations and possible complications; when a patient understands that certain sequelae or risks can occur, the patient will be better prepared to manage any difficulties during recovery from surgery.
- Hematoma is the most common complication. Understanding the causes and creating a plan to prevent hematoma as well as management, such as blood pressure control and the use of hemostatic treatments is critical to minimize this risk.
- Understanding the facial anatomy and high-risk areas of the face can help minimize risk to sensory and motor nerves.
- The dissatisfied patient can be secondary to postsurgical complications, a poorly informed patient about their surgical course and risks, unsupportive family or friends, unrealistic expectations, or a personality disorder.

INTRODUCTION

If you perform surgery, no matter your level of skill or experience, you will have complications. If you have not had a complication, you haven't done much surgery, yet. The vast majority of procedures and operations are performed by well-trained and properly credentialed facial plastic surgeons and have excellent outcomes and happy patients. Our patients are a distinct group of individuals. They are healthy, of a good mindset, and are ready to make a serious investment in their appearance. They expect a high level of consideration and pampering, and are quite knowledgeable about the procedures. They expect to fly First Class. It is important for the surgeon to think beyond the "sell," beyond the booking, the bandages and drains, and beyond the next patient. It is important to establish a good rapport with each patient. Doing so, will create a relationship with your patient that will make her journey through the process of rejuvenation surgery friendly and her confidence in your abilities strong. If a complication should arise, dealing with it will be with understanding rather than contention.

Establishing Rapport

A prospective patient will have noticed how time's passage has become increasingly more evident on her face. She will have seen all the information on television, in social media, in print, and even on billboards that bombard us with the wonders of facial rejuvenation. One day she may pick up the phone and call your office. Her phone call is the first contact with your practice and creates the first and last impression. To that end, the person answering the call must have a warm, friendly, and inviting demeanor. Your receptionist must have a good knowledge of your practice, and the procedures offered, and be able to answer a few basic questions. This starts an intricate and

[a] 193 Main Road, Westhampton, MA 01027, USA; [b] Private Practice, 299 Faunce Corner Road, 1st Floor, Dartmouth, MA 02747, USA
* Corresponding author.
E-mail address: bill.truswell@gmail.com

Facial Plast Surg Clin N Am 31 (2023) 239–252
https://doi.org/10.1016/j.fsc.2023.01.013
1064-7406/23/© 2023 Elsevier Inc. All rights reserved.

cautious dance that, if handled well, will convert that desire through the steps of consultation, surgery, and care to achieve the desired end for patient and surgeon both, happiness (**Fig. 1**). Her desire is to improve and rejuvenate her face. The consultation is made and the process started.

The patient will often have significant knowledge about procedures and surgeries. She will want to have confidence that she is choosing the right surgeon. Among her concerns are can she trust this surgeon? Will this surgeon listen to my concerns? How good is he/she? How much experience does this doctor have? Will I still look like me? What if I don't like the result? Will people notice? Will they stare? How long will it last? What does it cost? And, what if something horrible happens? The consultation is the opportunity to directly or indirectly answer all of these worries. The surgeon should be self-confident, humble, and show no conceit. Be friendly and show interest in her as a person not just a patient or, even worse, another face. Assess her needs, personality, self-awareness, and character. Ask "What brought you here?." Observe her hands. It is not unusual for a shy person who wants a facelift to answer, "I was thinking about Botox, or maybe fillers" while pushing her neck and cheek skin up and back with her hands. Use a mirror, ask if you may touch her face, and be gentle. Your hands are your most valuable asset and touch communicates a great deal about you. Imaging is a great tool. If you use it, do not show more than what you can realistically deliver. Share examples of your work, but don't just show your "home runs". Show more everyday faces rather than models.

Lastly, discuss sequelae and complications. This should not be done by quickly listing bullet points. The patient should know about sequelae, things that can be expected to happen. They will have some discomfort, a better word than pain. Pain is very subjective and often means pain pills. In our experience, most patients need mostly just acetaminophen. Swelling and bruising are variable. There will be fine scars that fade over time. Hypesthesia is common but disappears over time. Some folks will experience postoperative "blues" two or three weeks out. It is rare and mild in most cases. When a patient understands that certain things are likely to happen, she will have been forewarned and will weather them with greater ease.

Complications and mistakes are what we do not want to happen. It is very important to speak about the possibility of postoperative problems that weren't supposed to happen. Patient education is paramount. Just as trust starts with the first phone call so does education. Each surgeon has his/her own unique method of giving instructions to patients. The senior author's approach is to use the whole staff to communicate with the patient. As stated earlier, the receptionist answers basic questions about the surgeon's experience and all the procedures offered by the practice. Financial questions will be answered at the time of the consultation. The patient is given a one-page form about her health history to fill out. The office manager greets the patient and escorts her to a small office for photographs. During this time she engages the patient in conversation to learn what her concerns are and to assess her personality. She also can answer more detailed questions the patient may have. The formal consult is done in the doctor's office. The consultation allows the surgeon to assess the patient and learn if she is an appropriate candidate for surgery. The consultation, if done well, will build her confidence that she has chosen wisely. She will feel comfortable about putting her trust and her face in the surgeon's hands.

Once the patient's issues are discovered, imaging is done, and the route forward is chosen. Sequelae and complications are then discussed. A few weeks before surgery, the patient returns to the office and meets with the nurse or surgeon for preop instructions. All the pre-, post-, and perioperative issues are thoroughly discussed and written instructions are given to her. It is important that patients understand that they will have certain responsibilities to follow to achieve the best possible outcome. Engaging the patient so that she thoroughly understands what her journey to rejuvenation entails, creates a bond between her and the surgeon and his/her staff. The surgeon will operate to the best of his/her abilities and the patient's needs and desires will be met. The endpoint of happiness is achieved.

Cosmetic surgery done by the hands of even the most experienced surgeons can still be deviled by a complication even when nothing untoward happened. If the patient who experiences this has been chosen wisely, is well educated and trusts the surgeon and his staff, she will understand that problems can and do arise. She will know that the surgeon and his team will guide her through whatever correction is necessary and success will be delayed but will be accomplished. Dealing with these issues becomes a learning opportunity for the surgeon and staff. It must be reviewed with the staff. The steps surrounding the event need to be considered to learn if any protocol was breached. Was there a specific problem that could have been avoided? Was any intraoperative step overlooked?

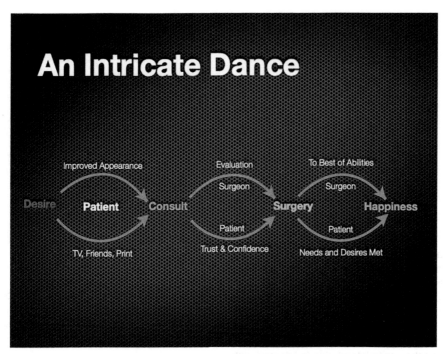

Fig. 1. An intricate dance guiding the patient on her journey through rejuvenation surgery.

All complications are difficult and anxiety-provoking to all involved. None are taken lightly. The three most difficult complications to deal with are hematoma, nerve injury, and tissue necrosis.

Hematoma

Postoperative bleeding is one of the most common complications of all surgeries. It is uncommon in facial plastic surgery but it is the most frequent complication in facelift surgery. It has been reported in 3% to 15% of all cases.[1-3] Male patients are at a greater risk of developing hematomas. Men have thicker skin, more pilosebaceous units, and a greater number of microvessels than do women.[4,5] It is important to elicit a thorough preoperative history from patients. The use of blood thinners is a relative contraindication of surgery. Prescriptive blood thinners should be stopped under the guidance of the primary care provider. If they cannot be halted for a few days, it might be prudent not to do the surgery. Over-the-counter medications such as aspirin, and nonsteroidal anti-inflammatory drugs should be discontinued for 7 to 14 days before and 7 days postoperatively. Numerous over-the-counter supplements including St. John's wort, ginkgo biloba, CoQ10, fish oil, garlic, and vitamin E all can contribute to increased bleeding.[6] A good rule of thumb is to have the patient stop all supplements for two weeks before surgery. Evidence based medicine has shown that the most effective method to reduce hematoma formation is preoperative blood pressure stabilization.[7] In addition, tissue sealants and tranexamic acid (TXA) are also effective. TXA is a low-cost additive with a good safety profile.[7,8] Pressure dressings, drains, and epinephrine as an additive to lidocaine or in wetting agents have not stood up to evidence-based scrutiny that they are of benefit in preventing hematoma formation.[7]

Hematomas most commonly occur in the first 24 hours after surgery. They can slowly develop or rapidly expand with alarmingly increasing pain accompanied by anxiety and agitation. They are usually unilateral in presentation, but with a complete elevation of the flaps bilaterally, the rapid expansion will cross the neck to the other side. This can ultimately cause airway compromise. If untreated hematomas can also compromise the blood supply to the flaps and lead to necrosis. Severe, rapidly increasing pain should be considered an emergency. The patient must be seen as soon as possible. The wound is opened and the hematoma is evacuated before hemostasis is achieved (Fig. 2). Intraoperative techniques are also preventative. Meticulous hemostasis is very important. Elevation of three separate flaps, two lateral cervicofacial, and one central will confine an expanding hematoma to its site of origin (Fig. 3). Hemostatic gauze (QuikClot hemostatic gauze, Z-Medica, Wallingford, Connecticut) is impregnated with

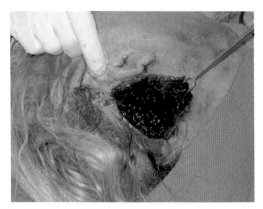

Fig. 2. Large right-side hematoma hours after surgery.

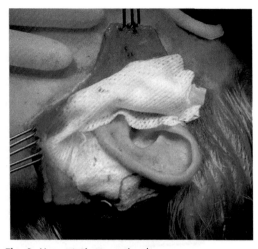

Fig. 4. Hemostatic gauze in place.

kaolin that initiates the clotting mechanism is quite useful. The senior author has used this for several years. Once the flap is elevated and sub cutaneous musculoaponeurotic system (SMAS) imbrication is attained, the gauze is placed on the SMAS (Fig. 4). The flaps are tacked with staples in front of and behind the auricle. The head is rotated and the contralateral side is injected with Lidocaine and epinephrine 1:1,000,000. Attention is returned to the first side. The gaze is removed. The wound will be absolutely dry (Fig. 5). Further bleeding is easily seen and dealt with as necessary.

Platelet-rich plasma (PRP) is also used. Blood is drawn from the patient, and spun in a centrifuge to separate the components. The buffy coat layer containing the platelets and growth factors is removed and placed in a double barrel syringe. The other barrel holds bovine collagen. This is then spread over the operative surfaces, the flap replaced and closure begun. Its effectiveness in hematoma prevention is marginal but bruising is

reduced.[1,9] The list of treatment options are many and worth trying. The best approach is to control the blood pressure before, during, and after surgery, and practice meticulous hemostasis.

NERVE INJURY
Facial Nerve

Motor or sensory nerve injury can lead to long-term palsy, unwanted paresthesia, or neuropathic pain resulting in an unhappy patient. Facial nerve injury has been reported with an incidence ranging from 0.3% to 2.6% with permanent nerve injury at 0.1%.[4,9–12] The most common motor branches injured are the frontal branch and marginal mandibular. Deficits can range from mild transient paresis to complete paralysis. Injury to the motor nerve can represent neuropraxia from traction, thermal injury from cautery, needle injury, or transection from deep dissection.

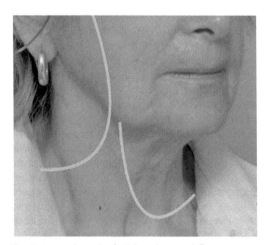

Fig. 3. Lateral cervicofacial and central flaps.

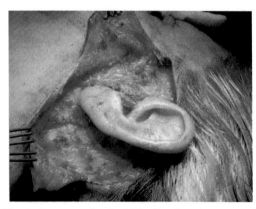

Fig. 5. Dry operative bed 10 min after placement of hemostatic gauze.

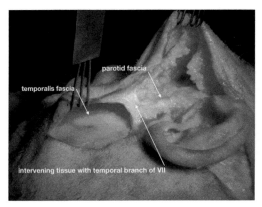

Fig. 6. Transition area from the parotid fascia to the temporalis fascia contains the temporal branch of the facial nerve.

The frontal branch has a consistent course extending from 0.5 cm below the tragus to 1.5 cm above the lateral brow. Dissection of the temporal portion of the facelift places the frontal branch of the facial nerve at risk. To minimize risk, dissection in this region should be in a subcutaneous plane. **Fig. 6** shows the area of transition from the parotid fascia to the temporalis fascia. The connecting tissue contains the temporal branch of the facial nerve. The buccal branches of the nerve travel from the edge of the parotid gland anteriorly just beneath the masseteric fascia, This fascia is very thin and the branches of the facial nerve can routinely be seen coursing forward (**Fig. 7**). **Fig. 8** shows paralysis of the right frontal branch. The danger zone for the marginal mandibular is from the angle of the mandible to its crossing by the facial artery and extends from the inferior border of the mandible to a parallel line 3 cm below.[12] The marginal branch is at risk when developing a posterior platysmal flap in the superior part of the neck, below the angle of the mandible; the nerve is located immediately beneath the muscle in this region. Injury to this branch results in inability to retract the lower lip (**Fig. 9**). Patients with atrophy of the platysma or undergoing secondary facelifts may have more fibrosis of the skin to the underlying platysma placing the nerve at greater risk during dissection. A second area of risk is in the region of the platysma over the submandibular gland. As the marginal mandibular nerve courses anteriorly, it may course in the fascia overlying the submandibular gland capsule. Thermal injury from cautery, through a thin or atrophic platysma can result in marginal mandibular nerve weakness. If facial dissection is too deep and the nerve injury is recognized, immediate repair with 6-0 nylon or finer suture should be instituted. Nerve recovery can take up to 2 years. **Fig. 10** shows the "danger

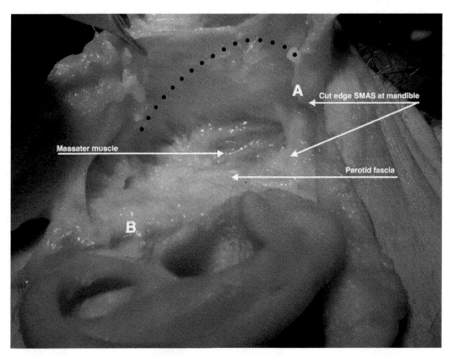

Fig. 7. Masseter muscle under its very thin fascia. (A) Cut and raised edge of the SMAS. (B) Cut edge of the SMAS anterior to the tragus.

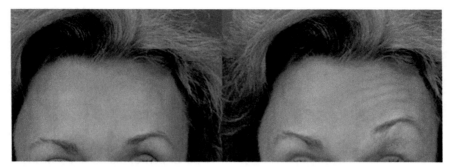

Fig. 8. Paralysis of the right front branch of VII.

zones" for the frontal, zygomatic, and marginal mandibular branches of the facial nerve and the approximate location of the greater auricular nerve.

When paresis is noted in the immediate postop period, wait. The chances are that it is from deep injection of the anesthetic and will in all likelihood resolve after several hours. Keep in mind that the facial nerve branches run below the muscle of facial animation. Maintaining dissection above the muscles is the safest way to prevent severing any branches. Adamson and colleagues[13] reported that up to 85% of facial nerve branches injured during surgery recover.

Great Auricular Nerve Injury

Most rhytidectomy patients experience transient paresthesia due to the transection of small sensory nerves with dissection in the periauricular region. The most common nerve injury during rhytidectomy is the great auricular nerve (GAN) with an incidence of up to 7%.[4,6] Injury to this nerve can result in permanent loss of sensation to the auricle and possibly pain. The GAN is not protected by the platysma muscle posteriorly and emerges on the posterior border of the sternocleidomastoid muscle (SCM) approximately 6.5 cm inferior to the external auditory canal (McKinney's point). In the elevation of the posterior flap, care must be taken to be in the subcutaneous plane, avoiding deeper dissection into the fascia or muscle of the SCM. Hydro-dissection with a local anesthetic may facilitate elevation of the flap that is often firmly adherent below the ear lobule and along the axis of the SCM.

Lesser occipital nerve injury

Lesser occipital nerve injury is rare but can occur if the posterior flap is in the subfascial plane and not the subcutaneous plane. This nerve emerges from the posterior border of the SCM, superior to the GAN and courses oblique-superiorly toward the ear and provides sensation to the superior one-third of the ear.[4]

Spinal accessory nerve injury

More posteriorly, deep dissection can result in injury to cranial nerve eleven. Erb's point, located on the posterior border of the SCM, approximately midway between the mastoid and clavicle, is a good landmark to bear in mind for the location of cranial nerve eleven, although it can exit from the posterior border 2 cm superior or inferior to Erb's point. Erb's point can also be estimated by drawing a horizontal line from the thyroid notch to the posterior border of the SCM.[2] Staying in a superficial subcutaneous plane and avoiding subfascial dissection can minimize risk.

Tissue Necrosis

The risk of flap necrosis is very low. It is elevated in smokers and diabetics. Cigarette smokers are asked to stop smoking from 2 to 4 weeks before and 2 weeks following surgery. It has been reported that smoking increases the overall risk of skin loss by a factor of 12 to 20 times.[9,10,14] Smoking creates both acute vasoconstriction and long-term changes to the microvasculature, increasing the likelihood of thrombogenesis, poor wound healing, and tissue hypoxia.[1] There is no hard and fast rule for how long one should abstain.

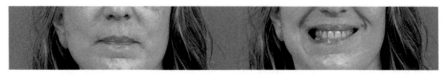

Fig. 9. Paralysis of the right marginal mandibular branch of VII.

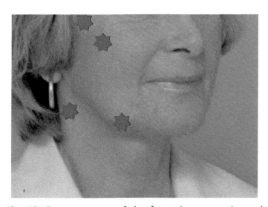

Fig. 10. Danger zones of the frontal, zygomatic, and marginal mandibular branches of VII and the greater auricular nerve.

Smokers are often disingenuous about how long or even if they have refrained from smoking. It is not unusual for a smoker to arrive on the day of surgery averring that they have not had a smoke. A urinary screening test for cotinine, a urinary metabolite of nicotine, can be used to confirm nicotine use within 7 days. This can aid the surgeon in determining whether to proceed with surgery or modify the plan.

The use of cigarette substitutes is not a choice. Nicotine gum, or patches and vaping must be avoided The question of whether or not to proceed is for the surgeon to determine. It is not unreasonable to proceed and not be as aggressive as one might be in a bona fide nonsmoker. Also, there is good reason to consider a deep plane procedure to protect the skin flaps. When full-thickness skin loss occurs, it is most likely in the pre- or postauricular area which often has the greatest tension placed on the skin flaps during closure.[10] If it should occur, the best procedure is to allow the area to heal by secondary intention.[1,6] The patient must be seen frequently for reassurance that it will heal with a much smaller area of a scar than they can imagine (Fig. 11). Referral to a friendly colleague for a second opinion is also a good idea.

Surgical missteps are often the cause of this potentially catastrophic complication. It is imperative to not use overly tight dressings. The use of cautery directly on the underside of the skin flaps should be avoided. Bipolar cautery is far safer than direct cautery. Avoid excessive tension on wound closure. If the flap edges are white on closure, release sutures until a capillary refill is evident. With signs of ischemia, efforts to increase blood flow should be considered including warm compresses which promote vasodilation and perfusion. Drugs such as sildenafil and tadalafil could also be considered because they encourage smooth muscle relaxation, dilate blood vessels, and increase blood flow. Consider nitroglycerine paste which is a vasodilator that increases blood flow and oxygen supply to ischemic tissue. Hyperbaric oxygen treatment helps wound healing by bringing oxygen-rich plasma to tissue starved for oxygen. It has the potential to deliver oxygen

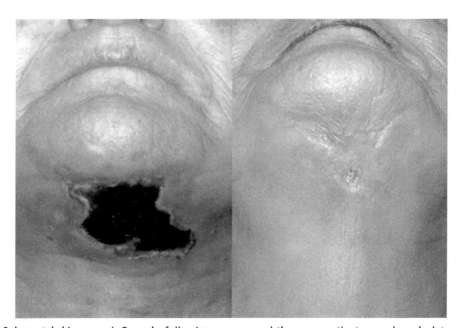

Fig. 11. Submental skin necrosis 3 weeks following surgery and the same patient several weeks later with the area healed by secondary intention. (*Courtesy of* Keith LaFerriere, MD, private practice, Springfield, MO.)

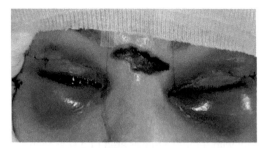

Fig. 12. Day 5 following pretrichial brow lift showing necrosis of the glabella tissues.

deep into the skin to oxygenate ischemic tissue, reduce edema, and promote angiogenesis. Hyperbaric O_2 has been shown to be effective even a day after the injury has incurred.[7]

The patient in **Figs. 12–14** underwent a pretrichial brow lift, upper lid blepharoplasty, and a mini lift under general anesthesia. The brow lift was performed first and electrocautery excision of the corrugator and procerus muscles was carried out. On the closure of the incision, the surgeon noticed that the electrocautery settings were double that which he requested. The glabella skin showed "signs of ischemia". Ice packs were applied and the rest of the procedures were carried out. Icing was continued for several days. On the fifth postoperative day the area showed signs of necrosis. This progressed to full-thickness loss of tissue with bone exposure. The figures show the patient at postop day 5, 3 to 4 weeks later, and 6 months later (see **Figs. 12–**

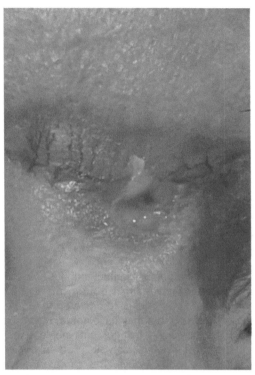

Fig. 14. Six months with scar tissue after secondary healing ensued.

14). This catastrophic problem could have been prevented had the surgeon checked the electric cautery settings his/her self before starting. The damage may have been curtailed if the surgery was stopped as soon as the ischemia was noticed, if ice were not applied contributing to vasoconstriction, and if the above methods were instituted. This complication is the result of mistakes.

Infection

Postoperative infections can be avoided and treated in most cases. The incidence of infection is low and reported to be 1%.[2] Good patient health, excellent blood supply of the face and neck, and a clean perioperative environment play a role. Many facial plastic surgery practices have their own private surgical suites. Unlike hospitals, the surgeon(s), his/her staff, and the patient are the only team populating the facility. Large institutions have a parade of surgeons, nurses, and ancillary staff all day long and every day of the week in and out of the rooms.

The use of perioperative antibiotics is debatable in elective surgery. This author uses antibiotic prophylaxis in facelift surgery administered the day before, the day of, and the day after surgery. In 45 years of doing facelift surgery, the infection

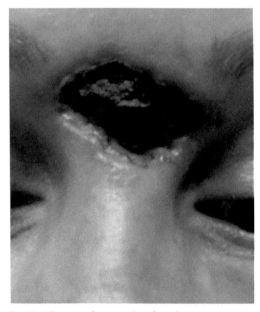

Fig. 13. Three to four weeks after the surgery.

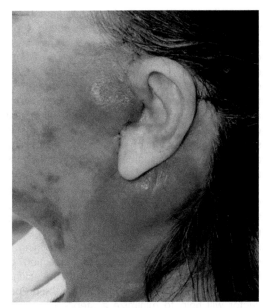

Fig. 15. Two of three abscesses on the fifth day after a facelift.

rate has been nil. Antibiotic coverage should take into consideration coverage for Staphylococcus, Streptococcus, and Pseudomonas.[2]

In addition to preoperative antibiotics, with one dose within 1 hour of incision time, consideration for the use of an antimicrobial wash of the patient's face and neck the day before or morning of the procedure can help reduce infection risk. Hibiclens (Molnlycke Health Care, Norcross, GA), can be used in the home setting by the patient before surgery, but the patient must be instructed to avoid

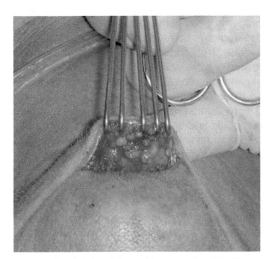

Fig. 16. Thin layer of fat is kept on the skin flap to camouflage small irregularities.

the periocular area as Hibiclens can be caustic to the eyes.

If infection does occur, wound cultures and prompt treatment are necessary. **Fig. 15** shows a patient who presented with abscesses involving bilateral cheeks and left neck. The infection occurred five days postop. The source of infection may have been due to poor wound care at home or a breakdown in the surgery protocols. In some cases, IV antibiotics and infectious disease consultation may be helpful.

Parotid Duct Injury

Injury to the parotid gland or duct may lead to sialocele, parotid fistula, or pseudocyst. Careful dissection deep into the SMAS can minimize injury. If injury to the gland occurs, careful bipolar cautery can be used to cauterize the ductules and minimize the risk of salivary extravasation. Alternatively, topical PRP sprayed over the surface of the gland and closure of the SMAS on top can be used.[2,6] If a parotid duct injury has occurred, Stenson's duct can be cannulated with a lacrimal probe or silicon tubing and the distal ends are approximated with 6-0 nylon sutures. The cannula or silicon tubing can be secured intraorally and removed at 2 weeks.

If a sialocele develops, serial aspiration and compression dressings can be done. If the sialocele persists or if a cutaneous fistula develops, the use of antisialogogues such as a scopolamine patch or oral glycopyrrolate may help reduce salivary flow. Neuromodulator injections in the parotid tissue have been shown to reduce salivary production and can also be considered.[15]

Contour irregularities

Contour irregularities can include dimpling, rippling of skin, persistent lumps, cobra deformity (a central hollowing in the submentum), pleating due to excess skin, or visible convexity along the jawline or submentum. Minor deformities may be avoided by leaving a thin layer of fat on the skin flaps. This affords a smooth contour and conceals unwanted irregularities[6] (**Fig. 16**).

Seroma formation, commonly seen in the submentum and occasionally secondary to parotid gland injury, can result in rippling of the skin if the seroma prevents the skin flap from adhering to the underlying tissue. Seroma can be treated with serial aspiration and pressure dressing application (eg, chin strap) or drain placement. If a drain is used, an oral antibiotic can be prescribed.

Post-seroma rippling may respond to frequent massage with or without the use of low-dose triamcinolone (5 or 10 mg/mL) over the course of 1 to 6 months. Occasionally, resolution may

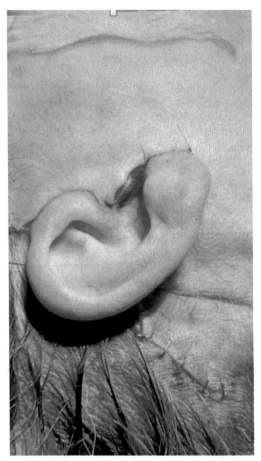

Fig. 17. Closing the skin without tension.

require wide undermining of the skin to provide better redistribution and skin contraction.

Over-aggressive liposuction or direct lipectomy may result in dermal injury and rippling as well. Ensuring that the cannula port is directed toward the platysma and away from the dermis can minimize the risk of dermal scarring to the underlying tissue. Taking care to feel or directly observe the thickness of the fatty layer can be helpful to determine the endpoint of lipo-sculpting. Dermal scarring irregularity can be more difficult to improve. Massage, low-dose triamcinolone injections or possibly fat grafting may aid in the reduction of the irregularities.

A cobra neck deformity may be due to aggressive midline subplatysmal fat and/or muscle resection, inadequate platysma plication, platysma dehiscence, or to an inadequate reduction of fat lateral to the midline. Avoidance of aggressive resection centrally can reduce the likelihood of this deformity. Treatment may require repeat corset platysmaplasty, fat grafting, filler treatment, or further lipo-sculpting.

Lateral neck, submandibular, or submental convexity or a fusiform deformity can occur within days to weeks after surgery. The most common cause of a postoperative "sausage" is simple subcutaneous tissue swelling and induration.[16] Fluid collections (seroma or hematoma) in the subcutaneous plane or the subplatysmal plane may also result in this deformity, with later development of fibrosis. Use of gentle compression with a chin strap, and early aspiration may be useful. Massage and serial low-dose triamcinolone injections may again be useful if fibrosis occurs.

Proper redraping of the skin and a minimal tension closure are key to limiting pleating, puckering, tethering, and dimple formation. Wide or focal undermining may be needed. The swoosh effect is often seen with extensive skin undermining in conjunction with limited deeper dissection or forceful misdirected re-draping of the skin.[9] Advancing and rotating the skin flap in the proper vector will help to minimize a stepped occipital hairline, abnormal pleating, or swoosh effect.[9] A releasing incision at the sideburn can minimize or prevent the loss of the sideburn with skin advancement.

Development of small lumps in the lateral cheek or neck skin can be due to dermal injury from cautery, aggressive flap elevation, or microseromas or hematomas that can form postoperatively. Being mindful of flap thickness and avoidance and minimizing cautery on the flap itself may reduce these focal areas of induration. Treatment involves tincture of time, frequent gentle massage, and/or low-dose triamcinolone injection.

Ear deformities

A "pixie ear" is the deformity associated with a downwardly stretched or elongated ear lobule. This is often caused by failure to inset the lobule properly, often with excessive inferior tension in this region.[9] Loeb has suggested to inset the earlobe "high and in a slightly backward position, toward the mastoid."[17] However, in the author's experience, redraping of the skin with no tension on the ear lobule and placement of supportive 5-0 vicryl fixation sutures in the flap posterior to the ear lobule and at the infra-tragal notch, has been helpful to minimize this risk. Repair of this deformity may require partial resection and/or a V-Y advancement technique.

Scarring and Poorly Designed Incisions

When done well, scarring should not be an issue in facelifting. Tissues should be handled with care and delicacy. Skin closure should be tension free (**Fig. 17**). Excessive tension on the skin flap can lead to depigmentation. This could involve an

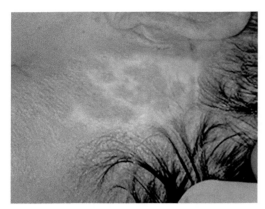

Fig. 18. Depigmented posterior flap skin from too much tension in closure.

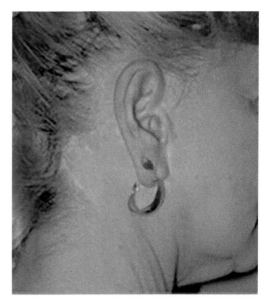

Fig. 20. Obvious "step off" deformity.

area too large to surgically remove (Fig. 18). All tension should be applied to the SMAS tissues. Dog ears and pleating are not acceptable. Closing the postauricular incision by running a 5-0 rapid dissolving plain gut suture from cervical skin to the connective tissue in the sulcus to the conchal skin assures that the scar will not migrate posteriorly to the neck over time (Fig. 19). Hairlines must be precisely aligned. Failure to do this will create a "step off" and women will be reluctant to wear their hair pulled back (Fig. 20). The skin flap on the tragus should be divested of most subcutaneous tissue to maintain its sharp contour[1] (Fig. 21). Failure to attend to these points are mistakes that do not rise to the standard of care expected of excellent facial plastic surgeons. Mistakes are not complications but they must be addressed.

Keloid and hypertrophic scars are problems that the surgeon has little control over. During the consultation, one should ask about scarring and ask to see any scars she might have. If she is prone to these types of scars, let her take responsibility for them should she proceed. If signs of these scars are becoming evident, encourage the patient to return as early as possible to begin treatment. Intralesional steroid injections, triamcinolone, 10 mg/mL or 40 mg/mL, are a mainstay of early treatment. Silicon sheets or gel are also helpful with early lesions. If the lesions are large (Fig. 22), excision is indicated.[6]

Lastly, hair loss is also problematic. It can be temporary or permanent. It is reported to occur in 8.4% of facelift cases.[18] Temporary loss is when the follicles enter the telogen effluvium a natural and normal phase.[19] This can happen due to trauma including surgery. It will recover over time. Permanent loss is almost always due to missteps by the surgeon (Fig. 23). Too thin skin flaps can destroy the follicles. Care must be taken

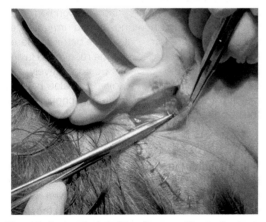

Fig. 19. Postauricular skin closure: skin to fascia to skin prevents migration of the scar.

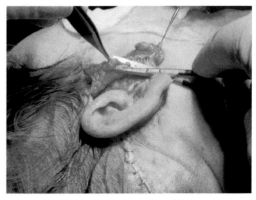

Fig. 21. Defatting the soon to be new tragal skin.

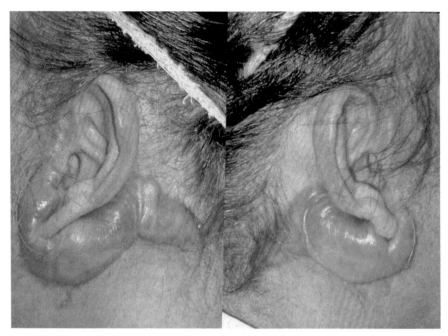

Fig. 22. Bilateral keloids after a facelift.

when using cautery on the undersurface of skin flaps in hair-bearing skin. Excessive tension on the flaps is another contributing factor.

Postoperative Depression

Postoperative blues or depression has been reported in up to one-third of female patients undergoing rhytidectomy.[20] The symptoms can be subtle, ranging from self-doubt and regret to more severe feelings of worthlessness, sadness, or loss of interest. Patients with a prior history of mood disorder or depression may be more vulnerable to experiencing these symptoms. The stress of surgery and the postoperative course with the

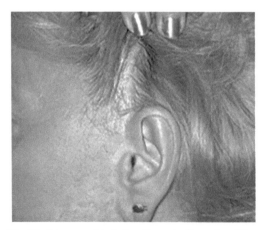

Fig. 23. Permanent hair loss 2 years after a facelift.

perceived distortion of swelling and bruising may be triggering factors.

It is important for the surgeon to be attuned to these symptoms and address their patients with empathy. Listening to the patient, seeing the patient frequently, letting the patient know that these symptoms are not uncommon and being encouraging can be helpful. If the symptoms are more severe, ask the patient if you could enlist the help of their PCP to aid them in the treatment of their depressive symptoms. In most cases, the symptoms are short-lived and resolve over the course of weeks postoperatively.

The authors believe that preoperative patient education is critical in helping to guide patients and set realistic expectations. Patients that have a good understanding and recognition that swelling, bruising, numbness, and irregularities will occur and are transient, will be better prepared to cope with the stressors of the recovery. Having patients return 6 to 8 weeks postoperatively with an aesthetician for a makeover can also help by making it a fun visit and restoring confidence in their appearance.

The Dissatisfied Patient

Patients undergo aesthetic surgery to improve their appearance and self-confidence. However, patient dissatisfaction can occur, even with a seemingly good outcome, even with the most experienced and capable facial plastic surgeon. Many factors can result in a dissatisfied patient.

- Surgical complication
- Unrealistic patient expectation
- Failure of the surgeon to inform the patient of risks, benefits, and outcomes
- Lack of supportive family and friends (eg, jealousy, hyper-critical comments)
- Unrecognized personality disorder or body dysmorphia

Regardless of the cause, it is important to try to maintain the confidence of that patient. Listening to the patient and scheduling frequent, supportive visits, may help to establish a more positive outlook and reset patient expectations. Unfortunately, even with an excellent result, some patients are unhappy. This type of patient may have had unrealistic expectations that were undetected preoperatively.

Preoperatively, the surgeon should explore what support mechanisms are available to the patient. Inquiring about how family or friends are receiving the patient's surgery (pre and postoperatively) may provide insight for the surgeon to address issues such as hyper-critical commentary or unsupportive family members or friends due to jealousy or other issues. Furthermore, patients with a personality disorder or body dysmorphic disorder may be adept at camouflaging this character trait.[6] The surgeon and ancillary staff must be diligent in recognizing patients with this problem and in doing so decline to accept them as patients.[6]

In many cases, time helps to resolve issues or concerns. However, it is important for the surgeon to acknowledge and accept that an outcome may be suboptimal and offer the patient a revision when indicated. It is important to put the patient and their concerns first.

SUMMARY

Sequelae are what will happen. Complications are what we do not want to happen. The patients must be educated on both. Intraoperative missteps can cause complications. Although mistakes should never happen, they do occur. Surgical complications are unfortunate and problematic. They must be recognized and immediately related to the patient. When they happen, a series of steps must be in place to remedy them. Educating the patient about all the perioperative events, both good and bad, expected and unexpected, will establish a mindset to let the patient understand and accept the problem. The patient will know that you and your staff will take care of the problem and do all in your power to address the situation, correct it, and end with a happy result.

CLINICS CARE POINTS

- Establishing good patient rapport and providing a thorough discussion of expectations and complications can better prepare a patient to manage difficulties arising from surgery.
- Hematoma prevention is best achieved through meticulous hemostasis and blood pressure control. Use of hemostatic gauze, tranexamic acid, and avoidance of blood thinning medications and supplements are helpful.
- Facial nerve injury can be minimized by understanding the anatomic locations of the individual branches and their danger zones. The majority of facial nerve injuries recover.
- Smoking increases the risk of tissue necrosis by a factor of 12 to 20 times.
- Patient dissatisfaction often stems from a surgical complication, but other factors such as unrealistic expectations, failure by the surgeon to adequately inform the patient of risks and outcomes, poor social supports, and unrecognized psychological disorders play a role.

DISCLOSURE

W.H. Truswell, nothing to disclose. A.J. Fox, nothing to disclose.

REFERENCES

1. Truswell WH. The facelift: a guide for safe, reliable, and reproducible results. In: Truswell WH, editor. Surgical facial rejuvenation a roadmap to safe and reliable outcomes. New York: Thieme Medical Publishers; 2008. p. 24–45.
2. Chaffoo RAK. Complications in facelift surgery: avoidance and management. Facial Plast Surg Clin North Am 2013;21:551–8.
3. Matarasso A. National plastic surgery survey: face lift techniques and complications. Plast Reconstr Surg 2000;106:1185–95.
4. Moyer JS, Baker SR. Complications of rhytidectomy. Facial Plast Surg Clin North Am 2005;13(3):469–78.
5. Rohrich RJ, Stuzin JM, Ramanadham S, et al. The modern male rhytidectomy: lessons learned. Plast Reconstr Surg 2017;139(2):295–307.
6. Truswell WH. Approaches to reducing risk in rhytidectomy surgery. Facial Plast Surg Clin North Am 2020;28:419–27.

7. Tiourin E, Barton N, Janis J. Methods for minimizing bleeding in facelift surgery: an evidence-based review. Wolters Kluwer Health, Inc. on behalf of the American Society of Plastic Surgeons. Plast Reconstr Surg Glob Open 2021;9e3765:1–7. Available at: www.PRSGlobalOpen.com.

8. Schroeder RJ II, Langsdon PR. Effect of local tranexamic acid on hemostasis in rhytidectomy. Facial Plast Surg Aesthet Med 2020;22:195–9.

9. Clevens RA. Avoiding patient dissatisfaction and complications in facelift surgery. Facial Plast Surg Clin North Am 2010;17:515–30.

10. Cristel RT, Irvine LE. Complications in Rhytidectomy. Facial Plast Surg Clin North Am 2019;27:519–27.

11. Baker DC, Conley J. Avoiding facial nerve injuries in rhytidectomy. Plast Reconstr Surg 1979;64:781–95.

12. Daane SP, Owsley JQ. Incidence of cervical branch injury with "marginal mandibular nerve pseudo-paralysis" in patients undergoing facelifting. Plast Reconstr Surg 2003;111(7):2414–8.

13. Adamson PA, Moran ML. Complications of cervicofacial rhytidectomy. Facial Plast Surg Clin North Am 1993;1:257–71.

14. Derby BM, Codner MA. Evidence-based medicine: face lift. Plast Reconstr Surg 2017;139(1):151e–67e.

15. Guintinas-Lichius O, Sittel C. Treatment of postparotidectomy salivary fistula with botulinum toxin. Ann Otol Rhinol Laryngol 2001;110(12):1162–4.

16. Feldman J. Neck Lift. Correcting problems from a previous neck lift. St. Louis, MO: QMP Inc.; 2006. p. 497–519, 1-57626-165-4.

17. Loeb R. Earlobe tailoring during facial rhytidoplasties. Plast Reconstr Surg 1972;49:485.

18. Leist FD, Masson JK, Erich JB. A review of 324 rhytidectomies emphasizing complications and patient dissatisfaction. Plast Reconstr Surg 1977;59:525–9.

19. Knuttel R, Torabian SZ, Fung M. Hair loss after rhytidectomy. Dermatol Surg 2004;30:1041–2.

20. Goin MK, Byron RW, Goin JM. A prospective psychological study of 50 female facelift patients. Plast Reconstr Surg 1980;65(40):436–42.

Reducing Surgical Risks for Otoplasty

Steven G. Hoshal, MD[a], Megan V. Morisada, MD[a], Travis T. Tollefson, MD, MPH[b],*

KEYWORDS

• Otoplasty • Complications • Mustarde sutures • Conchal setback

KEY POINTS

• Prominent ear is a common auricular deformity that can lead to psychosocial distress.
• Otoplasty is a well-tolerated procedure with high satisfaction and low complication rates.
• Adverse surgical outcomes are avoided by preventing hematoma and overcorrection.

INTRODUCTION

Prominauris (protruding or prominent ears) is a relatively common auricular deformity affecting up to 5% of the Caucasian population and inherited in an autosomal dominant pattern.[1] It is most often due to underdevelopment of the antihelical fold or overdevelopment of the conchal bowl. There is a wide range of what is perceived as within the spectrum of normal. Significant psychosocial distress may result from prominent ears,[2] leading to the development of a variety of surgical techniques over the years. A thorough understanding of the anatomy of both the normal and prominent ear is crucial for accurate analysis and surgical correction of the deformity.

History

Surgery on the protruding ear was first described in Vedas, an ancient Indian text from around 600 BC, with oral transmission of information preceding centuries before that. The text describes repair of the earlobe using cheek flaps, as performed by the potter caste.[3] In 1845, Dieffenbach was the first to describe suture fixation of the conchal bowl to the mastoid periosteum and postauricular skin excision for surgical repair of the post-traumatic protruding ear.[4] In 1881, Ely described the resection of postauricular skin along with a crescentic cartilage strip and concho-mastoid fixation suturing for correction of congenitally prominent ear, a procedure he staged by side.[5]

Luckett then introduced the concept of restoration of the antihelical fold in 1910 by breaking the cartilage with a skin–cartilage excision along the antihelical fold and horizontal mattress suturing.[6] In 1952, Becker described a cartilage-tubing technique to accentuate the antihelix to produce a more rounded result.[7] In 1963, Mustarde developed a popular technique to create the antihelical fold without needing cartilage incision using concho-scaphal mattress suturing, which resulted in less sharp edges and more natural contour in a manner that was easy to perform with lasting results.[8] Finally, in 1968, Furnas[9] introduced concha-mastoid suture fixation as a technique to reduce excessive conchal height and fix the cephalo-auricular angle, a technique that was later modified by Spira.

Anatomy and Embryology

Fundamental anatomic principles of the auricle will guide surgical principles and approaches to correction. The adult auricle measures 5.5 to 6.5 cm in length with ear width being 50% to 60% of length. Ear length growth is about 85% complete by the age of 3 years,[10] whereas ear width reaches maturity by age 7 years in

a Department of Otolaryngology–Head and Neck Surgery, University of California Davis, 2521 Stockton Boulevard, Suite 7200, Sacramento, CA 95817, USA; b Division of Facial Plastic and Reconstructive Surgery, Department of Otolaryngology–Head and Neck Surgery, University of California Davis, 2521 Stockton Boulevard, Suite 7200, Sacramento, CA 95817, USA
* Corresponding author.
E-mail address: tttollefson@ucdavis.edu

Facial Plast Surg Clin N Am 31 (2023) 253–261
https://doi.org/10.1016/j.fsc.2023.01.011

boys and age 6 years in girls.[11] The conchal depth is normally less than 1.5 cm,[12] and the antihelical fold is often a greater than 90° angle between the concha and scapha.[13] Cartilage stiffens with age, affecting the techniques selected such as cartilage bending versus resection.

With regard to auricular position, the axis of the auricle is about 20° posterior from vertical and sometimes parallels the slope of the nasal dorsum.[14] The base of the tragus starts about one ear length lateral to the lateral orbital rim, with the top of the helical rim roughly level with the lateral brow.[15] Protrusion can be measured from the scalp to the helical rim which is often 10 to 12 mm at the superior pole, 16 to 18 mm at the mid-pole, and 20 to 22 mm at the lobule.[10] The average auriculocephalic angle measures 25° in males and 21° in females,[11] which is another method to measure ear protrusion (Fig. 1).

Because of the stage of anatomic development and psychosocial distress that can arise from prominent ears with patient self-awareness and beginning of school socialization, intervention is often recommended from 3- to 6-year old. Optimally, waiting until the patient is mature enough to desire and actively participate in the postoperative care makes the process easier for both patients and their families.[2] Although an individual surgeon's algorithm and a variety of surgical techniques can be considered as part of one's arsenal, it is also important to pay attention to the patient and their family's individual request as well as to establish appropriate and realistic goals and expectations before surgery.

Preoperative Evaluation

Preoperative evaluation should involve measurements of the ear and protrusion, including conchal bowl depth, auriculocephalic measurements (superior helix, mid-helix, and lobule), scaphoconchal angle, and degree of helix development. The quality and stiffness of the auricular cartilage must be considered when considering cartilage-manipulating techniques. Asymmetry between the two sides must also be considered, with surgical correction often starting with the more prominent side and matching correction of the contralateral side. It is also important to assess motivation and readiness for surgery of the patient and their parents as part of the preoperative surgical workup.

Surgical Techniques

Anesthesia and preparation for surgery

We prefer to use a general anesthetic for pediatric patients. After intubation with a laryngeal mask airway, the patient is turned 180° from the anesthetist. The ears are carefully analyzed and standard measurements of auricular length, and distance of the upper, mid, and lower helix projection from the scalp are recorded. At this time, we make the final decision on the type of otoplasty techniques to use based on the morphologic features of the auricle and deformities present. Local anesthetic (1% lidocaine and 1:100K epinephrine) is infiltrated into the postauricular region in the planned incision as well as judicious use along the region of the planned anti-helical fold. Next, we fold the ear to create the desired anti-helical

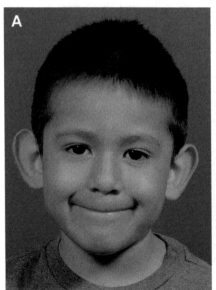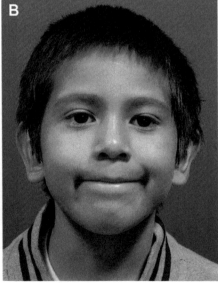

Fig. 1. Photograph of 7-year-old boy presenting with asymmetric prominent ears (A) before and (B) after otoplasty.

fold and tattoo the fold with methylene blue on 30-gauge needle. A sterile field is created including draping of the endotracheal tube circuit with a sterile ultrasound probe sheath to allow both ears to be in the field and visualized.

Cartilage Preserving Otoplasty: Mustarde Sutures

Patients with underdeveloped antihelical folds require surgical correction with Mustarde-type mattress sutures. The steps are as follows.

- Incision: A postauricular "dumbbell"-shaped incision is fashioned approximately 3 cm in length planned approximately half-way between the postauricular crease and the antihelical fold. The pre-op marking with methylene blue allows the design of the skin excision to be designed to ease the placement of the horizontal mattress (*Mustarde) sutures. Care must be taken to avoid over-resection of skin which can lead to hypertrophic scarring. After excising the full thickness skin, baby-double prong skin hooks are used for retraction and a supra-perichondrial plane is dissected sharply with a 15 blade and littler scissors to raise the anterior and posterior flaps. Visualizing of the tattooed antihelical fold requires adequate dissection in the anterior and posterior vector for suture placement.
- Cartilage scoring: Conservative posterior cartilage scoring with a 15 blade is performed to reduce cartilage memory.
- Mustarde suture placement: The transverse travel of the horizontal mattress sutures is approximately 16 or 8 mm on each side of the antihelical fold. Vertical travel of the mattress suture is 10 mm, and each mattress is spaced apart by 2 to 3 mm.[8,16,17] We have found that a PS-2 needle (19 mm length) on a 4-0 clear nylon suture achieves the 16 mm horizontal travel without difficulty. Three to five sutures are placed to create the desired effect. During suture placement, we visualize the anterior helix to ensure that there is no evidence of visible suture material passing through or just beneath the anterior skin to avoid suture extrusion/infection. After each suture is passed, they are placed on tension while visualizing the anterior helix to confirm the desired effect. Once confirmed, each suture is cut and tagged with a mosquito clamp until completion of all suture placement.
- Mustarde suture fixation: After completion of the mattress suture placement, they are serially tied down from superior to inferior to create the desired effect. Care must be taken

to ensure that skin and fascia are not tucked into the knot, as the suture is tied without visualizing the knot. Caution is required to avoid over-correction resulting in iatrogenic deformities (hidden helix, telephone ear, reverse telephone ear). When performed together with concha-mastoid sutures, the Mustarde sutures are secured first.
- Ensuring symmetry: Before skin closure on the second auricle, it is essential to compare the left to right ear to ensure symmetric cephalo-auricular angles are achieved at all levels of the auricle (upper, middle, and lower one-thirds) and that no iatrogenic deformities have been created.
- Skin closure: Skin closure is performed using buried interrupted 5-0 monocryl deep dermal sutures. Tension free skin sutures are critical to avoid hypertrophic scarring. The skin is approximated with a combination of running and interrupted 5-0 fast gut suture. We often apply octyl-2-cyanoacrylate (Dermabond) skin glue to the cranial half of the incision.

Cartilage Preserving Otoplasty: Furnas Conchal Setback

The Furnas technique (concha-mastoid sutures) is necessary to the deformity associated with over-developed conchal bowls.[9] Concha-mastoid mattress sutures are used to correct excessively deep concha by lowering and flattening the conchal bowl and decreasing the distance between the conchal cartilage and mastoid prominence. The steps are as follows.

- Incision: The postauricular incision is designed like the Mustarde incision if performed together. If Mustarde sutures are not part of the operation, the incision should be designed closer to the postauricular crease due to the need for dissection along the mastoid prominence.
- Flap elevation and mastoid fascia contouring: The anterior aspect of the incision is elevated to expose the posterior conchal cartilage. Through posterior incision, the posterior auricularis muscles are divided with monopolar cautery, and the posterior flap is raised as a musculo-areolar-cutaneous flap.[18] As the flap is raised posteriorly, a concave depression is created for the conchal cartilage setback care carefully excising mastoid fascia. Care must be taken to avoid clearance of excessive fascia atop the mastoid prominence because the periosteum/supra-periosteal fascia must be thick enough to hold concha-mastoid

suture tension. Inadequate fascial suturing may lead to failure/recurrent auricular prominence.

- Concha-mastoid Suture Placement: Given the tension on the concha-mastoid suture, we recommend a permanent suture—such as the Mustarde sutures (4–0 clear Nylon PS-2 needle). These sutures are passed with full-thickness bites through the posterior conchal cartilage, taking care not to penetrate the epidermis in the concha cavum. Suture placement requires thoughtful planning; placing the sutures too far forward will lead to the dreaded complication of narrowing of the external auditory canal (EAC), whereas placing them too far posterior will widen the transverse dimension of the concha. In the vertical vector, placement too cephalically may lead to over-flattening of the concha, whereas placement too caudally may lead to an ineffective suture.[19]
- Concha-mastoid suture fixation: The sutures are serially tied while carefully inspecting the auricle from the anterior view and comparing sides for symmetry and desired cosmetic changes balanced with facial proportions.
- Note: When Mustarde sutures are being performed together with concha-mastoid sutures, the Mustarde sutures should be completed and tied before cinching down the concha-mastoid sutures.

Cartilage Preserving Otoplasty: Furnas Conchal Setback Modification

A modification in the Furnas conchal setback was described by Spire and Stal.[20] They used a laterally based flap of cartilage sutured posteriorly to mastoid periosteum, arguing that this reduced the risk of narrowing the EAC while avoiding long-term anterior conchal cartilage irregularities.

Postoperative Dressings

Postoperative dressings play a crucial role in increasing the odds of a satisfactory postoperative course. After otoplasty, we dress the ears with bacitracin, Xeroform gauze, Telfa, a mastoid-type dressing for 3 days. This is secured in place applying pressure to the auricle for approximately 3 days. The patient leaves the dressings intact until their first postoperative visit. After the 3 to 5 days post-op visit and wound check, we encourage all patients to wear an athletic headband for 6 weeks after surgery to improve appearance and reduce the risk of recurrent auricular ear protrusion.

Reducing Surgical Complications

Early complications

Postoperative hematoma Despite a generally low incidence of auricular hematoma after otoplasty (0%–2.2%),[21] it is a dreaded complication that can significantly impact the patient's experience and surgical outcomes. The often-repeated quote in surgical training, "An ounce of prevention is worth a pound of cure" certainly is relevant in avoidance of complications in otoplasty surgery. Certain controllable/modifiable factors may improve outcomes. During initial consultation, it is important to elicit a thorough history to determine if the patient has any history of bleeding diatheses, easy bruising, or is taking medications or supplements that may lead to coagulopathy. During the operation, judicious use of cautery to avoid bleeding after vasoconstriction wears off is paramount as the auricle is well vascularized with multiple branches of the external carotid system.[22] The herald symptom of an auricular hematoma after otoplasty is unilateral pain. If a patient presents with pain out of proportion to examination, we recommend removing the dressings to inspect for hematoma. Untreated hematoma may lead to skin and cartilage necrosis with permanent deformity. As demonstrated in the prior section on postoperative dressings, we emphasize auricular pressure dressings to decrease the risk of hematoma/seroma.

Infection/perichondritis Postoperative wound infections will most likely manifest between days 3 and 5 after surgery. Signs and symptoms of infection include increasing pain, redness, warmth, tenderness to palpation, purulent discharge from the incision/fluctuant fluid collection, and fevers/chills. It is critical to treat an early skin soft tissue infection expeditiously to avoid the feared complication of perichondritis due to *Pseudomonas aeruginosa* species. In the setting of perichondritis, systemic anti-pseudomonal antibiotics are a necessity and if there is sluggish improvement, careful debridement of the wound or opening the incision may be beneficial. Poorly treated infection/perichondritis may lead to cartilage necrosis and permanent deformity.

Cartilage/skin necrosis As mentioned above, progressive hematoma and infection/perichondritis may lead to necrosis of the skin and deeper cartilage. Soft tissue handling techniques should include finesse in atraumatic grasping of tissues with fine forceps/double prongs, care to avoid overthinning of skin flaps, judicious use of electrocautery, and careful handling and scoring of the cartilage are all maneuvers that reduce the risks of cartilage or skin flap necrosis. This complication must be prevented at all costs as the patient may end up with a disfigurement worse than the presurgical auricular prominence.

Late complications

Hypertrophic scar/keloids Wounds closed with excess tension on the skin are at risk of hypertrophic or keloid scarring with higher incidence in patients with darker skin pigment. Keloid formation may be as high as 1.2% to 2.5%.[21] If a keloid or hypertrophic scar is inspected on postoperative evaluation, immediate treatment is offered including pressure dressings/silicone barriers and serial triamcinolone (10 mg/mL) or 5-fluorouracil injections. Isolated keloid in the posterior auricular incision can be predicted with family history or personal history of keloids, but certainly need to be discussed in the informed consent of all children. An isolated keloid should have excision and treatment immediately (**Fig. 2**). Appropriate counseling about the risks of intralesional steroids includes soft tissue atrophy, hypopigmentation, and pain. Disfiguring scars (**Fig. 3**) may require

re-excision and aggressive postoperative medical management. A frank discussion with the family should include the potential for recurrence regardless of the treatment. Rarely consideration of adjuvant radiation after discussion of risks and benefits may be necessary to abate recidivistic keloid growth once a patient has achieved adult age.[23]

Suture Extrusion

Suture extrusion is not infrequent after otoplasty with permanent sutures and should be part of the informed consent process. To avoid visibility of suture, we prefer using a 4 to 0 clear nylon. In our experience, this has led to less suture visibility than colored permanent sutures. In addition, permanent suture has better durability and lower risk of recurrence than absorbable suture.[24] In the setting of early suture extrusion, removal is necessary and depending on the shape of the ear may warrant revision otoplasty. In a delayed extrusion, if the ear has retained postsurgical shape revision may not be necessary and simple trimming of the suture will resolve the problem.

RECURRENCE

Cartilage memory may lead to recurrent auricular prominence which tends to have a higher incidence in suture only techniques up to 24%.[25,26] However, when cartilage scoring or excision techniques are performed, there may be improvement in recurrence rates[27] with the tradeoff of greater risk of contour irregularities and cartilage necrosis along the new antihelical rim.[28]

Esthetic Complications

Persistent or novel auricular deformities are caused by an abnormal relationship of the auricle to the scalp and abnormal shape of the auricle. Postoperative deformities include telephone ear/reverse telephone ear, overcorrection of the helix/hidden helix, auricular ridges, cartilage buckling, and narrowing of the EAC and meatus.

Inadequate Correction

If correction is not adequate this can be attributed to improper preoperative evaluation and diagnosis of the auricular deformity. For example, an auricle with overdeveloped conchal bowl will not have adequate correction with Mustarde-type sutures alone. On the contrary, a patient with an underdeveloped antihelical fold will not have adequate results with a Furnas conchal setback alone.

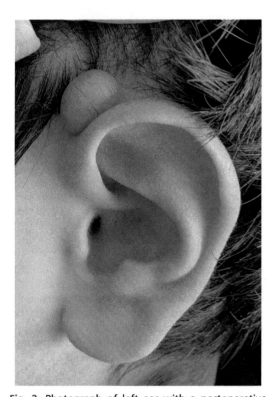

Fig. 2. Photograph of left ear with a postoperative isolated lobulated keloid in the superior most aspect of the posterior auricular incision after otoplasty. This was successfully treated with excision, triamcinolone, and 5-fluorouracil injections, and 6 weeks of pressure dressing.

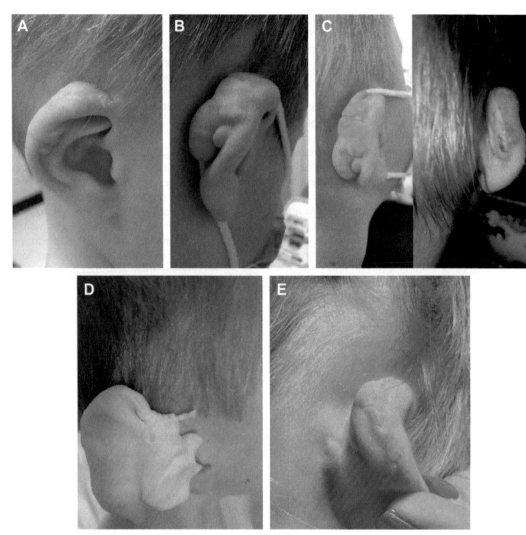

Fig. 3. Auricular cartilage deformity after otoplasty referred in from outside facility shown (*A*) right helical fold keloid with nodularity anteriorly, (*B*) large posterior auricular keloid, and (*C*) immediately after keloid excision, full-thickness skin grafting, steroid injection. (*D*) The pressure ear dressing shown was adapted to the ear for 1-week postoperatively. (*E*) Same ear shown 6 months after skin grafting while undergoing steroid injections every 6 weeks.

OVERCORRECTION

Over aggressive correction of the prominent ear may result in overcorrection of the auricle with flattening against the scalp resulting in a hidden helix deformity (**Fig. 4**). This must be prevented at the time of the primary surgery by careful measurement of the auricular prominence with each suture tightening.

Telephone Ear Deformity

Telephone ear deformity occurs when the middle one-third of the prominent auricle is overcorrected as may be seen in an overzealous conchal setback.

On the contrary, a reverse telephone ear deformity may develop when the upper and lower one-third is overcorrected with Mustarde-type sutures and the middle one-third conchal protrusion is not adequately addressed. Careful analysis and judicious maneuvers should be performed in the revision setting to avoid overcorrection.

Cartilage Buckling Deformity

Cartilage buckling develops when Mustarde-type sutures are spaced too far apart creating a buckling effect between the tension applied by the suture. Avoiding this type of complication requires careful   measurement   and   adherence   to

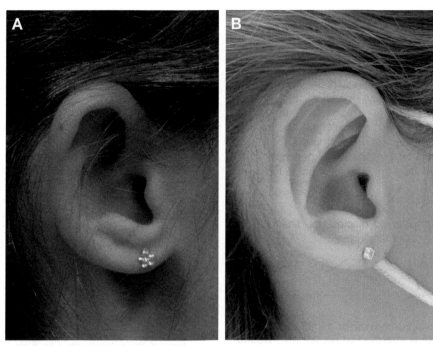

Fig. 4. Photographs of (A) pre-op and (B) post-op otoplasty with overcorrection of the Mustarde sutures leading to a prominent helical fold which looks unnatural.

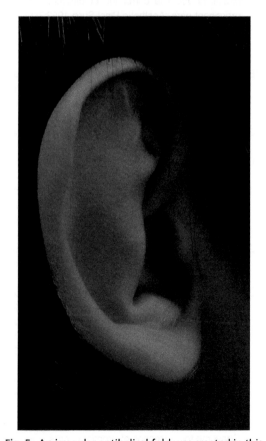

Fig. 5. An irregular antihelical fold was created in this otoplasty likely due to excessive scoring or cartilage excision during the Mustarde suture placement.

appropriate suture placement.[8,16,17] It is plausible that if the Mustarde sutures are placed with excessive scoring of the ear cartilage, an irregular antihelix can be created (Fig. 5).

Narrowing of the External Auditory Canal and Meatus

This cosmetic and functional iatrogenic deformity is associated with aggressive conchal setback.[29] Care taken to avoid the placement of the mastoid periosteal suture too anteriorly can reduce the risk of EAC narrowing; thoughtful placement of concha-mastoid sutures in the posterior vector will reduce this complication. In addition, partial conchal cartilage excision[29] or a lateral flap technique on which a laterally based flap of conchal cartilage is incised and secured to the mastoid periosteum may reduce EAC stenosis.[20]

Auricular Ridges

Abnormal auricular ridges are generally associated with cartilage cutting and scoring techniques. This complication can be avoided altogether by using cartilage preserving techniques, for example, Mustarde sutures and Furnas concho-mastoid sutures.

SUMMARY

Thankfully, the incidence of complications after otoplasty is relatively low, and the procedure is well tolerated, giving patients a renewed sense of confidence in their appearance after a successful operation. Careful preoperative evaluation and adherence to meticulous cartilage-sparing techniques will lead to good results and low complication rates. As in any operation, the informed consent process is emphasized to discuss esthetic changes and establish realistic expectations; if this is achieved both the patient and the surgeon will have a better experience in the journey to correct the prominent ear deformity.

DISCLOSURES

The authors have no disclosures, financial conflicts of interest or funding.

CLINICS CARE POINTS

- Early complications can be minimized through meticulous attention to hemastasis , wound closure, and dressings perioperatively.
- Subacute complications should be treated promptly and close follow up.
- Pre-operative measurements can help to avoid over or under-correction and adherence to appropriate anatomical standards.
- A thorough informed consent process should be reviewed and emphasized to establish realistic patient expectations.

FUNDING AND CONFLICTS OF INTEREST

None.

REFERENCES

1. Adamson PA, Strecker HD. Otoplasty techniques. Facial Plast Surg 1995;11:284–300.
2. Macgregor FC. Ear deformities: social and psychological implications. Clin Plast Surg 1978;5:347–50.
3. Davis JE, Hernandez HH. History of the aesthetic surgery of the ear. Aesthetic Plast Surg 1978;2: 75–94.
4. Dieffenbach J. Die operative chirugie. Leipzig: F A Brockhaus; 1845.
5. Ely E. A Classic reprint: An operation for prominence of the auricles (with two wood-cuts). Aesthetic Plast Surg 1987;11:73–4.
6. Luckett W. A new operation for prominent ears based on the anatomy of the deformity. Surg Gynecol Obstet 1910;10:635.
7. Becker OJ. Correction of the protruding deformed ear. Br J Plast Surg 1952;5:187–96.
8. Mustarde JC. The correction of prominent ears using simple mattress sutures. Br J Plast Surg 1963;16: 170–8.
9. Furnas DW. Correction of prominent ears by concha-mastoid sutures. Plast Reconstr Surg 1968;42: 189–93.
10. Adamson JE, Horton CE, Crawford HH. The growth pattern of the external ear. Plast Reconstr Surg 1965;36:466–70.
11. Farkas LG, Posnick JC, Hreczko TM. Anthropometric growth study of the ear. Cleft Palate Craniofac J 1992;29:324–9.
12. Rubin LR, Bromberg BE, Walden RH, et al. An anatomic approach to the obtrusive ear. Plast Reconstr Surg Transplant Bull 1962;29:360–70.
13. Pitanguy I, Muller P, Piccolo N, et al. The treatment of prominent ears: a 25-year survey of the island technique. Aesthetic Plast Surg 1987;11:87–93.
14. Nachlas NE. Otoplasty. In: Papel ID, editor. Facial plastic and reconstructive surgery. New York: Thieme; 2016. p. 351–63.
15. Tolleth H. Artistic anatomy, dimensions, and proportions of the external ear. Clin Plast Surg 1978;5: 337–45.
16. Mustarde JC. The correction of different types of prominent ears. Aesthetic Plast Surg 1983;7:163–8.
17. Mustarde JC. Correction of prominent ears using buried mattress sutures. Clin Plast Surg 1978;5: 459–64.
18. Horlock N, Misra A, Gault DT. The postauricular fascial flap as an adjunct to Mustarde and Furnas type otoplasty. Plast Reconstr Surg 2001;108: 1487–90. ; discussion 1491.
19. Furnas DW. Otoplasty for prominent ears. Clin Plast Surg 2002;29:273–88, viii.
20. Spira M, Stal S. The conchal flap: an adjunct in otoplasty. Ann Plast Surg 1983;11:291–8.
21. Limandjaja GC, Breugem CC, Mink van der Molen AB, et al. Complications of otoplasty: a literature review. J Plast Reconstr Aesthet Surg 2009;62: 19–27.
22. Zilinsky I, Erdmann D, Weissman O, et al. Reevaluation of the arterial blood supply of the auricle. J Anat 2017;230:315–24.
23. Ogawa R, Mitsuhashi K, Hyakusoku H, et al. Postoperative electron-beam irradiation therapy for keloids and hypertrophic scars: retrospective study of 147 cases followed for more than 18 months. Plast Reconstr Surg 2003;111:547–53. discussion 554-545.
24. Maslauskas K, Astrauskas T, Viksraitis S, et al. Comparison of otoplasty outcomes using different types of suture materials. Int Surg 2010;95:88–93.
25. Hyckel P, Schumann D, Mansel B. Method of Converse for correction of prominent ears: comparison of results. Acta Chir Plast 1990;32:164–71.

26. Tan KH. Long-term survey of prominent ear surgery: a comparison of two methods. Br J Plast Surg 1986; 39:270–3.

27. Schlegel-Wagner C, Pabst G, Muller W, et al. Otoplasty using a modified anterior scoring technique: standardized measurements of long-term results. Arch Facial Plast Surg 2010;12:143–8.

28. Ferzli G, Sukato D, Araslanova R, Romo Iii T. Cartilage-Sparing Otoplasty: A Systematic Review. Facial Plast Surg Aesthet Med 2020. https://doi.org/10.1089/fpsam.2020.0123.

29. Small A. Prevention of meatal stenosis in conchal setback otoplasty. Laryngoscope 1975;85: 1782–4.

Reducing Surgical Risks for Hair Replacement Surgery

Daniel E. Rousso, MD[a], Jaclyn A. Klimczak, MS, MD[a,b,*]

KEYWORDS

- Hair transplant • Androgenetic alopecia • Follicular unit • Follicular unit excision • Hair grafting
- Hair transplantation • Alopecia • Hair regeneration

KEY POINTS

- Hair replacement surgery has become widely popular and accepted as a meaningful and permanent solution to hair loss.
- Surgical complications, although uncommon, are largely due to insufficient surgical planning or questionable surgical techniques.
- A thorough preoperative evaluation of the patient is critical to increase the likelihood for a successful postoperative experience.

INTRODUCTION

Hair loss is a common problem that can affect both men and women and have significant effects on self-image and emotional well-being. The most common cause of hair loss between both genders is androgenic alopecia (AGA) but hair loss can be caused by a variety of factors that include, but are not limited to, trauma, infection, dermatologic diseases, systemic diseases, and stress. Hair replacement surgery (HRS) is widely popular and a sought out procedure with few complications when performed by a skilled and knowledgeable surgeon. HRS includes more historical techniques such as tissue expansion, scalp reduction, and skin flap surgery that today has essentially evolved into the more popular hair transplant surgery. The type of HRS mostly depends on the individual patient's needs. Although these techniques have been developed to achieve excellent cosmetic results, they are not without risks for potential complications even among the most highly skilled surgeon and assistant team. In this article, we discuss complications that can arise with HRS with a focus on hair transplantation. We present solutions and preventative measures that help achieve the best cosmetic results.

HISTORY OF HAIR REPLACEMENT SURGERY

The quest to combat hair loss has been a long and laborious road that traces back for thousands of years. Wigs and hairpieces were commonplace among the elites in ancient societies in 3000 BC highlighting the importance of their quality as a means of status. One of the earliest and simplest remedies dating back to ancient India developed the tradition of standing on your head to increase blood flow to the scalp.[1,2] However, it was not until 1553 BC when the earliest medical text, the Egyptian Ebers, Papyrus described treatments for hair loss using a mixture of iron oxide, red lead, onions, alabaster, honey, and fat from a variety of exotic animals including snakes, crocodiles, hippopotamuses, and lions. The mixture was to be swallowed while reciting a magic chant to their sun god in hopes of reversing the hair loss. If that effort fell short of delivering results, boiled porcupine hair was to be applied to the bald areas for 4 days.[1,3] Although these remedies expectedly failed,

There are no sources of funding to report. The authors state that there are no financial disclosures to report. The authors state there are no conflicts of interest.
[a] Rousso Adams Facial Plastic Surgery, 2700 Highway 280, Suite 300W, Birmingham, AL 35223, USA; [b] Nose and Sinus Institute of Boca Raton, 1601 Clint Moore Road #170, Boca Raton, FL 33487, USA
* Corresponding author.
E-mail address: Dr.jaclynklimczak@gmail.com

facialplastic.theclinics.com

different mixtures of animal products, herbs, spices, and natural oils were continuously used in the ancient Greek, Roman, Chinese, and Scandinavian cultures.

Hippocrates (460 to 370BC) eventually lost most of his hair, where the term androgenic hair loss is commonly referred to as "Hippocratic baldness." He went on to become the first to record a surgical solution to baldness in the "Aphorisms of Hippocrates," when he observed a parallel between testosterone levels/libido and hair loss. The observation came from the Persian Army eunuchs, who lacked testosterone from castration and retained their hair.[1] Although this surgical solution did not gain popularity, people such as Julius Caesar, King Henry VIII, and King Louis the IVX turned again to concoctions of animal byproducts and finally modalities that concealed their baldness with wreaths and wigs. Eventually, these ornamental replacements went on to signify power and affluence and were adopted up until the 1700s and the birth of America.

It was not until 1822 when the first written record of successful hair transplantation was introduced. A medical student named Diffenbach described in his thesis an experimental surgery performed with mentor Professor Dom Unger on the allotransplantation and autotransplantation of hair, feathers, and skin of animals. Although this technique did not become widely adopted by other surgeons, the use of skin flaps and free grafts for the treatment of traumatic alopecia were more commonly used in the late nineteenth century. The modern surgical techniques of hair transplantation were developed in 1939 by Japanese physician Okuda who described the successful transplantation of hair-bearing skin punch autografts from the posterior scalp to areas of balding on the frontal scalp, eyebrows, mustache, and pubic areas.[4] His success outside of Japan was overshadowed by World War II until 1959 when American Dermatologist Norman Orentreich reported the first successful hair transplant performed in the United States for male pattern alopecia. He is notably known as the founding father of hair transplant surgery.[5] Rapid developments in hair loss took off in the second half of the twentieth century with the advent of medications such as Minoxidil and Finasteride as well as an evolution of hair transplantation techniques such as scalp reduction, tissue expanders, and skin flap surgeries. It was not until the emergence of the follicular unit concept that modern HRS gave rise to the natural results we have today.[6,7] Hair loss continues to plague 65% to 85% of men and 30% to 40% of women and can be caused by a variety of genetic, endocrine, immune, and inflammatory processes.[8,9] Although hair transplantation and other restoration surgeries have been accepted as the gold standard for hair loss now for decades, advances in this field to minimize risk and create safe, consistent, effective, and natural-looking results are critical.

PREOPERATIVE EVALUATION

Setting the stage for a successful HRS begins in the preoperative period as there are many factors to consider that can influence the outcome of the surgery. The most common form of surgically treatable alopecia is AGA, which leads to male and female pattern baldness. However, other etiologies of alopecia should be considered during the patient evaluation such as infections, burns, traction, autoimmune diseases, neoplasms, radiation exposure, psychologic disorders, and hormonal imbalances to touch on just a few of the many causes of hair loss in humans. Many causes of hair loss are not amenable to certain types of HRS or surgery at all, which is why a comprehensive evaluation before developing a treatment plan is critical. Patients with inflammatory or autoimmune disorders such as frontal fibrosing alopecia for instance are not good candidates for hair transplantation because the transplanted hair will not survive in the long term. Patients who have been exposed to radiation or have significant scarring are at an increased risk for complications of undergoing any HRS because of the compromised blood supply to the scalp.

A thorough discussion and education on hair loss with patients is important to set expectations and achieve long-term success in the procedure before proceeding with a surgical treatment. A fundamental concept that needs to continuously be reiterated is that hair loss is a progressive process that will continue as the patient ages. Patients may consider or already be on medical therapies such as Minoxidil, Finasteride, or Spironolactone for their hair loss, and the use and discontinuation of these therapies should be discussed in length and documented.[10–12] Discussion of family history and patterns of hair loss among relatives gives the surgeon a better idea of what to expect as this patient ages and can appropriately develop a surgical plan that will continue to look natural as they potentially lose more hair. A long-term plan especially in younger patients who present with alopecia is crucial as they can develop unnatural hairlines and an "operated" look as they continue to lose hair with age. Younger patients are more likely to present with unrealistic goals and want an aggressive restoration, but this can lead to a cosmetically unfavorable graft distribution later in life. One way surgeons limit this risk is by limiting HRS for patients younger than 22 to 24 years old.

Establishing candid and trusting communication with the patient and openly discussing the quality of their hair are other essential components in managing expectations. This includes reviewing the shaft diameter, color, texture, follicular unit density, curl, and the telogen/anagen ratio of in situ donor's hair.[13] Hair color is of also great importance because the less contrast there is between hair and scalp color, the better potential for coverage. Ideal candidates include those with curly, coarse salt and pepper-colored hair. The patients' expectations of the surgery should be continuously reviewed. The surgeon should provide the patient with a stepwise treatment plan of what they will likely experience, their limitations postoperatively, and what to expect throughout the process. In the case of hair transplantation surgery where results are not immediate and can take many months, education, and setting expectations is imperative to a successful result.[14] The number of grafts needed to achieve a desired result is dependent on the patients' Norwood classification and may require multiple sessions depending on their donor site density to achieve substantial results. The type of HRS performed is also based on the patient personal preference and clinical circumstances. For instance, if a patient desires to keep their hair short (less than 0.5 inch), long incisional scars will be harder to hide and a follicular unit extraction (FUE) is best recommended. A complete knowledge of hair anatomy and thorough patient preoperative assessment can accurately predict the results the patient can expect.

Although discussing potential complications is difficult, it is necessary so proper action can be taken in a timely manner. This also allows the patient to be aware of what differences can exist between expected postoperative occurrences (pain, edema, scabbing/crusting, temporary thinning, and hypoesthesia) and complications are so they can be handled if and when they occur.

GENERAL COMPLICATIONS AMONG ALL HAIR RESTORATION SURGICAL TECHNIQUES
Bleeding

Bleeding is not uncommon after HRS and minor bleeding at the surgical site can often be stopped with continuous pressure application for 10 to 15 min. Preoperative evaluation and screening for a history of bleeding disorders or issues should be undertaken before surgery and the patient should be provided with a list of medications to avoid before and after their surgery. The most common agents include nonsteroidal anti-inflammatory medications, aspirin, vitamins, and supplements such as vitamin E, fish oil, Ginkgo biloba, ginseng, or other anticoagulative agents. A thorough review of the patient's medication list and discussion on safely stopping any medications that can affect coagulation should be discussed and cleared by their primary care doctor before surgery. The risk of significant bleeding is more common in skin flaps, scalp reduction, and at the donor site in strip harvesting for hair transplantation due to a larger area of undermining and the potential for vascular transection of scalp vessels. In these cases, bleeding can be controlled with bipolar or unipolar coagulation or suture ligation in the case of large caliber vessels. When controlling bleeding with coagulative devices, the surgeon must be careful to avoid follicular units that can be permanently affected by thermal injury. Small vessel bleeding at skin edges should therefore be controlled with epinephrine-containing anesthetic injection and meticulous wound closure.

Hematomas are exceedingly rare among HRS and are usually due to the transection of a large vascular branch of the occipital or superficial temporal artery. Maintaining awareness of anatomy and incisional depth are the best preventative measures at ensuring the avoidance of these vessels. If bleeding should occur, appropriate cauterization and/or suture ligation is warranted for control. Eliminating dead space with a multilayer closure is another technique to consider that aids in preventing postoperative fluid collection. A pressure dressing is appropriate for 24 h along the skin flap, scalp reduction incision line or donor site strip harvest suture line to control for potential bleeding. If a hematoma does occur, prompt recognition, drainage, and cauterization are essential in the first 24 h to prevent surgical site necrosis and wound healing complications.

Edema

Edema is an expected occurrence after HRS and oftentimes will migrate to the surrounding forehead and periorbital area. Although patients may associate swelling with a negative outcome, it should be discussed preoperatively in detail explaining this is a normal occurrence. Symptoms of edema will peak around postoperative during days 3 to 5 due to the third spacing of fluids. Patients who undergo a larger area of hair replacement are more prone to a larger area of edema due to the venous and lymphatic disruption caused by surgical trauma in addition to the cumulative anesthetic and tumescent fluid loads.[15] To combat edema, patients should be instructed to always maintain their head above their heart (30° to 45°) in the first 1 to 2 weeks of recovery. Cold compresses over the periorbital area can facilitate postoperative recovery most notably when performed diligently at 20-min intervals in the first 24 h postoperatively. Patients should be carefully instructed on where to place cold compresses and instructed to avoid areas such as skin flaps, which can produce devastating effects on tissue vascularity. Additional measures such as a postoperative systemic corticosteroid taper and low sodium diet can also prevent significant edema.

Infection

Surgical site infection is extremely rare following HRS (<1%) due to the rich vascular supply of the scalp. Serious infection is most notably caused by poor hygiene and excessive scabbing over the surgical sites that can be mitigated with thorough postoperative instructions given to the patient in writing and taught to the patient on their postoperative day 1 visit.[16] The teach-back method is one of the most effective measures in ensuring patients are comfortable with the postoperative care required to guarantee successful results. Significant crusting can be a nidus for bacterial proliferation increasing the risk of infection. Crusting over the donor site in FUE and the recipient site in all hair transplant modalities is expected and is the most common cause of postoperative infection. Grafts from hair transplantation will develop crusts over the recipient sites in the first 24 h and small crusts will continue to fall off naturally over the subsequent week. Frequent showering and shampooing to dislodge crusts and keep the scalp clean should be stressed to patients who are often apprehensive about touching their scalp after surgery. A spray bottle of witch hazel is recommended to patients for periodic spraying over the graft zone to aid in dislodging the crusts followed by gently shampooing. Prevention of postoperative infections should be carried out with perioperative antibiotics with good skin flora coverage such as cephalexin or ciprofloxacin in patients with an allergy to cephalosporins and taken for 7 days postoperatively.[17]

Even so, infections may occur and a high suspicion should be maintained by the surgeon and staff when patients complain of symptoms such as pain, swelling, and erythema out of proportion to the procedure, as well as fever, or discharge from the surgical site. Prompt discovery and implementation of appropriate treatment is imperative to result in a complication-free solution.

Infections over incisional areas are more likely to occur after high-tension closures and subsequent vascular compromise. In the immediate period, this can be combated with suture/staple removal. If any signs of infected fluctuance are noted, the area should be opened, drained, and thoroughly irrigated. Packing may be required in some cases where there is a risk of re-accumulation.

WOUND COMPLICATIONS AND SCARRING IN HAIR TRANSPLANTATION SURGERY
Wound Dehiscence

Wound dehiscence most commonly occurs due to increased tension along the incision line (**Fig. 1**). Appropriate preoperative planning to determine scalp elasticity and direction of elasticity is essential before proceeding with any HRS that requires incisions. Preoperative scalp relaxation exercises can be used and taught to the patient to perform at least twice a day for 5 min each. Scalp exercises improve scalp laxity and increase the mobility of the available tissue, allowing the surgeon to close the donor area with more ease. The more laxity the tissue has the less tension there will be in the closure which facilitates better healing and potentially allowing more grafts to be harvested. Sutures are typically removed between 10 and 14 days following surgery when the tensile strength of the wound can maintain an approximation of skin edges. If removal is noted to be premature, the surgeon should promptly address it with resuturing of the site. If there is tension noted upon reapproximating the wound edges a few techniques can be used to improve elasticity. This includes undermining the wound edges in the deep subcutaneous layer, performing galeotomies, and/or placement of towel clamps for a few minutes to achieve mechanical creep. If the wound is under great tension despite efforts to gain elasticity, the decision should be made to close in a delayed fashion to prevent necrosis, hair loss,

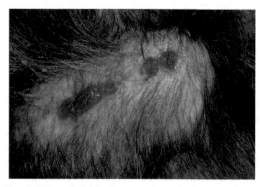

Fig. 1. Wound dehiscence at the strip harvest donor site after suture removal.

and additional scarring.[18] Wound dehiscence can be a cause of underlying medical problems such as diabetes, or from inappropriate patient management such as early physical activity or smoking. Patients should be medically optimized before surgery and educated on their restrictions in the perioperative period.

Necrosis

A feared complication that commonly derives from compromised vascular supply due to excessive tension along an incision is skin necrosis. Not only does it permanently damage the surrounding skin, but also its hair follicles. Patients who had previous surgery on their scalps are at a higher risk for necrosis due to greater tension and non-vascularized scar tissue. This should be noted upon their preoperative evaluation. Again, pre-existing conditions such as diabetes and habits such as smoking increase a patient's risk of necrosis and should be rectified before performing surgery. If necrosis does occur, prompt identification and management is essential. In the immediate period, application of topical nitroglycerin two to three times a day can potentially salvage a compromised vascular supply. If the area declares itself with an eschar, topical antibiotic ointments and conservative debridement should be carried out until vital tissue is apparent. Long-term management of these areas may require serial excisions or tissue expansion.

In hair transplantation surgery the recipient area and donor site area for FUE can also be at risk for ischemia and necrosis. One of the potential causes is the excessive vasoconstrictor effect injected with the tumescent solution. If areas of concern show blanching with slow or no regain of capillary fill, the surgeon should cease performing any additional grafting or injection or epinephrine-containing anesthetics to the area. This is more commonly seen in patients with previous hair transplant surgeries or previous scars from surgery or scarring alopecia.[14] Surgeons should also be cognizant of how densely they pack their recipient grafts and the depth of the recipient site as a compromised vascular supply can ensue from leaving little to no space between the sites.

Scarring

The goal of all HRS techniques is to create a natural-looking result free of obvious scarring. Many factors are involved in wound healing as described above, and all require participation from the surgeon and patient to adhere to strict wound care guidelines to prevent gross scarring.

As hair loss is often a progressive process, the surgeon must be aware of incisional placement and effective wound management to optimize scar camouflaging. Incisions should be placed in areas of greatest hair density where loss is less likely to widen from tension. Poor wound healing and wound care can lead to wide scars, crosshatched scars, and/or hypertrophic scars and keloids (**Fig. 2**).

Incisions for donor site strip harvesting should place the knife blade parallel to hair follicles in a trichophytic fashion to reduce follicle transection and allow hair growth through the future scar[19] (**Fig. 3**). Tumescence, after local anesthetic infiltration, aids in straightening out the hair follicles as well as limiting injury to the underlying nerves and vessels. Dissection is carried out in the subcutaneous plane above the galea to avoid transection of the underlying blood supply, nerves, and disruption to the surrounding hairs (**Fig. 4**). Meticulous tension-free closure should be carried out with a running locking 2 to 0 Prolene with care to avoid deep bites and only reapproximate wound edges. Superficial suture depth avoids the portion of the hair follicle to which the arrector pili muscle attaches thereby preventing deep follicle damage (**Fig. 5**). This important region captured the interest of surgeons because it is where follicular epithelial stem cells have been identified.[13,20] Although multilayered closures are also advocated, the essence of minimizing the risk of poor scarring depends largely on meticulous tissue handling and a tension-free closure. Injecting platelet-rich plasma (PRP) at the time of HRS can facilitate tissue

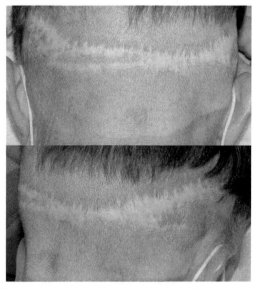

Fig. 2. Patient who underwent strip harvest hair transplantation with donor site scar widening.

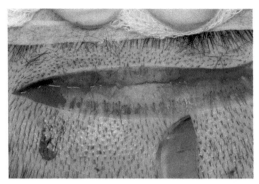

Fig. 3. Proper demonstration of beveling the 10-blade in a trichophytic fashion during strip harvest follicular unit transplantation.

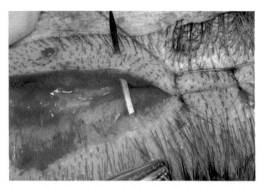

Fig. 5. Closure of the strip harvest donor site with a 2 to 0 running locking prolene showed at the precise level to avoid hair follicle damage and strangulation.

regeneration and stimulate new capillary growth potentially improving wound healing.[21] With subsequent strip harvesting, removal of the old scar should be included in the harvest to avoid multiple scars and facilitate scalp elasticity as scars limit tissue flexibility. Avoid placing the incision lower than the nuchal ridge to prevent migration to a more visible area.

Even in the best hands, wound healing is not over when the incision is closed. Patient management is extremely important. Patient education

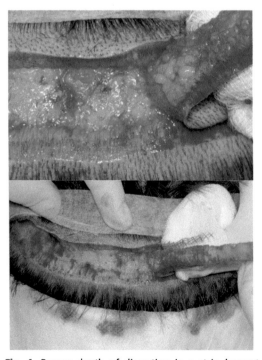

Fig. 4. Proper depth of dissection in a strip harvest follicular unit transplantation in the subcutaneous plane.

should include wound care instructions such as scalp cleaning with baby shampoo and decrusting with witch hazel while limiting physical activity for 2 weeks postoperatively. Neck flexion should be minimized to avoid additional pulling on the incision line. The consequences should be clearly described to patients.

Scarring is less likely to occur in FUE but careful planning and extraction techniques need to be used to prevent the risk of an unnatural appearance. Although the 1-mm punch in FUE heals in such a pattern that the scars are largely invisible, aggressive donor site harvesting can lead to areas of depletion and increase the risk of long-term visible scarring (**Fig. 6**). This complication is predominately due to poor surgical planning and poor implementation of techniques. Placement of FUE harvest and assessment of hair quality and density can easily avoid the complication of depletion. Hypopigmentation of the donor site in FUE can also be of concern that leads to an unnatural appearance in patients who keep their hair very short. This risk can be avoided by ensuring the punch is sharp thereby not traumatizing the surrounding tissue and, again, not overharvesting from the area.

Visible scarring is challenging to correct. Although serial excisions and scalp tissue expansion can be considered, the risk of a worse scar after revision remains a possibility. Potential treatment options include microdermal pigmentation to the affected area, tissue expansion, and skin flap or hair transplantation along the scar line to correct the defect (**Figs. 7** and **8**).

TELOGEN EFFLUVIUM

Telogen effluvium (TE) is categorized among the nonscarring alopecia's and is defined as diffuse hair thinning and shedding that occurs about 3 to

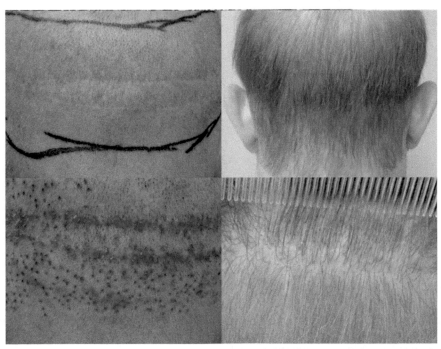

Fig. 6. Donor site depletion and scarring from multiple prior strip harvesting corrected with FUE to the donor site area. (Photographs courtesy of James E. Vogel, MD, FACS Associate Professor of Surgery, Department of Plastic Surgery, The Johns Hopkins Hospital and School of Medicine.)

4 months after a triggering event[22] (**Fig. 9**). Patients undergoing hair transplant surgery are counseled that it is normal to shed the grafted hairs after surgery, with no effect on the follicular unit itself. However, additional loss of non-transplanted hair can be devastating in the postoperative period. Thinning can occur anywhere along the HRS incision lines or near the recipient sites for

hair transplant surgery and is likely due to regional edema, inflammation and trauma causing the hair follicles to go into a synchronized resting phase. Patients during this time need frequent counseling that this is a temporary condition. Although there is no known preventative measure to combat TE, topical minoxidil may speed follicular recovery over the area of thinning.[23] Topical minoxidil can

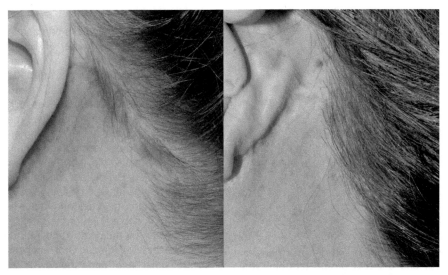

Fig. 7. Postoperative scarring and alopecia after a rhytidectomy is corrected with FUE to the area.

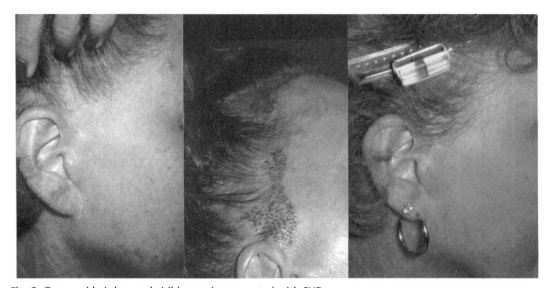

Fig. 8. Temporal hair loss and visible scarring corrected with FUE.

be started as early as 24 to 48 h after surgery and may aid in the prevention of TE although more research is needed. Additional measures that could help prevent TE include meticulous tissue

handling, limitation of cautery, and tension-free incision lines.

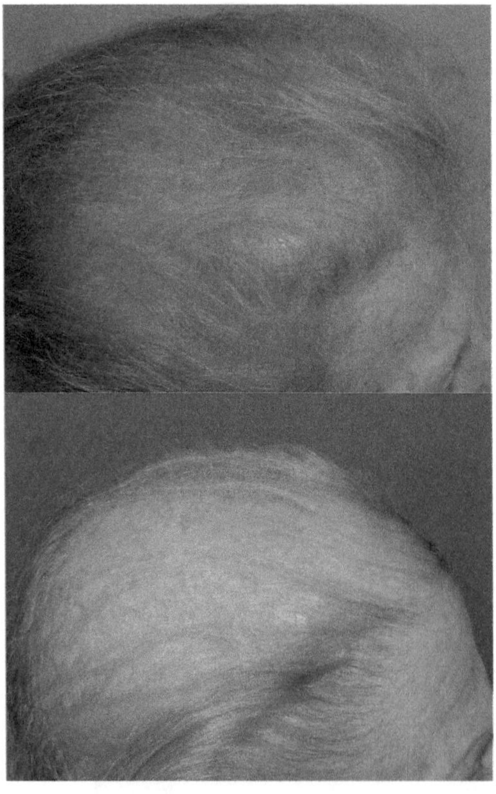

NERVE INJURY

Hypoesthesia of the scalp is common after HRS, and patients should be counseled that this can last 6 to 12 months after surgery. Permanent numbness however is uncommon and most likely due to complete nerve transection of the greater occipital, lesser occipital, or auriculotemporal nerves. Prevention of this compilation can be easily managed by controlling the depth of the incision during donor site strip harvesting with care to not violate the galea.

FOLLICULITIS, CYSTS, AND INGROWN HAIRS

Folliculitis and ingrown hairs can commonly occur in the first few weeks after HRS. Although the cause of folliculitis is not clear theories include a foreign body reaction from a trapped hair follicle at the recipient or donor site.[24] Although they can be painful for patients, most folliculitis pustules and cysts are sterile on culture medium. Prevention of folliculitis includes ensuring a hair-free incision line before closing and careful placement of recipient grafts into their newly created sites. Once identified, the patient should initiate aggressive scalp hygiene with cleaning using chlorhexidine gluconate or povidone-iodine shampoos. The surgeon should unroof the pustule and apply a thin layer of antibiotic ointment until healed over the active lesions. Oral antibiotics have a controversial role and should be reserved in more severe and resistant cases where the

Fig. 9. Preoperative photograph of a hair transplant patient (top) and 6 weeks postop (bottom) when they experienced telogen effluvium.

infection is suspected. Warm compresses can also provide symptomatic relief to the patient. Active management and frequent follow-up is recommended as chronic folliculitis can destroy recipient grafts and cause scarring.

Posttransplant epidermoid cysts can arise from technical areas caused in both the recipient and donor sites of FUE HRS. At the recipient site, the graft may become buried by creating a site that is too deep or plaining the graft over a previously placed graft. A fragment of ectopic epidermal cells can also be accidentally implanted by the 18-gauge hypodermic needle used for making the micrograft recipient track or by the punch used at the donor site, especially when the instruments used are dull. Careful graft harvesting and placement of grafts, with close inspection of the donor and recipient sites can be time well spent to avoid a postoperative complication. If an epidermal cyst does develop, it can be tender and erythematous causing great discomfort to the patient. The surgeon should incise or excise and drain the entrapped sebaceous debris and hairs, and instruct the patient to apply warm compresses and antibiotic ointment to the area until resolution. Systemic antibiotics may be needed for more severe infections and excision of the cyst should be done if it recurs.

POOR GROWTH OF HAIR
Low Graft Survival

The handling, placement, and creation of graft sites are the most important and meticulous parts of HRS. One of the most disappointing complications is getting a low graft yield from the donor site during either strip harvest or FUE. FUE has a higher chance of low graft survival because it is more technically demanding and time-consuming than strip harvest. Follicle transection can occur because the motorized punch should be set to the appropriate depth and angled to the hair exiting the scalp which can be challenging especially for novice surgeons. The angle of the emergent hair is more acute than the angle of the follicle in the dermis and this anticipation must be understood to obtain healthy grafts[25] Tumescence of the donor scalp elevates the follicles above the deep subcutaneous arteriolar plexus, aiding in the extraction of grafts. Coaxing the remainder of the graft with the punch or forceps should be done in a short twisting motion with a stable hand. A back-and-forth motion or pulling with forceps can lead to unnecessary transection. Transection rates range from 1.3% to 10%, whereas strip harvesting has an approximate transection rate of 1% to 2%.[26] Small micro-adjustments in depth and angle when harvesting can avoid long-

term potential problems. Strip harvest dissection requires dividing the donor strip into single rows and then diving them using a straight blade into individual grafts (**Fig. 10**). Although the technician has more control during a strip harvest, the grafts can be overly manipulated or improperly trimmed leading to failure. Careful sectioning and handling of the grafts under high power magnification is essential to their survival.

Once the grafts are harvested and prepared, they should be placed in cold sterile isotonic saline. Dehydration or placement of the grafts in another solution can render them unviable. Solutions that are toxic to grafts include sterile water and povidone-iodine.[14,27] Recent studies have advocated the use of PRP as a preservative for hair grafts, or to be injected over the recipient area before graft placement with potential improvement in hair density, graft uptake, and quality although more research is warranted in this area.[28]

POOR COSMETIC OUTCOME

One of the complications of HRS is a poor cosmetic outcome or an unhappy patient. This can be due to improper graft placement, poor hairline/shaping design, or graft type error.

Poor Design

The first principle in designing the recipient sites is developing a strategic plan with the patient that would continue to look natural even with progressive hair thinning. The hairline is typically 7.5 and 9.5 cm above the glabella. In men, the forelock pattern hair transplant that includes the area bounded anteriorly by the frontal hairline, posteriorly by the anterior crown region, and laterally by the parietal fringe, is commonly maintained.[13,15] This pattern holds stable for both the younger patient in the beginning stages of hair loss to stabilize

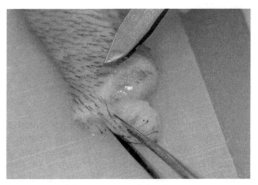

Fig. 10. Careful sectioning of the donor strip into single rows preserving all follicular units.

their frontal hairline and frame their face as well as the older patient with more extensive baldness. Creating a lower hairline in younger patients risks potential loss behind the newly implanted hair and thus an unnatural result as time goes on.[29,30] The frontal hairline should also have natural breaks or waves, and care should be taken to avoid creating straight unnatural lines (**Fig. 11**).[31]

Women with female pattern hair loss tend to have a more stable frontal hairline and diffuse thinning. Concentrating the grafts diffusely over the areas of thinning is most appropriate to stabilize their loss.[32] A more rounded temporal infill and lower hairline is more appropriate for women. Women with a high hairline who are candidates may also benefit from a hairline advancement surgery.[33] This should be performed at a separate time due to potential vascular supply compromise.

Recipient Site Creation and Placement

Recipient sites should be meticulously created at angles that follow the natural pattern of growth to the surrounding hair. Despite the numerous instruments that can be used from needles to knife blades, the technique should match the size of the individual recipient site with the length and width of the patient's follicular unit. We find that using an 18 gauge needle bent at two 90° angles

allows for better control of the recipient site depth and accounts for the degree of upward lift of the graft as they grow in **Fig. 12**. These needles will have to be changed accordingly as they dull (typically after 200 sites are made), and a highly skilled surgeon should be cognizant of its ease of insertion with the surrounding scalp. Blades can also be used to create precise recipient sites and although less cost-effective, the use of either the blade or needle should be at the comfort of the surgeon doing the procedure. The frontal hairline is the most unforgiving area when it comes to revealing technical error in graft placement and choice, therefore some smaller caliber single hair grafts should be inserted to create a natural appearance. Placement of grafts requires an efficient, skilled technician that can place the grafts atraumatically while maintaining their hydration. Handling the grafts with a forceps held only by the surrounding fat cuff and never on the hair shaft itself can avoid the risk of crushing or overmanipulating the graft which can lead to kinky hair growth (**Fig. 13**). When the appropriate angle is made, the grafts should sit in their recipient site 1 mm above the skin so when edema resolves it settles flush to the scalp (**Fig. 14**). If the graft sits flush with the skin or below, the patient is at risk for pitting and if placed too high, cobble stoning can occur.

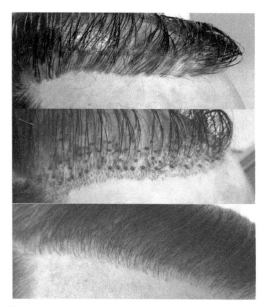

Fig. 11. Common complication of an unnatural straight hairline created with plugs (top) is corrected with the excision of previously transplanted hair and replaced with FUE. (Photographs courtesy of James E. Vogel, MD, FACS Associate Professor of Surgery, Department of Plastic Surgery, The Johns Hopkins Hospital and School of Medicine.)

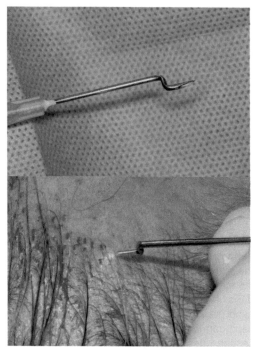

Fig. 12. Our 18-gauge needle can be bent to control the exact depth of the hair follicle and is used to make recipient sites.

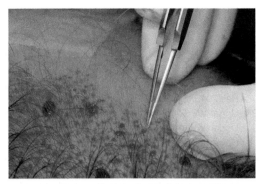

Fig. 13. Gentle handling of the grafts with forceps for precise insertion of each follicular unit. Grafts are adequately spaced to preserve the surrounding blood supply.

Both these technical errors are difficult to fix without completely removing the grafts. Camouflaging of the area can be done with subsequent HRS.[18]

POSTOPERATIVE CARE

Grafts sit gently in their recipient site and are therefore at risk for dislodgement in the immediate postoperative period. Significant stability and crust formation is seen between 3 and 4 days, but can occur as early as 24 h. Patients should be instructed to avoid tampering with the graft areas during this time period to prevent accidental dislodgement.[15,34] This includes rubbing, scratching, combing, brushing, or styling the hair. If a graft becomes dislodged, patients should be instructed to place it on a clean cool gauze moistened with saline and brought promptly to the office for reinsertion. Although this in theory seems promising, most grafts become dried out and unviable by the time of evaluation for reimplantation.

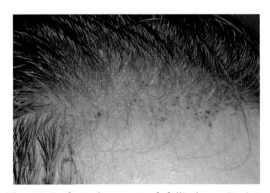

Fig. 14. Perfect placement of follicular units into recipient sites.

SUMMARY

HRS is a very safe procedure that provides an excellent means to treat many forms of alopecia in men and women. Although complications of HRS remain low, there still remain risks that can be easily prevented in the hands of a skilled surgeon and his/her team. Although the techniques in HRS have advanced to create natural appearing results, we continue to strive to make advancements in this field and limit the risks involved. Patient selection, evaluation, and clarifying expectations with the procedure are of the utmost importance in reducing risks and setting the stage for a successful treatment plan. Adhering to strong techniques for both the surgeon and technician as described in this article will lay the foundation for a successful HRS practice and mastery of this artistic surgical skill.

CLINICS CARE POINTS

- Hair replacement surgery requires a highly skilled and well-trained surgeon and staff to accomplish natural results devoid of complications.

- Although relatively safe, it is not without its risks of short- and long-term complications that can be related to the donor site and or recipient site.

- Careful preoperative planning and understanding preventative measures that can avoid these complications are key to successful results and satisfied patients.

REFERENCES

1. Trüeb RM. The difficult hair loss patient: a particular challenge. Int J Trichology 2013;5(3):110–4.
2. Giacometti L. Facts, legends, and myths about the scalp throughout history. Arch Dermatol 1967; 95(6):629.
3. Orentreich DS. The history of hair restoration. In: Stough D, Haber R, editors. Hair replacement. St Louis (MO): Mosby; 1996. p. 59–62.
4. Okuda S. Clinical and experimental studies of transplantation of living hairs. Jpn J Dermatol Urol 1939; 46:135–8.
5. Orentreich DS, Orentreich N. Hair transplantation. J Dermatol Surg Oncol 1985;11(3):319–24.
6. Bernstein RM, Rassman WR. The aesthetics of follicular transplantation. Dermatol Surg 1997;23(9): 785–99.

7. Limmer BL. Elliptical donor stereoscopically assisted micrografting as an approach to further refinement in hair transplantation. J Dermatol Surg Oncol 1994;20(12):789–93.

8. Norwood OT. Male pattern baldness: classification and incidence. South Med J 1975;68(11):1359–65.

9. Rose PT, Parsley WP. The science of hair line design. In: Haber RS, Stough DB, editors. Procedures in cosmetic dermatology. Hair transplantation. Philadelphia: Elsevier Saunders; 2006. p. 55–72.

10. Kaufman KD, Olsen EA, Whiting D, et al. Finasteride in the treatment of men with androgenetic alopecia. J Am Acad Dermatol 1998;39(4):578–89.

11. Leavitt M, David PM, Rao NA, et al. Effects of finasteride (1 mg) on hair transplant. Dermatol Surg 2006;31(10):1268–76.

12. Olsen KR, Hall DJ, Mira JC, et al. Postoperative surgical trainee opioid prescribing practices (POST OPP): an institutional study. J Surg Res 2018;229:58–65.

13. Vogel JE, Jimenez F, Cole J, et al. Hair restoration surgery: the state of the art. Aesthet Surg J 2013;33(1):128–51.

14. Perez-Meza D, Niedbalski R. Complications in hair restoration surgery. Oral Maxillofac Surg Clin North Am 2009;21(1):119–48.

15. Konior RJ. Complications in hair-restoration surgery. Facial Plast Surg Clin North Am 2013;21(3):505–20.

16. David PM. Complications in hair restoration surgery. Oral Maxillofac Surg Clin North Am 2009;21:119–48.

17. Leaper D, Ousey K. Evidence update on prevention of surgical site infection. Curr Opin Infect Dis 2015;28(2):158–63.

18. Lam SM. Complications in hair restoration. Facial Plast Surg Clin North Am 2013;21(4):675–80.

19. Marzola M. Trichophytic closure of the donor area. Int Soc Hair Restor Surg 2005;15(4):113–6.

20. Paus R, Cotsarelis G. The biology of hair follicles. N Engl J Med 1999;341(7):491–7.

21. Lacci KM, Dardik A. Platelet-rich plasma: support for its use in wound healing. Yale J Biol Med 2010;83(1):1–9.

22. Harrison S, Sinclair R. Telogen effluvium: telogen effluvium. Clin Exp Dermatol 2002;27(5):389–95.

23. Malkud S. Telogen effluvium: a review. J Clin Diagn Res 2015;9(9):WE01–3.

24. Unger WP. Complications of hair transplantation. In: Unger WP, editor. Hair transplantation. 3rd edition. New York: Marcel Dekker; 1995. p. 363–74.

25. Dua A, Dua K. Follicular unit extraction hair transplant. J Cutan Aesthet Surg 2010;3(2):76–81.

26. Harris JA. Follicular unit extraction. Facial Plast Surg Clin North Am 2013;21(3):375–84.

27. Parsley WM, Perez-Meza D. Review of factors affecting the growth and survival of follicular grafts. J Cutan Aesthet Surg 2010;3(2):69–75.

28. Abdelkader R, Abdalbary S, Naguib I, et al. Effect of platelet rich plasma versus saline solution as a preservation solution for hair transplantation. Plast Reconstr Surg Glob Open 2020;8(6):e2875.

29. Bernstein RM, Rassman WR. Follicular transplantation. patient evaluation and surgical planning. Dermatol Surg 1997;23(9):771–84 [discussion: 801–5].

30. Jimenez F, Ruifernández JM. Distribution of human hair in follicular units: a mathematical model for estimating the donor size in follicular unit transplantation. Dermatol Surg 1999;25(4):294–8.

31. Norwood OT, Taylor BJ. Hairline design and placement. J Dermatol Surg Oncol 1991;17(6):510–8.

32. Cousen P, Messenger A. Female pattern hair loss in complete androgen insensitivity syndrome: female pattern hair loss. Br J Dermatol 2010;162(5):1135–7.

33. Orme S, Cullen DR, Messenger AG. Diffuse female hair loss: are androgens necessary?: non-androgenic diffuse female hair loss. Br J Dermatol 1999;141(3):521–3.

34. Rose P. Hair restoration surgery: challenges and solutions. Clin Cosmet Invest Dermatol 2015;8:361.

Reducing Risks for Local Skin Flap Failure

David B. Hom, MD*, Benjamin T. Ostrander, MD, MSE

KEYWORDS

- Local flaps • Flap salvage • Reconstruction • Facial plastic surgery • Mohs surgery
- Plastic and reconstructive surgery

KEY POINTS

- Good surgical technique, careful monitoring, and numerous strategies throughout the care pathway can be used to reduce the risk of skin flap failure and ensure favorable outcomes.
- The intrinsic vascularity and perfusion of a flap are the most critical determinants of successful transfer. Anything that impacts perfusion will affect the overall outcome of the flap.
- Recognizing the etiology of flap compromise is the first step in salvaging a failing flap. Careful monitoring with attention to color, capillary refill, bleeding, flap temperature, and firmness will help identify issues promptly.
- Etiologies of flap failure can be broadly classified as venous, ischemic, tension-related, hematologic, and infectious. Common contributory causes of flap compromise include kinking of the flap or pedicle, hematoma, pressure or tension on the flap, systemic patient factors, poor surgical technique, or cool topical temperature.
- Ischemic compromise can be either primarily arterial or venous in nature. Swift action to restore perfusion or venous outflow, such as relieving tension, repositioning the pedicle, or applying heat, may be helpful. For arterial comprise, hyperbaric oxygen therapy is a consideration. For venous congestion, leeches may be helpful. Vasodilating agents and aggressive wound care can be used as adjuncts in specific cases.

BACKGROUND

Introduction

Local tissue rearrangement through the targeted manipulation of local tissue flaps is a fundamental technique in facial reconstruction. A flap is a unit of tissue that maintains its own blood supply while being transferred from a donor site to a recipient site.[1] Local flaps are obtained from tissue in the immediate region of the defect to be reconstructed. They can be transferred using a variety of methods including advancement, transposition, rotation, and interpolation. Small and moderate-sized facial cutaneous defects are very often reconstructed with local flaps.

The intrinsic skin vascularity of a local flap is the most critical determinant of successful transfer[2] (Figs. 1 and 2). Fortunately, the head and neck cutaneous regions are richly vascularized, with significant redundancy of the vascular system. Perfusion is dictated by major distributing vessels along septocutaneous and musculocutaneous perforators, which lead to a densely interconnected network of dermal and subdermal plexuses[3] (Fig. 3). One concept used to understand perfusion is that of the angiosome, proposed by Taylor and Palmer, whereby the body is said to be comprised anatomically of multiple three-dimensional composite tissue blocks, consisting of muscle, fascia, subcutaneous fat, and skin, that are supplied by particular source arteries.[4] The head and neck region has 13 angiosomes supplied mostly from branches of the external carotid, internal carotid, and subclavian arteries,

Department of Otolaryngology–Head and Neck Surgery, University of California San Diego, 9300 Campus Point Drive, MC 7895, La Jolla, CA 92037-7895, USA
* Corresponding author.
E-mail address: dbhom@health.ucsd.edu

Facial Plast Surg Clin N Am 31 (2023) 275–287
https://doi.org/10.1016/j.fsc.2023.01.006

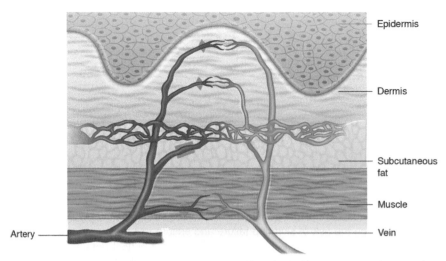

Fig. 1. Skin contains precapillary sphincters (designated by *triangle*), which regulates blood perfusion by local stimuli and preshunt sphincters (designated by *square*) which regulates thermoregulation. (Borrowed with permission from Local Flaps in Head and Neck Reconstruction, Figure 2.1, page 14.[51])

which form the theoretic basis for the design of tissue flaps. It is this redundant network that allows for the creation and survival of local flaps. Local flaps are often classified based on their vascularity. McGregor and Morgan classified cutaneous flaps as random flaps, axial pattern or reverse-flow axial pattern flaps, and island flaps.[5] Random flaps are based on the subdermal plexus and traditionally limited to 3:1 length-to-width ratios, although this is region dependent and can be theoretically extended to 4:1 in the well-perfused head and neck regions.[2] Axial pattern flaps contain a single direct artery within the longitudinal axis of the flap.

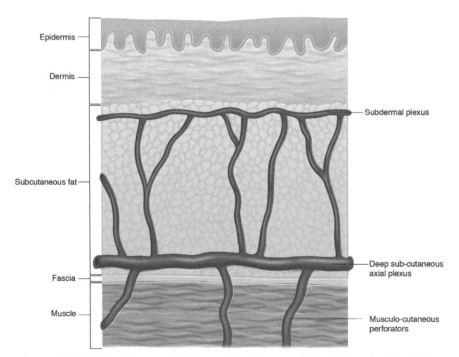

Fig. 2. Vasculature of facial skin. (Borrowed with permission from Local Flaps in Head and Neck Reconstruction, Figure 26.10, page 700.[51])

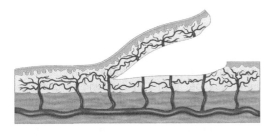

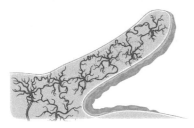

Fig. 3. Overlapping vascular skin regions from multiple perforating vessels that interconnect to maximize skin perfusion. (Borrowed with permission from Local Flaps in Head and Neck Reconstruction, Figure 2.4, page 16.[51])

Common etiologies of flap failure

Complications are an inherent and inevitable part of surgery, and learning how to prevent them, as well as manage them when they occur, is essential. As the face is a complex region with critical esthetic and functional purposes, complications during reconstruction of this region can result in disfiguring and functional consequences.[6,7]

Complications from reconstruction with local flaps can take many forms. Etiologies of skin flap failure include tension-related, ischemic, hematologic, and infectious causes.[6] Complications may arise intraoperatively or may not occur until the early or late postoperative phases. Flap perfusion is paramount, and strict evaluation of perfusion is essential to prevent, recognize, and treat impending complications.[2] Common causes of flap compromise include systemic patient factors such as comorbidities (diabetes, malnutrition, conditions of poor wound healing and immunosuppression), concurrent smoking, recreational drug or medication use, hypovolemia, hypotension, and anemia.[1] In addition, poor surgical technique, cool ambient room temperature, kinking of the flap or pedicle, hematoma, and pressure on the flap may also lead to flap failure.[8] Therefore, careful preparation and excellent technique are critical for a successful outcome.

SURGICAL TECHNIQUE
Patient Preparation

Having a consistent perioperative routine for skin flap care is the first step in reducing complications.

Avoiding complications begins in the preoperative period with a thorough patient history and physical examination. Every patient should be preoperatively optimized and comorbidities should be actively managed. Numerous comorbidities have a significant impact on wound healing. These include age, functional status, diabetes, renal disease, cardiac disease, liver failure, peripheral vascular disease, tobacco use, vasculitis, malnutrition, immunosuppression, obesity, inherited blood dyscrasias, inflammatory skin conditions, history of hypertrophic scarring or keloids, and history of radiation to the site.[2,6,7] The overall nutrition of the patient, including the presence of nutritional and vitamin deficiencies (eg, albumin <2.5 mg/dL), can significantly alter the wound healing pathway.[9] Although some of these factors may be optimized, others are not modifiable. Nonetheless, knowledge of their presence is helpful and may impact surgical approaches and modify the risk of skin flap failure.

Medications may impact the outcome of local flap reconstruction. Patients should be questioned about the use of medications and herbal supplements that reduce clotting or contribute to immunosuppression before surgery, with clear instructions regarding reducing these substances if possible, in the perioperative period. These include nonsteroidal anti-inflammatory drugs, commonly used anticoagulants such as warfarin, aspirin, and clopidogrel, and steroids.[1] In addition, the use of herbal supplements should be queried. Ginkgo biloba, ginseng, ephedra, kava, St. John's wort, echinacea, garlic, valerian, and vitamin E are among the more commonly used herbal supplements and can exert substantial effects on coagulation.[10]

Alcohol and tobacco use both significantly increase the risk of local flap complications. Heavy alcohol use modulates liver function, which affects the clotting cascade and drug metabolism, increasing risks for excessive bleeding or hematoma formation.[11] Tobacco use has a well-documented detrimental effect on tissue perfusion.[2] Smoking one cigarette reduces tissue perfusion by more than 30% within 45 min in some regions of the body.[12] The injurious effects of nicotine seem to increase with prolonged exposure.[13] The mechanism whereby tobacco or nicotine lowers flap survival is believed to be direct endothelial damage or vasoconstriction secondary to catecholamine release or local concentrations of prostaglandins. Smoking impairs flap healing by causing vasoconstriction from nicotine and increased levels of carboxyhemoglobin, which limits oxygen delivery. In addition, smoking decreases neutrophilic function and decreases collagen synthesis.[14,15] Nonsmokers produce 1.8 times more collagen compared with smokers.[15] Interestingly, the role of nicotine and its relationship to tissue hypoxia is not fully known, as nicotine transdermal patch use did not have comparable effects on wound healing compared with tobacco smoking in one clinical trial.[14]

Smoking has been associated with an increased incidence of flap necrosis in facelift operations.[16] Exposure to tobacco smoke resulted in increased flap necrosis of dorsal flaps in rodents.[17] In a retrospective study of 91 patients with facial skin defects reconstructed with local flaps, of which 38 (42%) were active smokers, complications occurred in 23 patients (25%; 37% in smokers, 17% in ex-smokers, and 17% in nonsmokers; $P < .03$), and all full-thickness skin losses and all cellulitis occurred in active smokers. The authors concluded that active smokers are at a higher risk for complications in facial skin flap surgery and that ex-smokers had a complication rate similar to that of nonsmokers.[18] In a study examining the association between cigarette smoking and necrosis of flaps and full-thickness grafts in 220 patients, a review of a series of 916 flaps and full-thickness grafts revealed 44 patients in whom some degree of tissue necrosis occurred. Current high-level smokers (those smoking one or more packs per day) had necrosis developed approximately three times more often than never-smokers, low-level smokers (less than one pack per day), or former smokers (95% confidence interval [CI], 1.2 to 8.2). Former smokers (relative risk, 1.4; 95% CI, 0.6 to 3.2) and low-level smokers (relative risk, 1.1; 95% CI, 0.2 to 6.1) were not at increased risk for necrosis compared with never-smokers. Once tissue necrosis developed, the median percent of the visible flap or graft tissue that necrosed was approximately threefold greater among current smokers than never smokers.[19] These studies suggest that part of smoking's adverse effect on skin flaps may be an acute phenomenon, and that smoking cessation for shorter (<1 year) periods of time before surgery may have a beneficial effect.

Smoking also results in a higher incidence of surgical site infection (SSI). This effect is present even for small, clean wounds.[14] Preoperative smoking abstinence reduces postoperative wound infections.[20] Poor wound healing and infection may be detrimental to local flaps and can lead to flap failure, especially when perfusion to flap tissue is tenuous.

The optimal duration of preoperative abstinence from smoking is debated. In one study, 4 weeks of abstinence reduced the wound infection rate to the level of never-smokers.[14] The wound healing process itself may require a longer time of abstinence. Smoking cessation for at least 4 to 6 weeks

is recommended before skin flap surgery.[1,21] Medications such as varenicline (Chantix) may assist in smoking cessation. Other strategies, such as the electronic cigarette or nicotine replacement therapy (eg, transdermal nicotine patch, nicotine gum) may be helpful in reducing smoking and improving flap outcomes, although do not entirely eliminate nicotine from the body.

Whenever possible, avoid flap transposition in previously irradiated regions due to decreased vascularity. In addition, if the patient has a previous history of surgery at the operative site, one needs to be cognizant as to whether vascularity has already been compromised.

Intraoperative Strategies

Good surgical technique is critical to the success of local flap reconstruction. The reconstructive surgeon should always remember that "blood supply is king." Techniques that promote maximal preservation of blood supply and the highest levels of perfusion will decrease flap failure. Various fundamental principles and techniques intraoperatively should be used to increase the probability of success.

This starts with an appropriate flap design. Excessive tension on the flap should be avoided, which is dependent first and foremost on selecting an effective flap design. When designing a flap, relaxed skin tension lines and facial subunits should be also taken into consideration. Placement of incisions parallel to relaxed skin-tension lines and along esthetic subunit borders allows for maximal extensibility and camouflage of the resultant scar.[6] Tension should not distort surrounding landmarks, especially mobile and functional ones such as the nose, eyelids, and lips. The flap should be designed such that excessive stretch is not required for closure, and the pedicle will not be kinked during inset. It should be noted that increasing the pedicle width does not necessarily ensure adequate perfusion to the distal flap.[22] In fact, raising a thicker flap with deeper subcutaneous vessels is more beneficial than making a wider flap base (Fig. 4). The old adage "measure twice, cut once" is essential in flap design.

When administering subcutaneous local anesthesia, avoid excessive injection of vasoconstrictors such as epinephrine around the vascular pedicle and underneath the flap. During second stage skin flap surgery or delaying a flap, consider using a 1:200,000 epinephrine concentration due to increased sensitivity of the precapillary sphincters. During surgery, gentle flap manipulation, delicate tissue handling, and avoidance of pressure, especially at the distal edge of the flap, will help preserve tissue viability. For example, the surgeon can place a single retraction suture at the distal end of the flap instead of grasping the flap with forceps to minimize pressure on the flap. For axial flaps, the feeding vessel must be preserved, or the flap will not survive. Excessive distal flap thinning should be avoided to maximize perfusion especially if the patient is a smoker.[23]

Hemostasis can be improved by injection 5 to 10 min before making the incision. Bleeding is most often encountered during the initial incision or while undermining the flap. Meticulous hemostasis and good technique help avoid postoperative hematoma formation. Undermining in a uniform plane at the correct depth minimizes blood loss. Vessel identification with the precise use of bipolar electrocautery is helpful.[6] Overly aggressive electrocautery should be avoided, since the dermal and subdermal plexuses contribute to flap perfusion. Larger (>1 mm) arterial

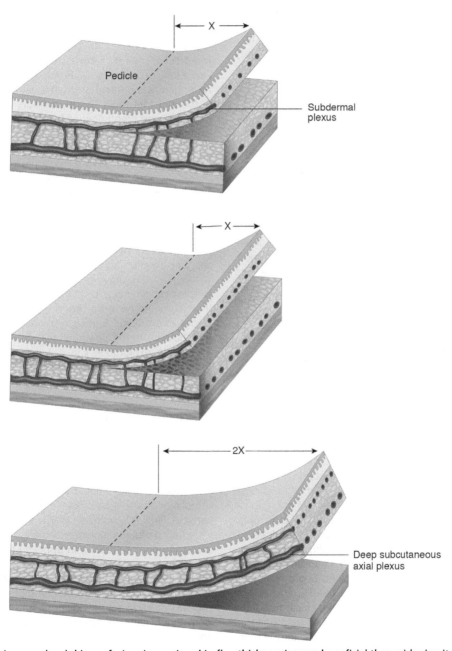

Fig. 4. To improve local skin perfusion, increasing skin flap thickness is more beneficial than widening its pedicle. (Borrowed with permission from Local Flaps in Head and Neck Reconstruction, Figure 26.11, page 701.[51])

vessels should be ligated. Copious irrigation with sterile water and gently blotting with gauze can help define bleeding vessels. If it is not contraindicated by the anesthesia team, maintain systolic blood pressure <105 mm Hg during the flap procedure to minimize flap vascular oozing.

Once adequate hemostasis is achieved, attention is turned to closure. A tension-less closure is important for reducing the risk of flap failure and improving the functional and esthetic result. Tension decreases perfusion and distorts critical landmarks. In one study, there was a statistically significant increase in flap necrosis for those flaps closed with greater than 250 g of tension.[24] Extensive surrounding undermining may be necessary to help achieve tension-less closure, with anchor sutures placed more deeply to assist in closure. In some instances, "delaying" a skin flap may be beneficial to prime and lengthen the random portion of the skin flap in preparation before flap transposition. Delaying a skin flap can be especially important in increasing skin flap survival if prior medical co-morbidities exist (such as diabetes or conditions of poor healing). Skin flap "delay" involves making the skin flap peripheral incisions 2 weeks before raising and transposing the flap. In this way, it primes the distal region of the skin for improved tissue perfusion. When an interpolated flap is transposed to a slow healing region, pedicle detachment of the flap may require 6 to 8 weeks for formation of adequate blood supply. To test a flap before detachment in a poor healing bed, a vascular loop tourniquet can be applied for 10 min. If cyanosis is apparent, flap detachment should be delayed.[7]

MANAGEMENT STRATEGIES WHEN SKIN FLAP COMPROMISE IS RECOGNIZED POSTOPERATIVELY

Attentive postoperative monitoring is critical for identifying flap compromise and recognizing potential complications early. Thus, periodic postoperative flap inspections are important. The sooner a problem is recognized, the higher probability of successful salvage of the skin flap. Flaps can be clinically monitored using a variety of indicators, including color, capillary refill, punctate bleeding, temperature, and firmness. Healthy flaps will be pink in color, have less than 4 s capillary refill after light manual pressure, will bleed bright red blood upon poking the skin with a needle, and will be soft with modest turgor.[7] Microvascular free flaps (not covered in this article) can also be monitored using Doppler, pulse oximetry, pH, temperature sensors, and laser angiography with indocyanine green.[6,25] However, for local skin flaps, there is

no widely accepted device to monitor skin flap perfusion besides clinical inspection.

Once skin flap compromise is recognized, ideally within hours after surgery, the next step is to determine the underlying etiology of compromise. Identifying the underlying cause for skin flap compromise is essential to determine the best clinical management. Common etiologies for flap compromise include ischemic (arterial or venous), hematologic, and infectious causes (**Fig. 5**).

Ischemic compromise

Ischemia is defined as inadequate perfusion to meet tissue needs. Causes of ischemia may be reversible or irreversible. Fortunately, significant redundancy is present in the perfusion system. It is thought that most tissue can survive on 10% of its average blood flow.[7] Most flaps can endure arterial insufficiency for up to 13 h, but venous congestion can kill a flap within 3 h.[7] Blood supply is essential for flap survival. Thus, prompt recognition of ischemic compromise is extremely important for preventing flap failure.

Several clinical indicators are helpful to detect skin flap compromise. In an arterial compromise, the flap may exhibit pale color, slow capillary refill (>4 s), slow or absent pinpoint bleeding, cool temperature, and/or low turgor. In a venous compromise, the flap may exhibit a mottled blue to purple cyanotic color, brisk dark pinpoint bleeding, increased temperature, and/or increased turgor (tense or swollen).[8] Evidence of arterial or venous insufficiency in the postoperative period requires immediate exploration within 4 h to salvage the local flap.

Arterial compromise

If skin flap ischemia is suspected, immediate methods to increase flap perfusion should be instituted. Arterial ischemia can be attributed to pedicle tension or torsion, vessel plaque, arterial spasm, pressure on the pedicle, technical error with pedicle injury, flap too large for its blood supply, or small-vessel disease (eg, smoking, diabetes).[26] Initial immediate responses to improve skin flap perfusion include releasing flap torsion, removing tight sutures, and applying topical heat to help restore arterial perfusion.[8]

Pharmacologic interventions sympatholytics, corticosteroids, calcium channel blockers, rheological drugs, direct vasodilators, and free radical scavengers (such as dimethyl sulfoxide) to salvage the flap with arterial insufficiency have been attempted, with inconclusive results.[27] Arterial ischemia can be caused by vessel occlusion from

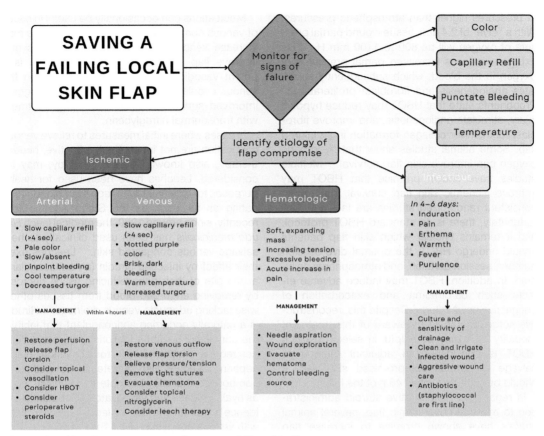

SAVING A FAILING LOCAL SKIN FLAP

Monitor for signs of falure

- Color
- Capillary Refill
- Punctate Bleeding
- Temperature

Identify etiology of flap compromise

Ischemic

Arterial
- Slow capillary refill (>4 sec)
- Pale color
- Slow/absent pinpoint bleeding
- Cool temperature
- Decreased turgor

MANAGEMENT
- Restore perfusion
- Release flap torsion
- Consider topical vasodilation
- Consider HBOT
- Consider perioperative steroids

Venous
- Slow capillary refill (>4 sec)
- Mottled purple color
- Brisk, dark bleeding
- Warm temperature
- Increased turgor

Within 4 hours! MANAGEMENT
- Restore venous outflow
- Release flap torsion
- Relieve pressure/tension
- Remove tight sutures
- Evacuate hematoma
- Consider topical nitroglycerin
- Consider leech therapy

Hematologic
- Soft, expanding mass
- Increasing tension
- Excessive bleeding
- Acute increase in pain

MANAGEMENT
- Needle aspiration
- Wound exploration
- Evacuate hematoma
- Control bleeding source

Infectious

In 4–6 days:
- Induration
- Pain
- Erthema
- Warmth
- Fever
- Purulence

MANAGEMENT
- Culture and sensitivity of drainage
- Clean and irrigate infected wound
- Aggressive wound care
- Antibiotics (staphylococcal are first line)

Fig. 5. Algorithm for management of an acute failing skin flap.

clotted blood. Given this, anticoagulant and thrombolytic agents have been used in an attempt to minimize or reverse arterial compromise. Heparin acts in conjunction with antithrombin III to inhibit thrombosis by inactivation of factor X, but it has been shown to be more effective at preventing venous thrombosis than arterial thrombosis.[2] Tissue plasminogen activator (tPA) and anisoylated plasminogen streptokinase activator complex (APSAC) exert their effects by cleaving fibrin within a thrombus. However, these agents will only improve flap perfusion if an arterial thrombus is the primary etiology of ischemia. Heparin and thrombolytic agents are more often used in free flap salvage, where the microvascular anastomosis is more susceptible to thrombotic ischemia.[28] In addition, the use of heparin is not without risk, as heparin can paradoxically lead to thrombosis via heparin-induced thrombocytopenia.

Aspirin has been used in reconstructive surgery as well. Aspirin acetylates the enzyme cyclooxygenase, thereby decreasing the synthesis of thromboxane A2, a potent vasoconstrictor in platelets, and prostacyclin, a potent vasodilator in vessel walls.[2] At low doses (eg, aspirin 81 mg) the effect

of aspirin is selective, with inhibition of cyclooxygenase, reduction in the formation of thromboxane, and less vasoconstriction. Despite these effects, there is no empiric evidence in the literature for using aspirin postoperatively.[29] Although aspirin is used empirically by some microvascular surgeons after free tissue transfer, in local tissue rearrangement the risks of bleeding from aspirin use outweigh any theoretic benefit on perfusion.

Avoidance of local hypothermia is an important adjunct to promote arterial profusion. Cold environments can provoke arterial ischemia. Temperature modulates blood vessel patency and resultant blood flow. In the range of 22° to 38° Celsius, the relationship between flap blood flow and the temperature was linear, with an increase in blood flow by 3.41% per degree Celsius.[30] All patients should be instructed to avoid ice or excessive surface pressure on the flap. If anything, light warm compresses may be used to increase vessel patency.

If arterial compromise is persistent despite efforts to resolve it, hyperbaric oxygen therapy (HBOT) can be considered as an adjunctive modality in a patient with an ischemic compromised skin flap. HBOT delivers oxygen concentrations at pressures higher than atmospheric pressures. With a "dive" of 2.4 atm, tissue wound partial pressure of oxygen will be 800 to 1100 mm Hg. This exposure induces increased partial pressures of oxygen in the blood, which subsequently stimulates angiogenesis and fibroblast proliferation.[31] Proponents state that HBOT may reduce hypoxic injury, stimulate angiogenesis, and improve fibroblast function for collagen formation in an injured flap. Some animal studies show that hyperbaric oxygen can improve skin flap survival.[32] Multiple studies have shown promise that HBOT may improve ischemic skin flap survival, but robust consistent randomized studies are lacking.[1] Unfortunately, there is no standard HBOT protocol, and it remains unclear which skin flap patients should undergo HBOT, the optimal dive session number, session duration, and atmospheres delivered. In addition, HBOT may induce adverse effects such barotrauma and exacerbation of congestive heart failure.[2] Despite this, reconstructive surgeons should be aware of this treatment modality as it may be helpful in select cases. If HBOT is considered an adjuvant therapy to salvage an arterial compromised skin flap, it should be instituted within 48 h of the flap insult.[33]

In regards to perioperative steroid administration to manage an ischemic flap, several animal studies have shown promise to increase flap viability[34,35] However, no large human study has been conducted.

Venous Compromise

Venous insufficiency can rapidly compromise flap viability. It can occur secondary to pedicle tension or torsion, flap edema, hematoma, or in the case of an island flap, tension within the tunnel.[27] Once venous outflow obstruction has developed, it can lead to erythrocyte extravasation, fibrin deposits in the perivascular regions, endothelial breakdown, microvascular collapse, arterial compromise, arteriovenous shunting away from the capillary bed, ischemia, thrombosis within the microcirculation, and ultimately flap death, which may occur within 8 h.[36]

Similar methods used in arterial compromise may be applied to suspected venous compromise in some scenarios. If venous congestion develops due to tension on the flap, torsion, or pressure on the venous outflow, appropriate measures to quickly restore the venous flow should be instituted. Pedicle or inset revision may be necessary in the case of axial or island flaps. Tight sutures should be cut, external pressure on the flap removed, hematoma evacuated, and/or tension or kinking on the pedicle corrected.

Medications can occasionally be useful in cases of venous compromises. Vasodilation agents may increase venous outflow in tenuous cases and improve flap survival. Topical nitroglycerin is a potent vasodilator with selective effects on the venous circulation. There is evidence to suggest improved survival of axial flaps using treatment with transdermal nitroglycerin.[37]

In cases where initial measures to relieve venous congestion are not immediately effective, hirudotherapy, also known as leech therapy, may be considered. Leeches have been used for health purposes for millennial, with reports of bloodletting dating as far back as the Stone Age.[26] More recently, since around 1960, the medical leech *Hirudo medicinalis* has been used clinically to help salvage venous congested skin.[38] Leeches exert their effect by injecting hirudin (an anticoagulant) at the site of their bite, reducing tissue necrosis by removing engorged blood from tissues otherwise lacking adequate venous drainage.[39] Hirudin is a naturally occurring anticoagulant that inhibits the conversion of fibrin to fibrinogen, but it does not require antithrombin III for activation, unlike heparin.[2] Leeches also secrete several additional compounds that may promote flap survival, such as hyaluronidase and vasodilators. Substantial evidence supports the use of leeches in skin flaps with venous congestion (**Fig. 6**).[38,40]

Importantly, hirudotherapy is considered a temporary modality to decrease skin flap venous congestion until further revascularization occurs for venous outflow.[38] It is not effective in the setting of arterial flow compromise or other nonvenous causes of flap failure.

There is no standard protocol for administering leech therapy in cases of venous compromise. One author recommends initiation of intervention within 2 to 3 h of the onset of venous congestion, as flap survival decreases precipitously within 8 h after onset.[26] Therapy is then continued until further angiogenesis has occurred and sufficient venous outflow is established, usually for 2 to 6 days, and guided by clinical improvement in flap metrics such as color, appearance, and capillary refill.[38] Hemoglobin should be monitored at regular intervals throughout therapy due to blood loss from the leeches.

Despite the possibility of flap salvage with leech therapy, its use is not without risks. Frequently cited disadvantages include the risk of infection, local reactions of pain and itching, the need for serial blood transfusions, anaphylaxis, bleeding, and scarring.[2,38] *Hirudo medicinalis* leeches are frequently associated with bacterial infection with *Aeromonas hydrophila*, thus antibiotic prophylaxis, commonly with fluoroquinolones, is always necessary.[38,41]

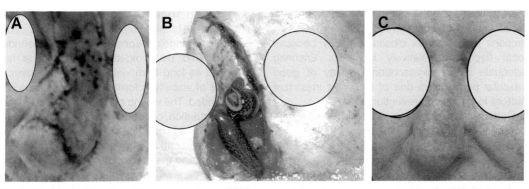

Fig. 6. (*A–C*) Example of a patient undergoing leech therapy salvage for venous congestion of a paramedian forehead flap to the left nose.

Hematologic Compromise

Hematologic compromise of flaps is related to excessive bleeding, which may cause hematoma, pressure, or poor perfusion. This is most often related to drug-induced coagulopathy and poor intraoperative hemostasis.[6,7] Uncontrolled hypertension, renal or hepatic failure, collagen vascular disorders, hematopoietic system malignancies, and excessive valsalva activity from vomiting or strenuous exercise in the immediate postoperative period are linked to bleeding complications.[7] Antiemetics can be prescribed to prevent postoperative nausea and vomiting, thereby decreasing forceful valsalva straining.

Aspirin, warfarin, and clopidogrel are the most implicated anticoagulants. In a retrospective review of patients taking clopidogrel and undergoing cutaneous surgery, severe complications were 6 times more likely with clopidogrel-containing anticoagulation and 8 times more likely with combined clopidogrel and aspirin than with aspirin monotherapy.[42] In a meta-analysis of complications attributed to anticoagulation following cutaneous surgery, patients taking warfarin were nearly seven times as likely to have a moderate-to-severe complication compared with controls (odds ratio [OR], 6.69; 95% CI, 3.03 to 14.7, $P < .001$).[43] However, cessation of anticoagulation may lead to serious thrombotic complications such as deep venous thrombosis, pulmonary embolism, myocardial infarction, or stroke. As such, the risks and benefits of cessation of anticoagulation must be carefully weighed, with the help of primary care or prescribing providers.

Hematologic compromise is frequently related to hematoma formation. Hematoma reduces perfusion and can lead to ischemia or necrosis by inducing vasospasm, stretching the subdermal plexus, or separating the flap from its recipient bed. Iron compounds from a hematoma may also promote local free radical production which can contribute to flap necrosis.[44] Early recognition of hematoma formation is imperative. Increasing flap tension, a soft expanding mass, excessive bleeding, and an increase in pain may all serve as indicators of hematoma. Aspiration of hematoma and pressure dressings may help control a small hematoma. However, pressure dressings can be difficult to place on the face and too much pressure can lead to ischemia. Wound exploration with hematoma evacuation and identification of the bleeding source may be necessary if conservative measures fail.[44] Within the first 48 h, hematomas are in liquid form. Over several days, as the clot becomes more solidified, it becomes more difficult to aspirate. If the hematoma is diagnosed more than 24 h after surgery, exploration may or may not be necessary, depending on the size of the hematoma and the status of the flap.[44] Hematomas may again liquefy from fibrinolysis in approximately 14 days.

Aside from deliberate and judicious intraoperative hemostasis, several postoperative measures can be used. These include elevating the head of the bed and administering antiemetics to prevent excessive nausea and vomiting (which can induce excessive hypertension leading to bleeding) and pain control to reduce elevated blood pressure. Patients should be instructed to avoid strenuous activity for at least 1 week after surgery to reduce the risk of bleeding.

Infectious Compromise

Infection is a risk with any procedure, and local flaps are no exception.[7] Fortunately, postoperative infections after clean cutaneous facial surgery are rare (<3% in one study).[45] However, reconstruction is not always performed on the same day as resection, which may result in an initially clean wound becoming a clean-contaminated one, thereby increasing the risk of infection. Moreover, facial wounds of local flaps are more prone to infections than wounds closed primarily because local flaps are relatively ischemic. Ensuring adequate tissue oxygenation by way of good vascular perfusion is one of the most important factors for infection prevention.[7,45,46]

Certain anatomic areas of the face have high bacterial colonization, such as the nose, ears, and lips, which predisposes wounds to higher bacterial loads.[45] Good aseptic and antiseptic techniques are fundamental preventive strategies, and prevention is the most effective strategy.[7] Importantly, antibiotic treatment is not directly correlated with infection eradication. Perioperative antibiotics are not required in clean wounds. For clean contaminated wounds, such as those that involve the oral cavity or intranasal mucosa, prophylactic antibiotics are at the discretion of the provider, as their utility in preventing postsurgical infection remains controversial.[6] Most surgeons will administer a perioperative antimicrobial prophylaxis dose for clean-contaminated cases or in revision cases, typically with a first-generation cephalosporin such as cefazolin. Systemic antibiotics are ideally administered 1 h before incision time to obtain adequate blood concentration at the time of surgery.[7]

Infection typically manifests four to 8 days following surgery and can occur despite every preventive effort. If an infection does develop, as evidenced by induration, erythema, pain, wound warmth, and/or purulence, wound drainage should be sent for culture and sensitivities, to determine which antibiotics should be initiated. Antistaphylococcal antibiotics, with consideration for methicillin-resistant strains, when applicable, are first line. The infection should be fully cleared before any attempts at revision reconstruction are done to prevent further tissue loss. Application of an antibiotic ointment over incision lines may be beneficial to prevent infection, however, keeping the incision covered with any moisture-retentive ointment is important to assist in the incision closure. Bacitracin/polymyxin B ointment is associated with less allergic reactions than neomycin-containing ointments and is therefore preferred.[7] Hydrogen peroxide application can be used at wound edges to reduce heavy crusting and local bacterial wound load.

Wound Care (Partial Thickness Versus Full Thickness Loss)

Flap complications can range from superficial epidermolysis to full-thickness necrosis. This necessitates effective wound care to promote good healing and minimize the consequences from flap loss. Management of tissue loss from ischemic changes is conservative. Early debridement should be avoided until the tissue has declared its long-term viability. After a demarcation line of viability is formed, necrotic tissue can be debrided. The wound can be left to heal by secondary intention, or another reconstructive surgery (skin flap or skin graft) can be planned, depending on the size, location, and functional importance of the defect and the patient's expectations.[6,7]

Wound care with moist ointments, antimicrobial prophylaxis, and vacuum-assisted closure (VAC) may expedite the process for open wounds to granulate from secondary intention. Maintenance of a moist environment along flap edges promotes epithelialization and serves a fundamental strategy for minimizing scarring.[9,47] Silicone gels can begin 1 month after the flap incision to minimize flap incision scars. Excessive scarring 1 month postoperatively may be managed with intralesional 0.5 to 1 mL triamcinolone acetonide (10 to 40 mg/mL) injections every 6 weeks until a desired effect is reached. Verapamil, bleomycin, and 5-fluoriuracil have also been used in more severe cases of hypertrophic scarring. Postoperative application of pressure dressings, silicone sheeting, cryotherapy, and laser therapy may be used as adjuncts.[48,49] Surgical scar revision should not be performed until after 6 months to allow for full healing to take place, unless the developing scar is causing a functional deformity.

For poor healing open wounds and multiple skin flap failures, VAC is an option to increase the granulation of an open wound bed for skin grafting or skin flaps. The VAC is an open-cell polyurethane foam dressing sealed with an adherent dressing subjected to sub-atmospheric pressure by a connected vacuum pump. The device functions by removing unwanted wound fluid, decreasing edema, increasing the production of granulation tissue and decreasing bacterial counts in wounds.[50] Negative pressure is applied continuously for 48 h and then intermittently. The VAC should not be used in contact with vessels or in the nasal and oral airways and should be used very carefully when in proximity to the eyes and ears. Mobile or highly contoured skin areas, such as the neck, may make the vacuum placement more challenging to achieve a seal. Other experimental modalities are currently being investigated to enhance skin flap viability (**Fig. 7**).

SUMMARY

Avoiding skin flap complications begins in the preoperative period with a thorough patient history,

INCREASE BLOOD SUPPLY   PROLONG TISSUE VIABILITY

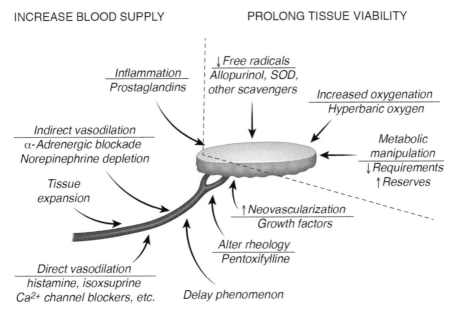

Fig. 7. Research modalities to try to improve skin flap survival. SOD, superoxide dismutase. (Borrowed with permission from Local Flaps in Head and Neck Reconstruction, Figure 2.11, page 14.[51])

including relevant medications, and physical examination. Every patient should be preoperatively optimized and comorbidities should be actively managed. Intraoperatively, the good surgical technique will reduce the risk of failure. This includes optimal flap design, delicate tissue handling, judicious hemostasis, and tension-less closure, with the aim to promote maximal preservation of blood supply. Postoperatively, careful monitoring of the flap is paramount. Recognizing the etiology of flap compromise is the first step in salvaging a compromised flap. Common causes of flap compromise include systemic patient factors such as concurrent drug or medication use (eg, anticoagulants), hypovolemia, hypotension, and anemia. In addition, poor surgical technique, cool ambient room temperature, kinking of the flap or pedicle, hematoma, and pressure on the flap may also lead to flap failure. Etiologies of flap failure can be broadly classified as tension-related, ischemic, hematologic, and infectious. In the case of ischemic arterial compromise, performing appropriate responses and rapidly restoring perfusion are essential. Commonly used interventions include adjusting the tension on the flap or pedicle and applying heat. HBOT is an adjunctive modality that may promote the healing of an ischemic flap. When venous compromise is identified, swift action to restore venous outflow is required. Additional measures such as administering leech therapy and possible vasodilators can help reduce venous congestion. Hematologic complications are most often related to drug-induced coagulopathy and poor intraoperative hemostasis. If a hematoma is identified postoperatively, it should typically be evacuated to relieve pressure on the flap. Although infection after facial reconstruction is uncommon, good aseptic techniques are important. Standard wound care and antimicrobial therapy may be used if an infection does develop.

CLINICS CARE POINTS

- Although flap compromise can occur, good surgical technique, careful monitoring, and numerous strategies throughout the care pathway can be used to reduce risk and ensure positive outcomes.

- The intrinsic vascularity and perfusion of a flap are the most critical factors for successful skin flap transfer. Anything that impacts perfusion will affect the overall outcome of the flap.

- Avoiding complications begins in the preoperative period with a thorough patient history, including relevant medications and herbal supplement use, as well as physical examination. Every patient should be preoperatively optimized and comorbidities should be actively managed.

- Recognizing the etiology of flap compromise is the first step in salvaging a failing flap.

Careful monitoring with attention to flap color, temperature, capillary refill, bleeding, and firmness will help identify issues promptly.

- In an arterial compromise, the flap may exhibit cool temperature, pale color, slow capillary refill (>4 s), slow or absent pinpoint bleeding, and/or low turgor. In a venous compromise, the flap may exhibit increased temperature, blue to purple cyanotic color, brisk capillary refill (>2 s), brisk dark pinpoint bleeding, and/or increased turgor (tense or swollen).

- Etiologies of flap failure can be broadly classified as tension-related, ischemic, hematologic, and infectious. Common causes of flap compromise include systemic patient factors such as comorbidities that reduce perfusion or healing, concurrent drug or medication use, hypovolemia, hypotension, and anemia. In addition, poor surgical technique, cool ambient room temperature, kinking of the flap or pedicle, hematoma, and pressure on the flap can also lead to flap failure.

- Good surgical technique is critical to reducing the risk of flap compromise. Fundamental principles include good aseptic and antiseptic techniques, optimal flap design, delicate tissue handling, judicious hemostasis, and tension-less closure

- Ischemic compromise can be either arterial or venous in nature. Swift action to restore perfusion or venous outflow, such as relieving tension, revising the pedicle, or applying heat, may be helpful. Hyperbaric oxygen therapy, vasodilating agents, leech therapy, and aggressive wound care can be used as adjuncts in specific cases.

DISCLOSURE

The authors have no financial or commercial conflicts of interest to disclose. No funding sources were used to complete this work.

REFERENCES

1. Baker SR. Local Flaps in Facial Reconstruction. Netherlands: Elsevier; 2021.
2. Janis JE. Essentials of Plastic Surgery. United States. Thieme Medical Publishers, Incorporated; 2014.
3. Honrado CP, Murakami CS. Wound healing and physiology of skin flaps. Facial Plast Surg Clin North Am 2005;13(2):203–14.
4. Taylor GI, Palmer JH. The vascular territories (angiosomes) of the body: experimental study and clinical applications. Br J Plast Surg 1987;40(2):113–41.
5. McGregor IA, Morgan G. Axial and random pattern flaps. Br J Plast Surg 1973;26(3):202–13.
6. Woodard CR. Complications in facial flap surgery. Facial Plast Surg Clin North Am 2013;21(4):599–604.
7. Vural E, Key JM. Complications, salvage, and enhancement of local flaps in facial reconstruction. Otolaryngol Clin North Am 2001;34(4):739–51, vi.
8. Brown DL, Brown DL, Borschel GH, et al. In: Michigan manual of plastic surgery, In: *Lippincott manual series*. 2nd edition. United States: Wolters Kluwer Health; 2014. p. 45–6.
9. Ondrey FG, Hom DB. Effects of Nutrition on Wound Healing. Otolaryngology-Head Neck Surg (Tokyo) 1994;110(6):557–9.
10. Collins SC, Dufresne RG Jr. Dietary supplements in the setting of mohs surgery. Dermatol Surg 2002;28(6):447–52.
11. Salem RO, Laposata M. Effects of alcohol on hemostasis. Am J Clin Pathol 2005;123(Suppl):S96–105.
12. Jensen JA, Goodson WH, Hopf HW, et al. Cigarette Smoking Decreases Tissue Oxygen. Arch Surg 1991;126(9):1131–4.
13. Forrest CR, Pang CY, Lindsay WK. Dose and time effects of nicotine treatment on the capillary blood flow and viability of random pattern skin flaps in the rat. Br J Plast Surg 1987;40(3):295–9.
14. Sorensen LT, Karlsmark T, Gottrup F. Abstinence from smoking reduces incisional wound infection: a randomized controlled trial. Ann Surg 2003;238(1):1–5.
15. Jorgensen LN, Kallehave F, Christensen E, et al. Less collagen production in smokers. Surgery 1998;123(4):450–5.
16. Rees TD, Liverett DM, Guy CL. The Effect of Cigarette Smoking on Skin-Flap Survival in the Face Lift Patient. Plast Reconstr Surg 1984;73(6):911–5.
17. Craig S, Rees TD. The Effects of Smoking on Experimental Skin Flaps in Hamsters. Plast Reconstr Surg 1985;75(6):842–6.
18. Kinsella JB, Rassekh CH, Wassmuth ZD, et al. Smoking increases facial skin flap complications. Ann Otol Rhinol Laryngol 1999;108(2):139–42.
19. Goldminz D, Bennett RG. Cigarette smoking and flap and full-thickness graft necrosis. Arch Dermatol 1991;127(7):1012–5.
20. Møller AM, Villebro N, Pedersen T, et al. Effect of preoperative smoking intervention on postoperative complications: a randomised clinical trial. Lancet 2002;359(9301):114–7.
21. Gottrup F. Trends in surgical wound healing. Scand J Surg 2008;97(3):220–5. ; discussion 225-6.
22. Milton SH. Pedicled skin-flaps: the fallacy of the length: width ratio. Br J Surg 1970;57(7):502–8.

23. Koopmann CF Jr. Cutaneous wound healing. An overview. Otolaryngol Clin North Am 1995;28(5): 835–45.

24. Larrabee WF Jr, Holloway GA Jr, Sutton D. Wound tension and blood flow in skin flaps. Ann Otol Rhinol Laryngol 1984;93(2 Pt 1):112–5.

25. Woodard CR, Most SP. Intraoperative angiography using laser-assisted indocyanine green imaging to map perfusion of forehead flaps. Arch Facial Plast Surg 2012;14(4):263–9.

26. Utley DS, Koch RJ, Goode RL. The failing flap in facial plastic and reconstructive surgery: Role of the medicinal leech. Laryngoscope 1998;108(8): 1129–35.

27. Pang CY, Forrest CR, Morris SF. Pharmacological augmentation of skin flap viability: a hypothesis to mimic the surgical delay phenomenon or a wishful thought. Ann Plast Surg 1989;22(4):293–306.

28. Barhoum F, Tschaikowsky K, Koch M, et al. Successful free flap salvage surgery with off-label use of Alteplase: A case report, review of the literature and our free flap salvage algorithm. Int J Surg Case Rep 2020;75:398–402.

29. Carroll WR, Esclamado RM. Ischemia/reperfusion injury in microvascular surgery. Head Neck 2000; 22(7):700–13.

30. Awwad AM, White RJ, Webster MH, et al. The effect of temperature on blood flow in island and free skin flaps: an experimental study. Br J Plast Surg 1983; 36(3):373–82.

31. Tibbles PM, Edelsberg JS. Hyperbaric-Oxygen Therapy. N Engl J Med 1996;334(25):1642–8.

32. Friedman HIF, Fitzmaurice M, Lefaivre JF, et al. An Evidence-Based Appraisal of the Use of Hyperbaric Oxygen on Flaps and Grafts. Plast Reconstr Surg 2006;117(7S):175S–90S.

33. Zhou YY, Liu W, Yang YJ, et al. Use of hyperbaric oxygen on flaps and grafts in China: Analysis of studies in the past 20 years. Undersea Hyperbar M 2014;41(3):209–16.

34. Eclamado RM, Larrabee WF, Zel GE. Efficacy of steroids and hyperbaric oxygen on survival of dorsal skin flaps in rats. Otolaryngol Head Neck Surg 1990;102(1):41–4.

35. Kuru B, Dinç S, Çamlibel M, et al. Efficacy of postoperative steroids on ischemic skin flap survival in rats. Eur J Plast Surg 2003;26(2).79–01.

36. Kerrigan CL, Wizman P, Hjortdal VE, et al. Global flap ischemia: a comparison of arterial versus venous etiology. Plast Reconstr Surg 1994;93(7): 1485–95. ; discussion 1496-7.

37. Rohrich RJ, Cherry GW, Spira M. Enhancement of skin-flap survival using nitroglycerin ointment. Plast Reconstr Surg 1984;73(6):943–8.

38. Welshhans JL, Hom DB. Are leeches effective in local/regional skin flap salvage? Laryngoscope 2016;126(6):1271–2.

39. Dabb RW, Malone JM, Leverett LC. The use of medicinal leeches in the salvage of flaps with venous congestion. Ann Plast Surg 1992;29(3):250–6.

40. Yousef A, Solomon I, Hom DB. Can Hyperbaric Oxygen Salvage a Compromised Local/Regional Skin Flap? Laryngoscope 2022. https://doi.org/10.1002/lary.30160.

41. Nguyen MQ, Crosby MA, Skoracki RJ, et al. Outcomes of flap salvage with medicinal leech therapy. Microsurgery 2012;32(5):351–7.

42. Cook-Norris RH, Michaels JD, Weaver AL, et al. Complications of cutaneous surgery in patients taking clopidogrel-containing anticoagulation. J Am Acad Dermatol 2011;65(3):584–91.

43. Lewis KG, Dufresne RG Jr. A meta-analysis of complications attributed to anticoagulation among patients following cutaneous surgery. Dermatol Surg 2008;34(2):160–4. ; discussion 164-5.

44. Diaz DD, Freeman SB, Wilson JF, et al. Hematoma-Induced Flap Necrosis and Free Radical Scavengers. Arch Otolaryngol Head Neck Surg 1992; 118(5):516–8.

45. Sylaidis P, Wood S, Murray DS. Postoperative infection following clean facial surgery. Ann Plast Surg 1997;39(4):342–6.

46. Pearl RM, Arnstein D. A vascular approach to the prevention of infection. Ann Plast Surg 1985;14(5): 443–50.

47. Sasaki A, Fukuda O, Soeda S. Attempts to increase the surviving length in skin flaps by a moist environment. Plast Reconstr Surg 1979;64(4):526–31.

48. Ledon JA, Savas J, Franca K, et al. Intralesional Treatment for Keloids and Hypertrophic Scars: A Review. Dermatol Surg 2013;39(12):1745–57.

49. Sherris DA, Larrabee WF, Murakami CS. Management of Scar Contractures, Hypertrophic Scars, and Keloids. Otolaryng Clin N Am 1995;28(5): 1057–68.

50. Hom DB. New Developments in Wound Healing Relevant to Facial Plastic Surgery. Arch Facial Plast Surg 2008;10(6):402–6.

51. Hom DB, Goding G. Chapter 2: Skin Flap Physiology. In: Baker SR, editor. Local flaps in head and neck reconstruction. 4th edition. Mosby; 2022.

Reducing Risks of Graft Failure for Composite Skin–Cartilage Grafts

Alisa Yamasaki, MD*, Sarah M. Dermody, MD, Jeffrey S. Moyer, MD

KEYWORDS

- Composite skin graft • Chondrocutaneous graft • Cartilage graft • Skin graft • Nasal reconstruction
- Facial reconstruction • Mohs reconstruction • Skin cancer

KEY POINTS

- Composite skin–cartilage grafts are a well-suited option for small defects of aesthetically sensitive areas such as the ear, eyelid margin, nostril margin, columella, and nasal lining.
- Patients should be optimized preoperatively for smoking status, diabetes, nutritional deficiencies, metabolic/thyroid abnormalities, and anticoagulation before the use of composite grafts.
- Composite grafts are commonly harvested from the auricular concha and limited to 1 cm in size, though this may be modified using adjunctive techniques.
- Composite grafts are slightly oversized to maximize contact between perichondrium and recipient tissue.
- Postoperative techniques to decrease the metabolic demand of the composite graft include hypothermia, steroids, and hyperbaric oxygen therapy, which may be used in combination to optimize graft survival.

INTRODUCTION

Facial skin defects pose unique challenges for the reconstructive surgeon. Ideally, the color, texture, and contour of skin defects are recreated, whereas scars are camouflaged and the procedural burden for patients is minimized. Achieving these reconstructive goals can be particularly challenging in aesthetically complex areas involving a free margin such as the ear, eyelid, columella, columella–lobule interface, soft tissue triangle, alar rim, and internal nasal lining, where secondary soft tissue contracture can lead to a very poor cosmetic outcome. In these cases, composite grafts offer an ideal combination of soft tissue coverage and structural rigidity, all accomplished in a single-stage surgery (Fig. 1). Facial composite grafts are most commonly composed of skin, subcutaneous, perichondral, and cartilage layers from an auricular donor site. For small full-thickness nasal defects, three-layered composite grafts—with subcutaneous fat and skin on either side of the cartilaginous components—can also be used.

Composite grafts are often underused in facial reconstructive surgery due to the tenuous blood supply and high reported rates of graft failure.[1–4] Grafts are initially nourished through imbibition, in which exudate from the wound bed supplies the graft tissue. Vascular inosculation occurs by 18 to 24 hours after transfer, as random vessel connections between graft and recipient tissues occur.[5] Neoangiogenesis and capillary ingrowth occur by 72 hours, at which point the likelihood of graft take becomes apparent.[5] Composite graft failure rates range from 47% to 70%, though studies are limited by small sample size and lack of uniform graft size, donor site, and recipient

Division of Facial Plastic and Reconstructive Surgery, Department of Otolaryngology–Head and Neck Surgery, University of Michigan Medical Center, 1500 East Medical Center Drive SPC 5312, 1904 Taubman Center, Ann Arbor, MI 48109-5312, USA
* Corresponding author. 1500 East Medical Center Drive, Ann Arbor, MI 48109.
E-mail address: ayamasa@med.umich.edu

Facial Plast Surg Clin N Am 31 (2023) 289–296
https://doi.org/10.1016/j.fsc.2023.01.007
1064-7406/23/© 2023 Elsevier Inc. All rights reserved.

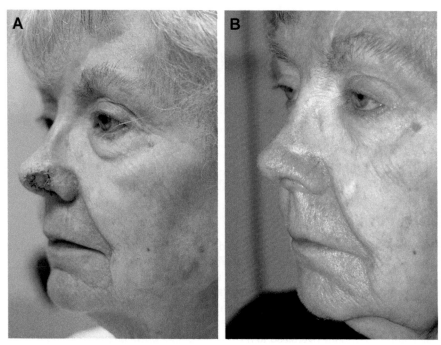

Fig. 1. (*A*) Postoperative healing of composite graft reconstruction of the left nasal soft tissue triangle. (*B*) Final postoperative appearance after healing is complete.

location.[3,4,6,7] Composite grafts are associated with higher complication and graft failure rates than single-tissue grafts (eg, full-thickness skin graft) due to the higher metabolic demands of composite tissue and the additional tissue bulk that must be traversed for nutrient diffusion during graft ingrowth.[8,9] Although vascular compromise and graft failure are the most problematic complications of composite grafts, additional complications include excessive secondary graft contracture, postoperative infection, dyspigmentation, and poor cosmesis. Robust data on the incidence of these complications do not currently exist in the literature.

The success of composite grafts does not simply hinge on graft size, as the reconstructive outcome can be impacted by a combination of perioperative, intraoperative, and postoperative factors. In this article, the authors review the aspects of patient selection, surgical technique, and postoperative wound care that can be used to optimize composite graft survival for facial reconstruction.

Preoperative Optimization

Patient selection is an important initial step to determine a patient's candidacy for a composite graft. Patient factors that portend poor wound healing such as smoking, diabetes, uncontrolled hypertension, coagulation disorders, thyroid disease, nutritional deficiencies, history of radiation, and history of prior surgery at or adjacent to the current defect should be evaluated. As with any elective surgery, modifiable risk factors should be optimized preoperatively. This should include a psychosocial screening process to ensure that patients have the appropriate mindset, expectations, and social support to undergo surgery.

Smokers should receive smoking cessation counseling. Smoking has been significantly associated with an increased risk of postoperative complications in facial reconstruction and has been strongly associated with graft loss in various types of reconstructive surgery.[9–15] Smoking status is a particularly important for composite grafting, as nicotine-induced vasoconstriction and inflammation can significantly impact nutrient diffusion and the likelihood of graft take. Studies have shown that self-reported smoking behavior is often inaccurate, and surgeons may consider nicotine testing preoperatively.[16] Nicotine metabolites such as cotinine have a half-life of 13 to 19 hours and can be tested in blood or urine.[17]

For patients on anticoagulation and antiplatelet therapy, evaluation of the risks and benefits of therapy cessation should be performed in collaboration with the prescribing physician. For patients taking daily aspirin, rates of bleeding and infection have not been shown to be higher during facial plastic surgery.[9] Warfarin, antiplatelet agents,

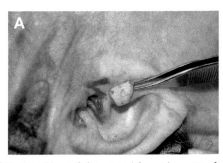 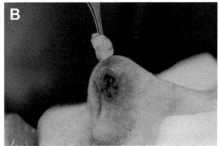

Fig. 2. (A) Composite graft harvested from the root of the helix. (B) Composite graft placed next to a freshened wound bed. The graft is oversized to accommodate anticipated graft contracture.

and direct factor inhibitors each vary in their onset of action with variable implications for surgery that are not well established for facial procedures. A therapeutic plan for these agents should be determined on a case-by-case basis. Multiple studies on cutaneous facial reconstruction have found that the use of anticoagulation or antiplatelet therapy does not increase the risk of postoperative complications, and therefore, continuing medically necessary anticoagulant and antiplatelet medication is recommended for cutaneous surgery.[9,18–20] However, no data exist specific to composite grafts, which are particularly susceptible to compromised blood flow from poor graft take and complications such as hematoma formation.

In cases where there are non-modifiable patient risk factors such as a compromised wound bed from prior surgery or radiation, delayed reconstruction may improve graft success.[21] In a retrospective study of 320 full-thickness skin and composite graft Mohs reconstructions, delayed reconstruction (ie, >6 days after Mohs) had a protective effect on postoperative complications including hematoma, infection, dehiscence, epidermolysis, and graft necrosis.[21] Delaying reconstruction by 2 to 3 weeks can be considered but should be balanced with the potential for scar contracture over time. If reconstruction is delayed, the newly formed scar is excised to include the subepithelium and the composite graft is oversized by 2 mm circumferentially to counteract further wound contracture.[22]

Surgical Technique: Defect Preparation

Preparing the recipient bed is critical for nutrient diffusion, neoangiogensis, and graft uptake. Meticulous sterile technique is used to avoid early postoperative infections that can compromise graft survival. Wound edges are freshened and inward beveled edges corrected to facilitate uniform thickness and skin eversion. Wound thickness should guide selection of the graft site. Aesthetic unit borders are marked for reference, but the

subunit principle is not typically followed in structurally sensitive areas such as the eyelid margin, alar margin, soft tissue triangle, and columella.[23–25] In these cases, non-aesthetic defect boundaries are tolerated in favor of preserving as much soft tissue and vasculature as possible to mitigate excessive soft tissue contraction.[26,27] If multiple facial subunits are involved, each is reconstructed individually. Once the defect perimeters are finalized, a subcutaneous pocket is developed for graft placement that maximizes contact between the native tissue and cartilaginous components of the graft.

Surgical Technique: Graft Harvest

The auricle is the most common composite graft donor site for facial reconstruction. The thin quality of the skin matches delicate areas such as the eyelid margin, nostril margin, soft tissue triangle, and columella.[28–31] The tight adherence between the skin and cartilage mimics that of the fibrofatty alae and soft tissue triangles and provides structural control that avoids slippage between tissue layers. The ear also has very low donor site morbidity. Scar lines are typically inconspicuous and cartilage removal results in minimal auricular distortion when using proper technique.[28–32] The specific site on the ear is selected based on the color, thickness, and cartilage contour of the defect. Common sites include the conchal bowl (cymba concha favored over concha cavum), helical root, helical rim, and tragus, though the antihelix, antitragus, and fossa triangularis can also be used if necessary (Fig. 2A).[22,32] Conchal bowl grafts are often an excellent contour match for the nasal ala, and in cases of larger grafts, the conchal bowl tends to heal well by secondary intention.[22,29–33] An anterior approach is typically favored given the tight adherence between the anterior auricular skin and cartilage. The thick subcutaneous fat layer of the posterior auricular skin is also avoided as its thickness is theorized to compromise graft viability.[22,34]

One centimeter is classically referenced as the maximal diameter for composite grafts to limit the theoretical diffusion distance between the graft and native tissue capillaries to no greater than 0.5 cm.[1,8,25] However, the optimal size for composite grafts has not been experimentally established. Three-layered grafts are more strictly limited to 1 or 1.5 cm given their complete reliance on a marginal blood supply.[35] Larger two-layered grafts have been described with the use of additional technical modifications. In a case series of 50 patients, an extended dermal pedicle was used for composite grafts of up to 2.0 cm.[36] The dermal pedicle was designed to be at least two times the defect size and was tunneled into a subcutaneous pocket to increase native tissue contact and incoming blood supply.[36] For defects greater than 1.5 cm, 24-hour of postoperative cooling was additionally used. Although patients were described as having tolerated the procedure well with good cosmesis, quantitative outcomes of this modified composite graft technique were not measured and no control group was used.[36] Grafts as large as 6.5 cm (approximately 30 cm^2) have also been described in the literature, though defects of this size are typically addressed using a combination of multistage techniques (eg, forehead flap with cartilage grafts).[37]

Once a donor site has been selected, local anesthesia is injected circumferentially around the graft margin but not within the skin paddle. Injecting local anesthesia into the skin paddle can compromise the composite graft by hydrodissecting the skin off of the cartilage.[34] The soft auricular cartilage must also be handled with care to avoid tearing or cracking. Perichondrium should be left on the exposed cartilage of the graft to minimize warping and resorption and also facilitate cartilage healing and neocartilage formation.[38,39] We routinely size composite grafts at least 2 mm larger than the defect to allow for adequate graft/recipient tissue overlap and compensate for expected graft contraction (**Fig. 2**B).[40] The cartilaginous portion of the composite graft is designed slightly wider than the cutaneous component so the cartilage can serve as a stabilizing strut that extends underneath the adjacent nasal skin in a "tongue in groove" fashion.[34,41–43] This maximizes the direct contact between native tissue and the cartilage layer that is required for initial survival via imbibition.[38] Some surgeons will perforate the cartilage using a 2-mm punch biopsy or needle, in which case care should be taken to avoid violating the skin or cracking the cartilage.[34] Once the graft is harvested, it can be stored in a cool, moist sponge, or saline until ready for inset. When closing the graft donor site, cartilage wedge resection and/or management of standing cutaneous deformities may be required to preserve the esthetic contours of the ear.[32]

Surgical Technique: Graft Inset

Several inset techniques can optimize graft survival by promoting contact between the graft and native tissue. When insetting the graft, delicate tissue handling is of paramount importance to avoid damaging the periphery of the graft and/or defect, which could jeopardize graft uptake. Tissue manipulation is similarly minimized. Meticulous hemostasis is achieved to prevent hematoma formation while also avoiding excessive cautery of the wound periphery, either of which may compromise graft perfusion and uptake.[37] The minimum number of simple interrupted sutures are used to precisely secure the graft skin to the native skin while avoiding obstruction of vascular ingrowth channels.[22] For larger composite grafts, simple sutures may also be placed between the graft cartilage and native cartilage/wound bed. For nasal reconstruction, an intranasal dental roll may be used to apply pressure and decrease fluid accumulation that can compromise blood flow.[22] External bolsters and pressure dressings may be used per surgeon preference to minimize the dead space between the graft and recipient bed, though excess pressure must absolutely be avoided.[22]

Special Considerations for Full-Thickness Nasal Defects

Full-thickness nasal defects present a unique reconstructive challenge due to the need to reconstruct the skin, cartilage, and inner lining. Three-layered composite grafts may be used for defects smaller than 1 cm. For larger defects, forehead flaps and other regional flaps can be used to serve as "carrier" flaps for two-layered skin cartilage composite grafts.[44] No difference in cartilage viability has been demonstrated based on the timing of pedicle division, and therefore, the regional flap pedicle can be divided at the standard time when used in conjunction with composite grafts.[44] Park and colleagues[44] demonstrated that cartilage viability does not depend on skin viability, supporting the concept that the cartilage of composite grafts do not rely on the same peripheral microvasculature as the skin and the epidermolysis tends to have little consequence on long-term graft outcome.

Postoperative Care

Several techniques have been explored for composite graft wound care that aim to decrease the metabolic demands of the graft tissue and thereby increase the chance of graft survival. The use of postoperative hypothermia was first proposed by Conley to improve the success of composite grafting for nasal defects that had previously been compromised by radiation, atrophy, or scar.[45] Cooling was intended to decrease the metabolic demands of the reconstructed tissue and create a bacteriostatic environment for healing, after which warming to room temperature was resumed to facilitate hyperemia and further graft ingrowth.[45] Conley's cooling protocol used continuous ice compresses to the wound for 2 weeks postoperatively, resulting in the successful uptake of 10 out of 12 composite grafts ranging from 1 × 1 to 2 × 2 cm in size.[45] Since this time, the use of postoperative icing has become widely accepted but is typically applied for a shorter postoperative period. Although the literature for composite graft hypothermia is sparse, the 72-hour cooling regimen has emerged as a common practice that slows cellular degeneration during the critical period before neovascularization between postoperative days 3 to 5.[6] In a method described by Hirase, ice-water and aluminum foil were used to enhance survival in both nasal-alar and fingertip reconstruction.[6] At the conclusion of surgery, the entire surgical site was covered with aluminum foil, and a vinyl ice-filled bag was kept in contact with the foil for 72 hours.[6] Compared with a retrospective control group of patients undergoing composite grafting, the cooling group demonstrated a nearly fourfold increase in graft survival.[6]

Perioperative steroids have also been proposed to further decrease the metabolic demands of grafted tissue. The efficacy of corticosteroids has been explored in several animal models.[2,46,47] In a rabbit auricular composite graft model, perioperative methylprednisolone (daily 30 mg/kg IM doses on postoperative days 0 to 3) was associated with a greater graft survival area (75.4% in steroid group vs 41% in untreated control).[47] In another rabbit model, perioperative methylprednisolone (one dose of 30 mg/kg IM 1 hour preoperatively followed by daily doses for 7 days) was associated with a significantly smaller necrotic area (28.75%) compared with controls (76.69%).[46] The exact mechanism of corticosteroids' impact on graft survival has not been elucidated but likely involves inhibition of phospholipase and inflammatory mediators, stabilization of cell membranes, stimulation of gluconeogenesis, and reduction of lactic acid levels.[8,46] There is variability in steroid regimens, ranging from a 3-day course of methylprednisolone to a 7-day prednisone taper (eg, 60 mg to 5 mg, taper by 10 mg daily).[22,34,41] Our institutional practice is to use a 6-day methylprednisolone dose pack (ie, 48 mg to 4 mg, taper by 4 mg daily). Although these data support the use of corticosteroids postoperatively, corticosteroids have not been shown to be effective for graft salvage once necrosis is evident.[2]

Other pharmacologic agents such as heparin, topical nitroglycerin, allopurinol, melatonin, nonsteroidal anti-inflammatory drugs (eg, ibuprofen, indomethacin), and oxygen-free radical scavengers (eg, chlorpromazine, dimethylsulfoxide, superoxide dismutase) have been proposed to improve composite graft survival due to their antithrombotic, vasodilatory, and/or anti-inflammatory properties.[46–48] Animal studies have shown improvement in composite graft survival with chlorpromazine, indomethacin, and dimethylsulfoxide compared with untreated controls, though results were not as dramatic as those seen with methylprednisolone treatment.[46] More recently, platelet-rich plasma (PRP) has been proposed as a potential adjunctive agent. In a rabbit model, PRP was associated with a 46% survival area compared with 30% in the untreated control.[3] The regenerative medicine approaches such as the use of adipose-derived mesenchymal stem cells have been explored in animal studies, demonstrating improved composite graft survival when used during delayed defect reconstruction.[49] Additional human studies of such pharmacologic techniques are needed.

Hyperbaric oxygen (HBO) is another adjunctive therapy that has been suggested to enhance survival of composite grafts that are more tenuous due to size (eg, > 1 cm) or a compromised wound bed. HBO increases tissue oxygenation by delivering 100% oxygen inspiration at pressures greater than 1 atmosphere, thereby maximizing oxygen diffusion through tissues and wound healing capacity.[50] HBO has been found to increase fluid diffusion distance by up to fivefold and is used for chronic wounds, osteomyelitis, and post-radiation soft tissue complications.[51–53] For composite grafts, HBO is thought to increase oxygen diffusion through multiple dense tissue layers during the critical days immediately after surgery. However, data on the impact of HBO on graft viability are mixed. Rabbit auricular models have shown that a 10-day course of postoperative HBO resulted in a 15.94% graft survival rate compared with 0.31% in the untreated control group.[54] A similar study in rats demonstrated 82% graft uptake in composite grafts sized 1 × 0.5 cm^2 after a 6-day course of HBO (ie, 4 hours on postoperative day 1 followed by 6 hours for 5 days) compared with 26.5% graft uptake in the control group.[55] Some studies suggest that HBO may have greater efficacy for larger grafts. In another rabbit model, graft survival was higher for 2 cm composite grafts treated with HBO (mean survival rate 85.8 ± 15.7%) compared with untreated controls (mean survival rate 51.3 ± 38.5%), with no benefit seen for grafts less than 2 cm.[56] Other studies demonstrate no difference in graft viability with HBO therapy in animal models.[48] Human studies are even more limited. A retrospective case study demonstrated graft survival rates of at least 80% when postoperative HBO was used for pediatric patients ($n = 9$) undergoing composite grafting of facial soft tissue defects greater than 1.5 cm, though the study was limited by the small sample size and lack of control cases.[50] Further research is needed to determine the indications and efficacy of HBO therapy as well as the optimal regimen for clinical use.

SUMMARY

Composite skin–cartilage grafts are an invaluable approach for reconstruction of facial defects that can be otherwise difficult to reconstruct using standard techniques. Composite grafting offers the ability to successfully recreate the color, texture, and contour of a defect through a single-stage procedure. Although graft failure is the most challenging complication of composite grafting, reliable functional and aesthetic outcomes can be achieved with appropriate patient selection, surgical technique, and postoperative care.

CLINICS CARE POINTS

- Surgical candidates should be optimized preoperatively, including wound healing disorders, smoking status, and psychosocial factors. Delaying reconstruction by 1 to 3 weeks can be considered for patients with non-modifiable risk factors such as a compromised wound bed from prior surgery or radiation.

- Defect boundaries not adhering to conventional aesthetic units are often tolerated for composite grafting in order to preserve soft tissue and wound bed integrity and avoid excessive soft tissue contraction.

- One centimeter is conventionally accepted as the maximal diameter for composite grafts. Two-layered composite grafts may be sized slightly larger, particularly with the use of modified surgical techniques and postoperative adjuncts.

- The use of postoperative cooling and steroids is associated with increased graft survival, and a short course of wound icing with postoperative methylprednisolone or prednisone should be considered.

DISCLOSURE

The authors have nothing to disclose.

REFERENCES

1. Brown JB, Cannon B. Composite free grafts of two surfaces of skin and cartilage from the ear. Ann Surg 1946;124(6):1101.
2. Fann PC, Hartman DF, Goode RL. Pharmacologic and surgical enhancement of composite graft survival. Arch Otolaryngol Head Neck Surg 1993;119(3):313–9.
3. Jeon YR, Kang EH, Yang CE, et al. The effect of platelet-rich plasma on composite graft survival. Plast Reconstr Surg 2014;134(2):239–46.
4. Konig F. Ueber nasenplastik. Beitr Klinisch Chir 1914;94:515–29.
5. Maves MD, Yessenow RS. The use of composite auricular grafts in nasal reconstruction. J Dermatol Surg Oncol 1988;14(9):994–9.
6. Hirase Y. Postoperative cooling enhances composite graft survival in nasal-alar and fingertip reconstruction. Br J Plast Surg 1993;46(8):707–11.
7. Rees TD. The transfer of free composite grafts of skin and fat: a clinical study. Plast Reconstr Surg Transplant Bull 1960;25:556–64.
8. Harbison JM, Kriet JD, Humphrey CD. Improving outcomes for composite grafts in nasal reconstruction. Curr Opin Otolaryngol Head Neck Surg 2012;20(4):267–73.
9. Miller MQ, David AP, McLean JE, et al. Association of mohs reconstructive surgery timing with postoperative complications. JAMA Facial Plast Surg 2018;20(2):122–7.
10. Goldminz D, Bennett RG. Cigarette smoking and flap and full-thickness graft necrosis. Arch Dermatol 1991;127(7):1012–5.
11. Heistein JB, Cook PA. Factors affecting composite graft survival in digital tip amputations. Ann Plast Surg 2003;50(3):299–303.
12. Kinsella JB, Rassekh CH, Hokanson JA, et al. Smoking increases facial skin flap complications. Ann Otol Rhinol Laryngol 1999;108(2):139–42.
13. Nolan J, Jenkins RA, Kurihara K, et al. The acute effects of cigarette smoke exposure on experimental skin flaps. Plast Reconstr Surg 1985;75(4):544–51.
14. Segal KL, Nelson CC. Periocular reconstruction. Facial Plast Surg Clin North Am 2019;27(1):105–18.
15. Woodard CR, Park SS. Reconstruction of nasal defects 1.5 cm or smaller. Arch Facial Plast Surg 2011;13(2):97–102.
16. Payne C, Southern S. Urinary point-of-care test for smoking in the pre-operative assessment of patients undergoing elective plastic surgery. J Plast Reconstr Aesthet Surg 2006;59(11):1156–61.

17. Benowitz NL. Cotinine as a biomarker of environmental tobacco smoke exposure. Epidemiol Rev 1996;18(2):188–204.

18. Cook-Norris RH, Michaels JD, Weaver AL, et al. Complications of cutaneous surgery in patients taking clopidogrel-containing anticoagulation. J Am Acad Dermatol 2011;65(3):584–91.

19. Kraft CT, Bellile E, Baker SR, et al. Anticoagulant complications in facial plastic and reconstructive surgery. JAMA Facial Plast Surg 2015;17(2):103–7.

20. Kreicher KL, Bordeaux JS. Addressing practice gaps in cutaneous surgery: advances in diagnosis and treatment. JAMA Facial Plast Surg 2017;19(2): 147–54.

21. David AP, Miller MQ, Park SS, et al. Comparison of outcomes of early vs delayed graft reconstruction of mohs micrographic surgery defects. JAMA Facial Plast Surg 2019;21(2):89–94.

22. Baker SR. 3rd edition. Local flaps in facial reconstruction, xii. Elsevier/Saunders, Canada; 2014.

23. Burget GC, Menick FJ. Aesthetic reconstruction of the nose. St. Louis: Mosby Year Book; 1994.

24. Burget GC, Menick FJ. Nasal support and lining: the marriage of beauty and blood supply. Plast Reconstr Surg 1989;84(2):189–202.

25. Menick FJ. Nasal reconstruction. Plast Reconstr Surg 2010;125(4):138e–50e.

26. Rohrich RJ, Griffin JR, Ansari M, et al. Nasal reconstruction–beyond aesthetic subunits: a 15-year review of 1334 cases. Plast Reconstr Surg 2004; 114(6):1405–16.

27. Zopf DA, Iams W, Kim JC, et al. Full-thickness skin graft overlying a separately harvested auricular cartilage graft for nasal alar reconstruction. JAMA Facial Plast Surg 2013;15(2):131–4.

28. Chen C, Patel R, Chi J. Comprehensive algorithm for nasal ala reconstruction: utility of the auricular composite graft. Surg J (N Y) 2018;4(02):e55–61.

29. Klinger M, Maione L, Villani F, et al. Reconstruction of a full-thickness alar wound using an auricular conchal composite graft. Can J Plast Surg 2010; 18(4):149–51.

30. Manafi A, Babaki AES, Mehrabani G, et al. Can we add auricular composite graft to our rhinoplasty armamentarium? World J Plast Surg 2013;2(1):33.

31. Scheithauer MO, Rotter N, Lindemann J, et al. The auricle's cavum conchae composite graft in nasal reconstruction. Am J Rhinol Allergy 2013;27(2): e53–7.

32. Singh DJ, Bartlett SP. Aesthetic management of the ear as a donor site. Plast Reconstr Surg 2007; 120(4):899–908.

33. Gloster H Jr, Brodland D. The use of perichondrial cutaneous grafts to repair defects of the lower third of the nose. Br J Dermatol 1997;136(1):43–6.

34. Chua DY, Park SS. Two-layered, auricular composite grafts. JAMA Facial Plast Surg 2014;16(3):226.

35. Iorio CB, Christophel JJ, Park SS. Nasal reconstruction: defects that cross anatomical subunits. Facial Plast Surg 2020;36(1):91–101.

36. Chandawarkar RY, Cervino AL, Wells MD. Reconstruction of nasal defects using modified composite grafts. Br J Plast Surg 2003;56(1):26–32.

37. Avelar JM, Psillakis JM, Viterbo F. Use of large composite grafts in the reconstruction of deformities of the nose and ear. Br J Plast Surg 1984;37(1):55–60.

38. Davis WB, Gibson T. Absorption of autogenous cartilage grafts in man. Br J Plast Surg 1956;9(3): 177–85.

39. Duncan MJ, Thomson HG, Mancer JF. Free cartilage grafts: the role of perichondrium. Plast Reconstr Surg 1984;73(6):916–23.

40. Brenner MJ, Moyer JS. Skin and composite grafting techniques in facial reconstruction for skin cancer. Facial Plast Surg Clin North Am 2017;25(3):347–63.

41. Jewett BS. Repair of small nasal defects. Facial Plast Surg Clin North Am 2005;13(2):283–99.

42. Ratner D, Katz A, Grande DJ. An interlocking auricular composite graft. Dermatol Surg 1995;21(9): 789–92.

43. Weisberg NK, Becker DS. Repair of nasal ala defects with conchal bowl composite grafts. Dermatol Surg 2000;26(11):1047–51.

44. Park SS, White GJ, Cook TA, et al. Cartilage viability with interpolated skin flaps: an experimental study. Otolaryngol Head Neck Surg 1997;116(4):483–8.

45. Conley JJ, VonFrankel PH. The principle of cooling as applied to the composite graft in the nose. Plast Reconstr Surg 1956;17(6):444–51.

46. Aden KK, Biel MA. The evaluation of pharmacologic agents on composite graft survival. Arch Otolaryngol Head Neck Surg 1992;118(2):175–8.

47. Hartman DF, Goode RL. Pharmacologic enhancement of composite graft survival. Arch Otolaryngol Head Neck Surg 1987;113(7):720–3.

48. Lim AA, Wall MP, Greinwald JH Jr. Effects of dimethylthiourea, melatonin, and hyperbaric oxygen therapy on the survival of reimplanted rabbit auricular composite grafts. Otolaryngol Head Neck Surg 1999;121(3):231–7.

49. Yucel E, Alagoz MS, Eren GG, et al. Use of adipose-derived mesenchymal stem cells to increase viability of composite grafts. J Craniofac Surg 2016;27(5): 1354–60.

50. Camison L, Naran S, Lee WW, et al. Hyperbaric oxygen therapy for large composite grafts: an alternative in pediatric facial reconstruction. J Plast Reconstr Aesthet Surg 2020;73(12):2178–84.

51. Eskes AM, Ubbink DT, Lubbers MJ, et al. Hyperbaric oxygen therapy: solution for difficult to heal acute wounds? Systematic review. World J Surg 2011; 35(3):535–42.

52. Grim PS, Gottlieb LJ, Boddie A, et al. Hyperbaric oxygen therapy. JAMA 1990;263(16):2216–20.

53. Thom SR. Hyperbaric oxygen–its mechanisms and efficacy. Plast Reconstr Surg 2011;127(Suppl 1): 131S.

54. McClane S, Renner G, Bell PL, et al. Pilot study to evaluate the efficacy of hyperbaric oxygen therapy in improving the survival of reattached auricular composite grafts in the New Zealand White rabbit. Otolaryngol Head Neck Surg 2000;123(5):539–42.

55. Zhang F, Cheng C, Gerlach T, et al. Effect of hyperbaric oxygen on survival of the composite ear graft in rats. Ann Plast Surg 1998;41(5):530–4.

56. Li EN, Menon NG, Rodriguez ED, et al. The effect of hyperbaric oxygen therapy on composite graft survival. Ann Plast Surg 2004;53(2):141–5.

Reducing Risk in Facial Reanimation Surgery

Tammy B. Pham, MD, Jacqueline J. Greene, MD*

KEYWORDS

• Facial palsy • Facial paralysis • Risk reduction • Patient privacy • Gracilis free-tissue transfer

KEY POINTS

- Preoperative assessments of patients' medical comorbidities and risk stratification help to guide the choice of intervention and improve medical optimization before surgery.
- To reduce the risk of misaligned provider–patient expectations, the clinician should thoroughly discuss the goals of the surgery, choice of procedure, postoperative care, long-term healing timeline, and the possibility of needing revisions.
- Providers should use Health Insurance Portability and Accountability Act (HIPAA)-compliant databases or software to reduce the risk of patient privacy violations when storing clinical photos or videos.
- Intraoperatively, avoidance of long-term paralytics, use of handheld nerve stimulators, and strategies to reduce operative time are critical to reducing the risk of suboptimal outcomes.
- Finally, early recognition and counseling after facial nerve palsy will help reduce the risk of delayed facial reanimation.

INTRODUCTION

Facial reanimation surgery comprises multiple interventions that aim to improve not only resting and dynamic asymmetry, but address functional impairment and morbidity from facial palsy, such as exposure keratitis due to incomplete eyelid closure, nasal obstruction due to nasal valve collapse, difficulty with speech/articulation, and impaired oral competence.[1,2] Significant psychosocial morbidity is reported due to the inability to emote via facial expressions—many patients become socially isolated and avoid situations where their facial dysfunction may become apparent.[3]

Although facial reanimation interventions can greatly improve patient quality of life,[4] these procedures are not without risk. In addition to the general surgical risks, there are specific risks to the facial palsy population regarding privacy and protection of collected photographs and videos, which are necessary for preoperative planning and monitoring postoperative outcomes. Management of facial palsy patients can be complex; there is a critical risk of failing to meet patient expectations despite achieving objectives, particularly if the patient anticipates full recovery to their premorbid state or does not have realistic expectations for their surgery. Finally, there are real risks in delaying facial nerve procedures that must be discussed with patients, such as the risk of vision loss from exposure keratitis or the inability to reinnervate musculature with a nerve transfer. Given that facial paralysis manifests uniquely for each patient, restoration of facial symmetry and facial movements likewise demands an individualized approach. This review focuses on strategies to identify and reduce the surgical risks of facial reanimation.

Department of Otolaryngology–Head and Neck Surgery, University of California San Diego Health, 9350 Campus Point Drive, La Jolla, CA 92037, USA
* Corresponding author.
E-mail address: j2greene@health.ucsd.edu

Facial Plast Surg Clin N Am 31 (2023) 297–305
https://doi.org/10.1016/j.fsc.2023.01.008

PREOPERATIVE EVALUATION
Reducing Risks of Misdiagnosis and Missed Opportunities for Intervention

A thorough history of facial palsy including time course, etiology, and prior treatment history must be documented (**Box 1**).[1,5,6] There are multiple excellent studies detailing the management strategy and decision planning for facial reanimation surgery;[2,7,8] Hohman and Hadlock,[8] for example, describe detailed algorithms for diagnosis, workup, treatment, and reanimation. On the basis of the patient's history, the likelihood of native facial nerve regeneration without intervention should be assessed, as this is critical for deciding whether (and when) to proceed with surgery.

There are risks of delaying surgery, as patients who experience delays of 12 to 18 months have decreased chances of success after facial reanimation surgery due to prolonged neural and muscular degeneration.[9] For example, Albathi and colleagues[10] found no detectable intraoperative electromyography (EMG) responses in 19 patients undergoing facial nerve exploration and grafting after > 6 months of flaccid facial paralysis following cerebellopontine angle (CPA) tumor resection. Of the eight patients with House–Brackmann (HB) VI facial palsy 6 months following skull-based tumor resection and who declined facial reanimation surgery in this study, at best an HB V recovery was noted after 20 months. Patients with HB VI facial paralysis six months following surgical resection of a skull base tumor with preserved facial nerve anatomic continuity merit facial reanimation (ie, nerve transfer), as they are unlikely to recover significant function.[10,11] As there are no imaging or other tests that can accurately reveal ongoing or predict ultimate nerve regeneration and muscle reinnervation, this timeline and risk of poor recovery without intervention is critical to discuss with patients.

Box 1
Obtaining a thorough facial palsy history

Timeline of facial palsy

History of steroids/antivirals for facial palsy

Remaining facial nerve function

Most bothersome symptoms (eg, exposure keratitis, lack of smile, and/or oral incompetence)

History of any previous facial nerve surgeries

Facial sensation

Masseter function

Facial vessel patency

Preoperative Assessment of Surgical Risks and Medical Optimization

During the initial visit, one should evaluate the patient's overall health, and whether they have a history of prior complications with surgery or anesthesia, coagulopathy, or immunocompromise.[12] Facial reanimation procedures require meticulous dissection, so the patient should be assessed for any systemic conditions that would preclude, or increase the risk of, prolonged time under anesthesia. If the patient takes aspirin, nonsteroidal anti-inflammatory drugs, or blood thinners such as Coumadin or a direct oral anticoagulant, these should ideally be stopped 10 to 14 days before surgery to reduce risks of bleeding. In some cases, however, it is permissive and even advantageous to proceed with surgery even with anticoagulation on board; for example, this can reduce the risk of thrombosis in free flaps but may raise the risk of postoperative hematoma.

If the patient is on chemotherapy, immunotherapy, or steroids, these should be stopped as far out of surgery as possible to prevent poor wound healing, if permissible.[12] For example, patients with type 2 neurofibromatosis who are treated with bevacizumab should stop therapy 6 to 8 weeks before surgery and 4 weeks after surgery to prevent an increased risk of wound complications such as dehiscence, ecchymosis, surgical site bleeding, and wound infection.[13]

It is important to involve the patient's primary care physician, oncologist, and/or their prescribing physician regarding these medications and how a potential facial reanimation surgery might interface with the rest of their medical care. Patient age is also an important consideration, as older patients may have worse reinnervation outcomes (particularly over long distances such as cable-graft repair of gracilis by cross-face nerve graft[14]), likely due to axonal atrophy and slower rate of axonal regeneration.[15,16] However, older age alone is not an absolute contraindication to any facial reanimation procedure; generally, it is the discretion of the facial nerve surgeon whether to advise static or dynamic procedures with higher success rates for older patients.[17]

Reducing Risks of Misaligned Provider–Patient Expectations

Perhaps the most important aspect of the preoperative visit(s) is understanding what the patient is most concerned with respect to their facial palsy/paralysis. Unfortunately, because many of the terms used by clinicians during facial analysis tend to be harsh ("droop", "deformity", "hump," "snarl," etc.), it is important for the clinician to balance delicate inquiry into common facial palsy issues (eg, visual field obstruction, oral incompetence, lack of smile) with ensuring that the patient has the opportunity to reveal what most bothers them about their appearance and facial function. The senior author has found it valuable to offer but not insist upon reviewing photodocumentation or mirror views with patients, as this may also cause emotional distress in some patients.

It is important to set reasonable expectations for what can be achieved with surgery and to help align those expectations with the patient's stated goals. The clinician should discuss the advantages and disadvantages of various facial nerve procedures, the immediate postoperative course, the long-term healing timeline, and the possibility of needing revisions or additional procedures. For example, the patient should be educated about the difference between static procedures, which provide immediate functional benefit but do not address facial movement, and dynamic procedures, which may not take effect for many months, and which often do not perfectly reproduce natural premorbid kinetic movements (although advances in multi-vector gracilis are approaching a more natural smile).[18,19] Patients should be counseled on the differences between bite-driven and spontaneous smiles (the former often results in stronger oral commissure excursion, but require volitional effort; the latter may achieve smaller excursion but allow for spontaneous, un-premeditated emotional expression such as laughing), as well as what to expect from postoperative facial nerve physical therapy. Patients should understand that although facial reanimation procedures serve to improve resting and dynamic symmetry and improve function, perfection is not achievable. Furthermore, patients who express hesitation about surgery may benefit from subsequent visits which give them time to develop their goals and expectations.

Setting Expectations for Oncologic Patients

There are unique challenges to addressing the potential of facial nerve sacrifice in the oncologic patient, especially in a patient with intact facial function (HB I). When patients present pre-resection with tumors either involving or likely involving the facial nerve, one should evaluate for preoperative facial nerve weakness and discuss with the ablative surgeon the likelihood of facial nerve sacrifice. In such cases, planning a combined oncologic resection and facial reanimation is ideal, if possible,[20] as the most important determinates of successful reinnervation are the duration of facial muscle denervation and timeliness

of facial nerve intervention.[21,22] It is important to discuss with the patient the implications of facial reanimation (including the additional time under anesthesia), and to consider the patient's medical comorbidities that may influence the feasibility of facial reanimation surgery.[20] For patients with intact facial function in particular, it is critical to provide education about facial paralysis and set expectations regarding the possibility of facial nerve sacrifice (while reassuring them that the team will do whatever they can to preserve facial nerve function). This often involves a lengthy discussion and surgical consent for multiple "possible" procedures. Patients are often overwhelmed at this stage by medical terminology and taking time to slow the discussion and answer their questions is critical. It is helpful to reassure the patient that the road to facial nerve recovery is a long one, and that they will continue to be cared for by the facial nerve surgeon through their oncologic treatment and beyond.

Standardization of Physical Examination and Facial Nerve Assessment

Every patient with facial palsy or anticipated facial palsy (eg, upcoming ablative surgery) should have a documented standardized facial nerve photo and video series: face at rest, brow elevation, gentle eye closure, full-effort eye closure, gentle smile, full-effort smile, lip pucker, and lower lip depression.[7,23] The physical examination should comment on both static and dynamic asymmetries, as well as the presence or absence of synkinesis. A complete cranial nerve examination should be documented, including both sensory and motor functions of cranial nerve V. Standardized data to be collected for facial palsy patients has been generally accepted to include clinician-based assessments of facial palsy (HB, Sunnybrook, and eFACE) and patient-based quality of life measures (FACE instrument or Facial Disability Index).[24]

Quantitative and objective assessment of facial function has historically been challenging.[23,25] Unfortunately, there is no current laboratory test or imaging modality to definitively assess if neural regeneration and muscle reinnervation is occurring or if the nerve and muscle are simply undergoing atrophy. Ultrasound and magnetic resonance imaging assessments of muscle thickness and facial nerve diameter can provide critical information for the diagnosis of facial nerve disorders but have limited value in predicting ultimate functional outcomes.[26] Electrophysiologic testing such as needle electromyography and electroneuronography may have limited diagnostic and prognostic value,[27] but evidence of denervation changes is often captured too late for facial reanimation surgery with a nerve transfer. Furthermore, these modalities are invasive and may be uncomfortable for participants with facial palsy.

Researchers have developed various tools for grading facial asymmetry from photos[28] and videos,[29] and there have been significant advances in machine-learning algorithms that correlate well with subjective scores of facial symmetry both pre- and postoperatively. These algorithms may serve as novel tools for objective functional outcome evaluation after facial reanimation surgery, but they are not yet widely used and may be limited by bias when based on training sets composed of patients without facial palsy.[30] Automated assessment tools such as Emotrics may provide avenues for algorithms to aid in objective measurements of facial paresis in the clinical setting, but at this time such technologies rely heavily on high-quality photography and videography and user landmark adjustments.[31]

Reducing Risks of Patient Privacy Violations

Although photography and videography are essential for documentation and surgical planning, they put patients at risk of privacy violation and emotional distress if not securely stored in accordance with the Health Insurance Portability and Accountability Act (HIPAA). In 2020, more than a third of health care organizations reported that they had been targeted by ransomware attacks, and 65% of those reported that hackers were successful in corrupting health care files.[32,33] In smaller settings where patient photos may be stored in a local server (such as outpatient clinics), threats to publicly release sensitive photos can be extremely damaging to patients' privacy and erode trust in their physicians.[34]

It is critical to use tools built into one's institutional electronic medical record (EMR) system or an encrypted database consistent with institutional Information Security guidelines, rather than storing files in a local unprotected clinic server which may be subject to cyberattacks. Although HIPAA privacy rules outline methods for de-identification of medical data, in the case of facial palsy and facial plastic and reconstructive patients, there is truly no way to de-identify medical media, and no way to protect patient's data once released on the internet. The most common sharing and storage methods used by facial plastic surgeons, such as texting or local/portable storage on unsecured drives, are not HIPAA compliant and prone to data theft.[35] However, there exist many HIPAA-compliant services, such as those described by Thomas and colleagues,[35] HIPAA-compliant medical cameras (eg, CaptureProof),[36] and EMR media managers which provide secure options for medical photo storage.[37]

SURGICAL PLANNING AND INTRAOPERATIVE CONSIDERATIONS
Setting up for Success: Anesthesia and Patient Positioning

The surgeon should communicate with the anesthesiologist that the patient should not have muscle relaxation on board during the surgery; this allows for intraoperative facial nerve monitoring. Although some surgeons prefer short-acting agents such as succinylcholine when possible, the advent of sugammadex[38] has allowed for non-depolarizing agents as viable options for induction in facial nerve reanimation surgeries for patients who have contraindications to succinylcholine.

Patient positioning should be geared toward maximizing safety and facial symmetry. The endotracheal tube should be taped straight down at the midline using as little tape as possible or suture-secured to the nasal septum immediately after endonasal intubation. The eyes should be lubricated with ophthalmic ointment to reduce the risk of corneal abrasions (the most common ophthalmologic complication during nonocular surgery)[39] and taped symmetrically with clear tape to allow for visualization of the upper facial features. Diluted epinephrine (1:100,000) should be injected subcutaneously before sterile prep so that it has time to take effect before incision. The whole face should be prepared with the sterile prep of choice; often a head wrap or turban is useful to ensure complete exposure. Usage of needle EMG monitoring (NIM) in facial muscles is per surgeon preference; the senior author prefers using a handheld nerve stimulator (checkpoint or other) and continuous visualization of the patient's facial muscles.

Reducing the Risk of Nerve Regeneration Failure: Direct Primary Repair vs Interposition Nerve Grafting

Although there is much about nerve regeneration that is still unknown, several key factors are widely acknowledged as contributing to nerve regeneration failure: tension at the neurorrhaphy site, multiple neurorrhaphies, and delaying the repair. For patients undergoing planned oncologic resection, the facial reconstructive surgeon should discuss with the patient the possibilities of primary direct repair (unlikely in cases with large tumor involvement), interpositional/cable nerve graft repair, nerve transfers, and static procedures such as fascia lata suspension and eyelid weight placement.[20] Whenever possible, repair should be pursued as soon as possible after facial nerve transection.[40]

Among the minority of patients with facial paresis in which there is an acute disruption of the facial nerve (eg, resection during surgery, trauma), direct repair of the nerve/nerve branches via primary tension-free neurorrhaphy should be pursued. As Wallerian degeneration occurs within 24 to 48 h of the injury,[41] the repair should be done as soon as possible, ideally within 72 h, to maximize the chances of the successful recovery of neural function.[42] Prasad and colleagues[43] found that 50% of patients who underwent facial nerve sacrifice during CPA tumor removal with subsequent cable grafting during the same surgery had recovered to HB III by the end of the postoperative follow-up period. However, the 72-h timeline should not be taken as a limitation on the possible success of nerve repair beyond that time; thanks to handheld nerve stimulators, and the use of well-known anatomic landmarks to guide distal facial nerve exploration under a microscope even with non-stimulating nerve branches, an experienced facial nerve surgeon can repair an injured or transected nerve several weeks after an injury.

When the nerve gap is too lengthy for primary tension-free neurorrhaphy, nerve grafts (eg, from the greater auricular nerve or sural nerve) may be used to bridge the gap. To reduce the risk of coaptation failure, it is important to harvest as much donor nerve as possible to ensure enough graft length for redundancy and tension-free coaptation. At our institution, we often take at least 25 to 30 cm of sural nerve when multiple facial nerve branches require repair.

Difficult Choices: Patient Counselling and Reducing Risks of Suboptimal Outcomes Following Nerve Transfers and Cross-Face Nerve Grafting

Among patients with intact distal facial nerve branches, nerve transfers such as those from the masseteric or deep temporal branches of the trigeminal nerve (V to VII) or hypoglossal nerve (XII to VII) may be used.[5] After coaptation of the masseteric nerve to the buccal branch of the facial nerve followed by rehabilitation and retraining, patients with facial paresis can develop a bite-driven smile by activating the masseteric nerve.[44] The V to VII transfer has the advantages of minimal donor-site morbidity and ease of volitional triggering. Choice of recipient facial nerve branch is

critical as reanimation outcomes can result in more of a "grimace" than a smile if individual nerve branches are not thoroughly assessed with a nerve stimulator and an assistant monitoring facial expression. In the setting of non-stimulable facial nerves, the senior author favors a middle or superior facial nerve branch to smile muscles, as the inferior midfacial nerve branch typically routes to the lower lip depressors and risorius muscles.

Patients should be counseled that masseteric nerve transfers have excellent oral commissure excursion reliability, with >90% of patients achieving some degree of facial nerve function reactivation (7% HB I, 62% HB II, 21% HB II, 3% HB V, and 8.8% HB VI),[45,46] but at the expense of spontaneity,[47] although up to 40% of adults naturally contract their masseter muscle while smiling and thus may achieve some degree of spontaneous smile.[48] Nowadays, masseteric nerve transfers are generally preferred to hypoglossal nerve transfers as the latter runs the risk of tongue morbidity, dysarthria, dysphagia, and are thus contraindicated in patients with preexisting issues or other cranial nerve deficits (ie, CN IX, X, or XII palsies).[2,49,50]

Cross-face nerve grafting (CFNG) with a sural nerve extending from a branch of the contralateral healthy facial nerve directly to the affected facial nerve may be used to create a more spontaneous smile, but typically accomplishes less oral commissure excursion compared with V to VII or XII to VII transfers.[45] CFNG placement with direct coaptation to an affected facial nerve has additional limitations: there is a lower rate of success in patients over the age of 30.[2,22] Because of the risk of muscle atrophy on the paralyzed side while the CFNG takes months to mature, a two-stage "babysitter" approach—connecting the ipsilateral hypoglossal nerve to the paralyzed facial nerve at the time of CFNG in the first stage, followed by second stage coaptation of the now mature CFNG to the paralyzed facial nerve was described in 1988 by Terzis.[51] Single-stage options reanimation options such as CFNG with masseteric nerve[40] or mini-hypoglossal nerve innervation[52] may provide both improvements in resting tone as well as in smile excursion.

Reducing Surgical Risks of Regional and Free Gracilis Muscle Transfer

Finally, in patients with longstanding facial paresis for which reinnervation of native facial muscles is not possible, regional or free muscle transfers provide options for dynamic facial reanimation and have become the gold standard. Length of anesthesia, risk of thrombosis at the vascular

Table 1
Risk-reduction strategies in facial reanimation surgery

Risk	Strategies for Risk-Reduction
Preoperative considerations and risks	
Medical comorbidities	• Involvement of patients' primary care physician, oncologist, etc., in preoperative medical optimization
Misaligned provider–patient expectations	• Patient-guided history of what they are most concerned about: Set expectations for goals of the surgery including postoperative care, long-term healing timeline, the possibility of needing revisions • Set expectations and discuss the pros and cons of static versus dynamic procedures, bite-driven versus spontaneous smiles, etc.
Patient privacy violations	• Recognize that data breaches are extremely common in health care • Use HIPAA-compliant databases or software, tools built into the EMR • Avoid unsecured local or portable drives
Intra- and Postoperative considerations	
Suboptimal intraoperative facial nerve monitoring	• Avoid long-term paralytics, or reverse with sugammadex when short-acting agents are not available
Incorrect choice of recipient facial nerve branch	• Use of handheld nerve stimulators to ensure a thorough assessment of individual nerve branches
Corneal abrasion	• Use ophthalmic ointment and clear tape to lubricate and protect the eyes.
Delayed facial reanimation	• Attempt primary repair within 72 h of injury whenever possible although repair with an experienced facial nerve surgeon and a microscope allows for repair several weeks after injury • In the setting of complete flaccid HB VI facial palsy, offer facial reanimation (ie, nerve transfer) at 6 months. • Counsel patient regarding decreased change of muscle reinnervation success after 18 months
Gracilis-specific risks	
Prolonged operative time	• Use of two surgical teams whenever possible
The sacrifice of healthy facial nerve branches during CFNG	• Confirmation of the redundancy of the donor facial nerve branches to smile musculature before the placement of the CFNG
Excessive bulk	• Superficial debulking of the gracilis muscle
Flap compromise	• Screen for risk factors that increase risk of vascular supply compromise (eg, coronary artery disease, diabetes, smoking, peripheral arterial vascular disease). • Admit to ICU for q1 hour flap checks with bedside Doppler for 24 h, followed by decreased frequency (ie, q4 hour checks) thereafter.

Abbreviations: CFNG, cross-face nerve graft; HB, House–Brackmann.

anastomosis site, donor-site morbidity, smile vector, and significant timeline for reinnervation are all risks that must be recognized and discussed preoperatively with the patient. The free gracilis muscle transfer (FGMT) is by far the most common method of free-tissue facial reanimation and is known for its ease of harvest, adequate length, and minimal donor-site morbidity (in a study of

104 patients after FGMT to the face or limbs, only 10 had donor-site complications in the postoperative period).[1,53] Among patients who are not ideal candidates for free muscle transfer, regional muscle transfers using the temporalis muscle provide a lower-risk option; however, risks of temporal contour changes and temporomandibular joint instability must be discussed with patients.[1,5]

Facial reanimation via free-tissue transfer can occur via single-stage (innervation by ipsilateral masseteric nerve) or two-stage (first-stage CFNG followed by second-stage free-tissue transfer after the CFNG has matured) procedures. In addition to the risks of nerve transfer or CFNG as described previously, free-tissue transfers add several additional risks related to the increased operative time and associated risks of deep vein thrombosis/pulmonary embolism, bulk of the flap, vascular anastomosis, and delay in muscle function.[5]

To reduce the risks of prolonged operative time, the second-stage gracilis transfer should ideally use two surgical teams, one for dissection at the head and one for harvesting the muscle, although this is not possible for all facial nerve teams. To reduce the risk of excessive bulk and exaggerated commissure displacement, the gracilis muscle should then be trimmed along its superficial surface.[7] In general, the gracilis weight should be lower if the donor nerve is the masseteric nerve (19 to 43 g, mean 31.7 g) than if the CFNG is used (20 to 50 g, mean 33.9 g).[54] Finally, to reduce the risk of flap compromise, patients should be admitted for q1 hour flap checks with bedside Doppler for 24 h, followed by decreased frequency (ie, q4 hour checks) thereafter. Patients with history of coronary artery disease, diabetes, smoking, peripheral arterial vascular disease, and hypertension are at 9.3 times increased risk of vascular compromise compared with low-risk patients[55]; therefore, these factors should be considered when selecting patients for gracilis free flap transfers, though they are not absolute contraindications.

One disadvantage of the gracilis by CFNG is that it requires dissection of the contralateral, healthy facial nerve and sacrifice of a single branch, with resulting risk to many patients only working facial nerve. In patients with unilateral facial palsy, contralateral facial weakness can be devastating, and patients electing to undergo CFNG should be extensively counseled on this risk. This dissection of intact, distal facial nerves should be treated with the utmost precaution by experienced facial nerve surgeons, with confirmation of the redundancy of the donor facial nerve branches to smile musculature before the placement of the CFNG. Donor nerve selection for CFNG is critical, as incorrect selection can lead to noticeably suboptimal results, such as a smile triggered by contralateral eye closure.[56] Finally, the sensory deficit from sural nerve harvest must be discussed with patients preoperatively. The use of endoscopic vessel harvesting systems has been shown to reduce operative times and minimize lower extremity trauma to a single 1.5 cm incision.[57]

SUMMARY

Strategies to reduce risk in facial reanimation surgeries are summarized in **Table 1**. A systematic and thorough history and physical will help guide surgical planning and patient selection. Photo and video documentation throughout the clinical evaluation process should be stored in a secure and HIPAA-compliant manner to reduce the risks of patient privacy violations. A candid, nonjudgmental, and patient-centered discussion of their goals for facial rehabilitation is critical for establishing trust, setting appropriate expectations, and preempting possible postoperative complications or setbacks—this includes a thorough discussion of the various reanimation options available to the patient (eg, static vs dynamic, or both; bite-driven versus spontaneous smile reanimation) and their benefits/drawbacks.

CLINICS CARE POINTS

- During the pre-operative assessment, obtain a thorough facial palsy history and exam and elicit from the patient the symptoms that are most bothersome to them. Avoid using harsh terms such as "droop" or "deformity" during this assessment.

- Thoroughly discuss the goals of the surgery, choice of procedure, post-operative care, long-term healing timeline, and possibility of needing revisions. Emphasize that perfection is not achievable. Patients who express hesitation may benefit from additional visits to further develop their goals and expectations.

- Use HIPAA-compliant databases or software when storing clinical photos or videos.

- Selection of facial reanimation techniques should take into account patient co-morbidities and expectations. When possible, take steps to reduce operative time.

ACKNOWLEDGMENTS/FUNDING

None to report.

CONFLICT OF INTEREST

None to report.

REFERENCES

1. Lindsay RW, Bhama P, Hadlock TA. Quality-of-life improvement after free gracilis muscle transfer for smile restoration in patients with facial paralysis. JAMA Facial Plast Surg 2014;16(6):419–24.
2. Garcia RM, Hadlock TA, Klebuc MJ, et al. Contemporary solutions for the treatment of facial nerve paralysis. Plast Reconstr Surg 2015;135(6):1025e–46e.
3. Jowett N, Hadlock TA. An evidence-based approach to facial reanimation. Facial Plast Surg Clin North Am 2015;23(3):313–34.
4. Nellis JC, Ishii M, Byrne PJ, et al. Association among facial paralysis, depression, and quality of life in facial plastic surgery patients. JAMA Facial Plast Surg 2017;19(3):190–6.
5. Pinkiewicz M, Dorobisz K, Zatoński T. A comprehensive approach to facial reanimation: a systematic review. J Clin Med 2022;11(10). https://doi.org/10.3390/jcm11102890.
6. Boahene K, Byrne P, Schaitkin BM. Facial reanimation. Discussion and debate. Facial Plast Surg Clin North Am 2012;20(3):383–402.
7. Jowett N, Hadlock TA. A contemporary approach to facial reanimation. JAMA Facial Plast Surg 2015;17(4):293–300.
8. Hohman MH, Hadlock TA. Etiology, diagnosis, and management of facial palsy: 2000 patients at a facial nerve center. Laryngoscope 2014;124(7):E283–93.
9. Funk EK, Greene JJ. Advances in facial reanimation: management of the facial nerve in the setting of vestibular schwannoma. Curr Otorhinolaryngol Rep 2021;9:177–87.
10. Albathi M, Oyer S, Ishii LE, et al. Early nerve grafting for facial paralysis after cerebellopontine angle tumor resection with preserved facial nerve continuity. JAMA Facial Plast Surg 2016;18(1):54–60.
11. Rivas A, Boahene KD, Bravo C, et al. A model for early prediction of facial nerve recovery after vestibular schwannoma surgery. Otol Neurotol 2011; 32(5):826–33. Available at: http://links.lww.com/MAO/A63.
12. Chaffoo RA. Complications in facelift surgery: avoidance and management. Facial Plast Surg Clin North Am 2013;21(4):551–8.
13. Gordon CR, Rojavin Y, Patel M, et al. A review on bevacizumab and surgical wound healing: an important warning to all surgeons. Ann Plast Surg 2009; 62(6):707–9.
14. Guntinas-Lichius O, Streppel M, Stennert E. Postoperative functional evaluation of different reanimation techniques for facial nerve repair. Am J Surg 2006; 191(1):61–7.
15. Verdú E, Ceballos D, Vilches JJ, et al. Influence of aging on peripheral nerve function and regeneration. J Peripher Nerv Syst 2000;5(4):191–208.
16. Weiss JBW, Spuerck F, Kollar B, et al. Age-related outcome of facial reanimation surgery using cross face nerve graft and gracilis free functional muscle transfer—A retrospective cohort study. Microsurgery 2022. https://doi.org/10.1002/micr.30896.
17. Lee AH, Liu RH, Ishii LE, et al. Free functional gracilis flaps for facial reanimation in elderly patients. Facial Plast Surg Aesthet Med 2021;23(3):180–6.
18. Boahene KO, Owusu J, Ishii L, et al. The multivector gracilis free functional muscle flap for facial reanimation. JAMA Facial Plast Surg 2018;20(4):300–6.
19. Ein L, Hadlock TA, Jowett N. Dual-vector gracilis muscle transfer for smile reanimation with lower lip depression. Laryngoscope 2021;131(8):1758–60.
20. Crawford KL, Stramiello JA, Orosco RK, et al. Advances in facial nerve management in the head and neck cancer patient. Curr Opin Otolaryngol Head Neck Surg 2020;28(4):235–40.
21. Boahene K. Reanimating the paralyzed face. F1000Prime Rep 2013;5. https://doi.org/10.12703/P5-49.
22. Kim L, Byrne PJ. Controversies in contemporary facial reanimation. Facial Plast Surg Clin North Am 2016;24(3):275–97.
23. Greene JJ, Guarin DL, Tavares J, et al. The spectrum of facial palsy: The MEEI facial palsy photo and video standard set. Laryngoscope 2020; 130(1):32–7.
24. Hadlock T. Standard outcome measures in facial paralysis getting on the same page. JAMA Facial Plast Surg 2016;18(2):85–6.
25. Fattah AY, Gurusinghe ADR, Gavilan J, et al. Facial nerve grading instruments: systematic review of the literature and suggestion for uniformity. Plast Reconstr Surg 2015;135(2). Available at: https://journals.lww.com/plasreconsurg/Fulltext/2015/02000/Facial_Nerve_Grading_Instruments__Systematic.45.aspx.
26. Gupta S, Mends F, Hagiwara M, et al. Imaging the facial nerve: a contemporary review. Radiol Res Pract 2013;2013:1–14.
27. Sillman JS, Niparko JK, Lee SS, et al. Prognostic value of evoked and standard electromyography in acute facial paralysis. Otolaryngol Head Neck Surg 1992;107:377–81.
28. Parra-Dominguez GS, Sanchez-Yanez RE, Garcia-Capulin CH. Facial paralysis detection on images using key point analysis. Appl Sci 2021;11(5). https://doi.org/10.3390/app11052435.

29. Monini S, Ripoli S, Filippi C, et al. An objective, markerless videosystem for staging facial palsy. Eur Arch Oto-Rhino-Laryngol 2021;278(9):3541–50.

30. Kollar B, Schneider L, Horner VK, et al. Artificial intelligence-driven video analysis for novel outcome measures after smile reanimation surgery. Facial Plast Surg Aesthet Med 2022;24(2):117–23.

31. Greene JJ, Tavares J, Guarin DL, et al. Clinician and automated assessments of facial function following eyelid weight placement. JAMA Facial Plast Surg 2019;21(5):387–92. https://doi.org/10.1001/jamaf acial.2019.0086.

32. Pifer R. More than 1/3 of health organizations hit by ransomware last year, report finds. Heathcare Dive 2021. Available at: https://www.healthcaredive.com/news/more-than-13-of-health-organizations-hit-by-ra nsomware-last-year-report-f/602329/. Accessed September 4, 2022.

33. Stop ransomware. Conti ransomware healthcare networks. 2021. Available at: https://www.cisa.gov/stopransomware/conti-ransomware-healthcare-networks. Accessed September 4, 2022.

34. Davis R. Urgent patient advisory. The center for facial restoration. 2019. Available at: https://davisrhinoplasty.com/patient-advisory.html. Accessed September 4, 2022.

35. Thomas VA, Rugeley PB, Lau FH. Digital photograph security: What plastic surgeons need to know. Plast Reconstr Surg 2015;136(5):1120–6.

36. Conroy M. CaptureProof: capture, organize, analyze - hipaa secure photos, videos, and case based chat. CaptureProof. Available at: https://captureproof.com/. Accessed September 14, 2022.

37. Nettrour JF, Burch MB, Bal BS. Patients, pictures, and privacy: managing clinical photographs in the smartphone era. Arthroplast Today 2019;5(1):57–60.

38. Nag K, Singh DR, Shetti A, et al. Sugammadex: a revolutionary drug in neuromuscular pharmacology. Anesth Essays Res 2013;7(3):302.

39. Grixti A, Sadri M, Watts MT. Corneal protection during general anesthesia for nonocular surgery. Ocul Surf 2013;11(2):109–18.

40. Bianchi B, Ferri A, Sesenna E. Facial reanimation after nerve sacrifice in the treatment of head and neck cancer. Curr Opin Otolaryngol Head Neck Surg 2012;20(2):114–9.

41. Griffin JW, Hogan MCv, Chhabra AB, et al. Peripheral nerve repair and reconstruction. J Bone Joint Surg 2013;95(23):2144–51.

42. Barr JS, Katz KA, Hazen A. Surgical management of facial nerve paralysis in the pediatric population. J Pediatr Surg 2011;46(11):2168–76.

43. Prasad SC, Balasubramanian K, Piccirillo E, et al. Surgical technique and results of cable graft interpositioning of the facial nerve in lateral skull base surgeries: experience with 213 consecutive cases. J Neurosurg 2018;128(2):631–8.

44. Buendia J, Loayza FR, Luis EO, et al. Functional and anatomical basis for brain plasticity in facial palsy rehabilitation using the masseteric nerve. J Plast Reconstr Aesthetic Surg 2016;69(3):417–26.

45. Bae YC, Zuker RM, Manktelow RT, et al. A comparison of commissure excursion following gracilis muscle transplantation for facial paralysis using a cross-face nerve graft versus the motor nerve to the masseter nerve. Plast Reconstr Surg 2006;117(7):2407–13.

46. Biglioli F, Colombo V, Rabbiosi D, et al. Masseteric-facial nerve neurorrhaphy: results of a case series. J Neurosurg 2017;126(1):312–8.

47. Gossett K, Chen D, Loyo M. Innervation options for gracilis free muscle transfer in facial reanimation. Plast Aesthet Res 2021. https://doi.org/10.20517/2347-9264.2021.69.

48. Schaverien M, Moran G, Stewart K, et al. Activation of the masseter muscle during normal smile production and the implications for dynamic reanimation surgery for facial paralysis. J Plast Reconstr Aesthetic Surg 2011;64(12):1585–8.

49. Coyle M, Godden A, Brennan PA, et al. Dynamic reanimation for facial palsy: an overview. Br J Oral Maxillofac Surg 2013;51(8):679–83.

50. Conley J, Baker DC. Hypoglossal-facial nerve anastomosis for reinnervation of the paralyzed face. Plast Reconstr Surg 1979;63(1). Available at: https://journals.lww.com/plasreconsurg/Fulltext/1979/01000/Hypoglossal_Facial_Nerve_Anastomosis_for. 11.aspx.

51. Terzis JK, Tzafetta K. The "babysitter" procedure: Minihypoglossal to facial nerve transfer and cross-facial nerve grafting. Plast Reconstr Surg 2009;123(3):865–76.

52. Terzis JK, Konofaos P. Nerve transfers in facial palsy. Facial Plast Surg 2008;24(2):177–93.

53. Azizzadeh B, Pettijohn KJ. The gracilis free flap. Facial Plast Surg Clin North Am 2016;24(1):47–60.

54. Braig D, Bannasch H, Stark GB, et al. Analysis of the ideal muscle weight of gracilis muscle transplants for facial reanimation surgery with regard to the donor nerve and outcome. J Plast Reconstr Aesthetic Surg 2017;70(4):459–68.

55. Lese I, Biedermann R, Constantinescu M, et al. Predicting risk factors that lead to free flap failure and vascular compromise: a single unit experience with 565 free tissue transfers. J Plast Reconstr Aesthetic Surg 2021;74(3):512–22.

56. Miller MQ, Hadlock TA. Lessons from gracilis free tissue transfer for facial paralysis: now versus 10 years ago. Facial Plast Surg Clin North Am 2021;29(3):415–22.

57. Hadlock TA, Cheney ML. Single-incision endoscopic sural nerve harvest for cross face nerve grafting. J Reconstr Microsurg 2008;24(7):519–23.

Reducing Risks for Midface and Mandible Fracture Repair

Néha Datta, MD[a,b], Sherard A. Tatum, MD[a,*]

KEYWORDS

- Midface • Maxillofacial • Craniomaxillofacial • Mandible fracture • Maxillary fracture • Safety
- Facial trauma • Fracture repair

KEY POINTS

- Hemorrhage may occur in the acute, intraoperative or postoperative period, requiring constant vigilance; therapeutic agents such as tranexamic acid and 4-factor prothrombin complex concentrate can aid in managing critical bleeding.
- Adequate exposure and precise fracture reduction are essential to help prevent postoperative complications.
- Staged reconstruction for critically ill patients involving initial fracture stabilization followed by definitive repair can reduce technical difficulty, and complications associated with prolonged operations.
- Early restoration/stabilization of the premorbid occlusal relationship can help prevent malreduction and malocclusion and aid in pain control.
- Attention must be paid to associated injuries and preexisting comorbidities to reduce complications associated with maxillofacial trauma.

INTRODUCTION

Traumatic fractures of the midface and mandible may result from motor vehicle collisions, interpersonal conflict including blunt or penetrating trauma, sports injuries, or falls. Midface and mandible fractures are often associated with other injuries; the maxillofacial surgeon must maintain a high degree of suspicion for ocular, intracranial, and/or spinal injuries.[1] In one series of 3950 patients with craniofacial fractures, 4.4% of patients with mandibular fractures had associated cervical spine injury (CSI), and this rate was higher for mandibular fractures with any midface fracture.[2]

The midface is composed of several structural subunits including the maxilla, lower orbit, zygomaticomaxillary complex (ZMC), nasal and nasolacrimal structures, palate, and upper dentition as well as their associated soft tissue components. The skull base unites with the midface through the pterygoid plates, medial and lateral orbital walls, and nasal septum; trauma in this region can result in life-threatening airway compromise and hemorrhage. The mandible is a single arch structural unit that may be subdivided into zones: symphysis, parasymphysis, body, angle, ramus, coronoid, condyle neck and head, and alveolar process. Mandibular fractures can result in debilitating trismus, malocclusion, malunion, or infection if not identified and treated in a timely manner. A thorough understanding of midface and mandible anatomy, fracture patterns, and a systematic approach to treating fractures in this region is essential to help reduce risks and complications of fracture repair.

[a] Department of Otolaryngology–Head and Neck Surgery, Upstate Medical University, State University of New York, 750 East Adams Street, Syracuse, NY 13210, USA; [b] Department of Plastic and Reconstructive Surgery, Johns Hopkins University School of Medicine, Baltimore, MD, USA
* Corresponding author.
E-mail address: tatums@upstate.edu

Facial Plast Surg Clin N Am 31 (2023) 307–314
https://doi.org/10.1016/j.fsc.2023.01.014
1064-7406/23/© 2023 Elsevier Inc. All rights reserved.

A detailed review of the technical aspects of facial fracture repair has been addressed in prior articles.[3,4] The following describes the major complications and unfavorable outcomes associated with these fractures, how to prevent their occurrence and how to manage them if they arise. Complications unique to each fracture region are also highlighted for consideration.

Complications Common to all Midface and Mandibular Fractures

Infection/osteomyelitis

Open fractures, where gingival, oral mucosal, or dentoalveolar disruption is present, should be treated with preoperative antibiotics to reduce the risk of infection. Postoperative antibiotic administration for patients with midface or mandible fractures is not supported by the literature[5] unless risk factors are present. It is important to note that although definitive fracture fixation may not be feasible in critically ill patients, every effort should be made to debride wounds and establish temporary occlusal reduction and stabilization. This can be accomplished at bedside in the critical care unit for patients who are sedated and may include bridle wires and maxillomandibular fixation (MMF). Teeth with significant caries near the fracture line should be considered for removal. Removal of healthy, stable teeth in the fracture is controversial. They can either aid or hinder reduction. They can either facilitate the seal of torn gingiva or, when pulled, provide an empty socket pathway for infection. Wounds and lacerations should be debrided and closed to help prevent the loss of tissue domain, improve long-term cosmesis, and help prevent infection. Fracture mobility from unstable fixation is an important risk factor for infection. Blood glucose control, tobacco cessation, and adequate nutrition also help mitigate infection risks. Management of acute wound/hardware infection includes cultures, antibiotics, wound washouts, possible hardware exchange, and/or bone debridement. Chronic infection with osteomyelitis requires hardware exchange (potentially more rigidity) bone grafting and cancellous bone grafting.

Soft tissue ptosis

Most maxillomandibular fractures are accessed via limited, hidden incisions. There is frequently significant subperiosteal elevation performed to provide adequate exposure for reduction and rigid internal fixation. Retraction, edema, and gravity can cause the soft tissue to redrape and distort the face even if the bony reduction is excellent. It is important to support the soft tissue at least with periosteal closure if not additional skeletally anchored sutures, particularly for the midface.

Malunion/nonunion

Improper technique, including inadequate fracture exposure, imprecise reduction and fixation, and not adhering to load-bearing/load-sharing principles can result in fixation failure with malunion or nonunion. Missed injuries can also lead to these complications, for example, in multiple-segment mandible fractures where one or more fractures is missed and loading forces are not appropriately addressed. Bone gaps more than a few millimeters should be addressed by early bone grafting, with autogenous bone preferred.

Hardware failure

Poor technique can contribute to interfragmentary instability, infection, and hardware failure, particularly in mandible fractures where continuous movement and devitalized bone can provide a substrate for pathogenic organisms.[6] Load-sharing fixation can only be used on simple fractures. Drilling must not be allowed to overheat or chatter away screw hole bone. The amount of bone holding the screw threads is a fraction of a millimeter. Stripped screw holes must have larger screws placed. Bending a plate too many times can weaken the metal to failure. Comminuted or defect fractures, and edentulous, atrophic mandibles should be treated with a heavy load-bearing reconstruction plate. Patients with partial dental arches can be treated with customized dental splints and MMF. Radiographic or clinical evidence of hardware failure should be addressed with revision including more rigid hardware.

Missed injuries

Missed injuries can include subtle craniofacial fractures or vascular injury not apparent on standard CT imaging. Ancillary physical examination findings such as Battle sign or periorbital ecchymosis may not be apparent in the acute setting and can take 24 to 48 hours to appear.[7] Patients with maxillofacial fractures have a 2% to 10% incidence of concurrent CSI especially in the setting of lower two-thirds facial fractures.[1–3] Missed injuries can have devastating consequences. Therefore, a high degree of suspicion must be maintained and cervical-spine precautions kept in place until CSI is definitively ruled out. In addition, blunt cerebrovascular injury (BCVI) can have serious complications such as stroke and may not manifest initial presentation. Dedicated multislice, multidetector CT angiography has been established as an equivalent gold standard for rapid diagnosis of BCVI compared with 4-vessel cerebral angiography and should be considered for any patient with significant facial fractures and/or spinal injury.[8] High-resolution, thin slice (1 mm or thinner) CT and 3 dimensional imaging can help resolve subtle fractures.

SYSTEMATIC APPROACH TO MIDFACE AND MANDIBLE FRACTURES
Trauma Assessment and Resuscitation

An organized, systematic approach to assessment and management of the patient with midface and mandible fractures is essential for reducing risks associated with repair. This begins with initial assessment and resuscitation following Acute Trauma Life Support (ATLS) guidelines. The ATLS program was developed by the American College of Surgeons Committee on Trauma and has been validated as a safe, reliable system to stabilize, resuscitate, and minimize risks of morbidity and mortality for the trauma patient. Following these established principles will reduce the risk of missed injuries.

Life-threatening injuries to the airway, central nervous system, and viscera are prioritized, and the patient is stabilized. Ancillary teams including Neurosurgery, Ophthalmology, and Orthopedic surgery are activated early, in addition to Otolaryngology, Plastic Surgery, and/or Oral Maxillofacial trauma surgeons managing the facial fractures. In facilities where advanced Interventional Radiology (IR) or Neurointerventional Radiology is available, it is essential to activate this team early in cases where intracranial and/or skull base hemorrhage is suspected. Preoperative history and physical examination is important but may not always be possible, such as the critically ill patient who cannot participate with examination. After the patient has been stabilized and resuscitated, a more thorough physical examination is performed. This includes comprehensive cranial nerve, sensory, motor, and dental examination.

Initial management

1. The cervical spine is stabilized while the airway is assessed and secured. Midface fractures are associated with skull-base injuries and present a relative contraindication to nasogastric tube placement and nasopharyngeal intubation; inadvertent intracranial placement is a well-documented complication and has resulted in mortalities. Advanced airway techniques are often required for patients with facial trauma and unstable airways; fiberoptic-guided orotracheal intubation or tracheostomy may be necessary to avoid manipulation of the cervical spine. Emergency tracheostomy indications include acute upper airway obstruction/ hemorrhage with failed endotracheal intubation, penetrating laryngeal trauma, and severe subcutaneous facial/neck emphysema. Elective tracheostomy is recommended for patients who are postcricothyrotomy, have panfacial fractures, and/or are expected to require mechanical ventilation longer than 7 days.

2. Breathing and ventilation are assessed and secured. Lower airway obstruction can result from inhalation of blood, teeth, or other debris. It is essential to carefully and thoroughly examine the nasal and oral airways to clear this material from the airway early and to obtain airway imaging.

3. Circulation is assessed and stabilized. Patients may have comorbid conditions predisposing them to uncontrolled bleeding after facial trauma. These can include coagulopathies, alcoholism, or hypertension. Trauma-induced coagulopathy is a known entity that can further worsen hemorrhage. Patients may be taking medications or supplements that impair normal coagulation. Consideration should be given to restoring blood volume and coagulation components with whole blood transfusion and clotting factors (such as 4-factor prothrombin complex concentrate [4F-PCC]), where available.[9-12] Patients with craniomaxillofacial trauma are more likely to have associated intracranial trauma and hemorrhage, constituting an emergency. Any delay in treatment can increase risk of major disability and death. Tranexamic acid (TXA) can reduce bleeding in trauma patients used systemically or topically. Several studies have demonstrated efficacy in reducing intraoperative blood loss[13-16] although its use in this setting remains off-label.

4. Causes of hemorrhage associated with facial trauma are essential for the craniomaxillofacial (CMF) surgeon to be aware of. These may develop in the acute or subacute setting, and vigilance is paramount. The vascular network of the head and face is robust, with multiple anastomoses and redundancies, making hemorrhage a significant concern. Midface fractures can be associated with disruption to the internal maxillary artery and its branches including the descending palatine arteries. Nasal septal hematoma may be present. Persistent, brisk epistaxis from both nares and/or the oropharynx may indicate either a posterior nasopharyngeal vascular disruption or an internal maxillary artery or ethmoidal artery laceration. Direct pressure with packing, cauterization, and ligation in areas with easy access can help abate hemorrhage. Hemorrhage from midface structures presents a unique challenge because direct pressure or suturing is often not

possible. Unstable patients with severe uncontrolled hemorrhage may require external carotid artery ligation. Attempting to control hemorrhage without adequate light and suction can lead to iatrogenic injury to adjacent structures. Intracranial and/or skull base hemorrhage is often best controlled by IR-access.

5. Definitive fracture repair is delayed until the patient has been resuscitated and stabilized. Patients should further undergo more refined physical examination and history collection. This includes sensory-motor examination, assessment of occlusion, and any relevant medical history. Injury-induced dysfunction must be documented before repair measures. Serial physical examination to assess for the evolution of trauma injuries must be performed consistently. Any changes should be documented and investigated; for example, carotid-cavernous sinus fistula can occur in patients with midface and skull base fractures and may not be readily apparent on an initial presentation.[17,18]

Imaging

The advent of high-resolution, thin slice computed tomography (CT) imaging has revolutionized the care of patients with facial fractures. Newer acquisition protocols reduce radiation exposure and contrast loads necessary for imaging. For patients suspected of having facial fractures based on physical examination and injury mechanism, CT imaging guides management and assists in surgical planning and has become the gold standard. Many centers have CT scanners within the trauma suite or ED to facilitate rapid, safe, early scanning. Subtle injuries may not be readily apparent on all views but could have significant influence on the management and risk reduction. Three-dimensional imaging adds improved visualization and perspective, although care should be taken to review the primary images for fidelity because small fragments may be erroneously fused to larger fragments in the 3D reconstruction. CT-guided intraoperative navigation has become more prevalent and may allow for more precise reconstruction in cases where severe comminution or tissue destruction is present.[19–21]

High-quality imaging is helpful to diagnose subtle but clinically significant findings; 1-mm or thinner CT tomographic images can identify fine fractures that may otherwise be missed. It is also important to consider associated cerebrovascular injury, which requires dedicated angiography of the vessels of the neck and skull base, as mentioned previously. Critically ill patients who are not suitable candidates for acute definitive operative fracture repair but are stable for CT scanning can benefit

from 3D modeling, virtual surgical planning, and creation of customized dental splints, which can aid in achieving temporary reduction of midface and/or mandible fractures with MMF.[22] This reduces the risk of malunion or nonunion and allows for minimal or simplified osteotomies during delayed fracture repair.

Intraoperative Considerations

Airway

Airway management of patients with facial trauma requires planning and sustained vigilance. In patients with midface fractures, nasotracheal intubation should be avoided if advanced airway skills are not present. The size, length, and geometry of the intubation tubing should be chosen carefully. Nasal or oral Ring-Adair-Elwyn (RAE) tubes are designed with a preformed bend that can facilitate facial surgery but they may make rescue maneuvers to resecure the dislodged airway difficult. Another disadvantage of RAE tubes is a predetermined depth of intubation based on the location of the bend, which may not be suitable for certain patients. Steel-reinforced tubing (anode or armored) can be more difficult to maneuver around; however, it is more resilient to collapse or inadvertent puncture.

Where possible, the airway circuit Fio_2 should be reduced to less than 35% when electrocautery is used, to reduce the risk of airway fires. Submental intubation should be considered when tube interference with occlusion is a concern. Sometimes, the tube can pass through dental defects or behind the posterior molars. Tracheostomy should be considered for patients meeting criteria as discussed above. Surgical airways established emergently should be inspected for collateral damage.

Blood loss management

Controlled hypotensive anesthesia has been studied in orthognathic surgery and found to be a safe and reliable method to reduce hemorrhage during dissection and exposure.[23,24] When this is combined with administration of a single preoperative dose of 10-20 mg/kg TXA in adults, blood loss can be significantly reduced.[13,16,25,26] Positioning the patient in reverse Trendelenburg, with the angle of the mandible above the level of the sternal angle helps prevent venous pooling in the operative field. The risk of air embolism must be considered if the skull is open, particularly in the presence of hypovolemia.

Special Considerations

Orbital complications potentially common to all midface fractures

- Telecanthus

- Nasolacrimal duct disruption
- Pulsatile ophthalmopathy
- Globe injury
- Retrobulbar hematoma
- Complete or partial vision loss
- Diplopia/periorbital/orbital entrapment
- Ectropion, entropion
- Enophthalmos, vertical dystopia, and diplopia
- Optic nerve/retinal ischemia

Nasomaxillary region

The blood supply to this region derives from a rich, interconnected network. Injury to the ethmoidal, sphenopalatine, and greater palatine arteries can be difficult to control locally; stable patients warrant urgent angiography and embolization. Unstable patients may require operative ligation of the external carotid artery.[27] The maxilla is a central keystone of the face, connecting the skull base with the orbit and occlusal plane. Orbital floor fractures, composed of the roof of the maxillary sinus, can lead to periorbital soft tissue entrapment. This can result in extraocular muscle dysfunction and/or volume loss. True muscle entrapment should be released urgently to avoid muscle fibrosis. A forced duction test must be performed at the beginning and conclusion of the procedure on all patients who undergo orbital floor repair to confirm the orbital soft tissue is freely mobile.[28]

Surgeons should be aware of the oculocardiac reflex, which can contribute to labile blood pressure due to bradycardia. The globe is vulnerable to direct and indirect injuries. A full ophthalmologic examination is indicated for fractures involving the orbit. Retrobulbar hematoma is a vision-threatening complication that should be recognized and intervened on emergently with lateral canthotomy/cantholysis. Blindness may be caused by direct optic nerve or optic canal injuries or by other causes including iatrogenic injury during facial fracture repair or retinal artery occlusion secondary to orbital compartment syndrome. Although rare, with postrepair blindness reported as low as 0.24% in a series of 1338 orbital fractures at one center,[29] the consequences are devastating for patients. Delayed vision loss may occur as late as a week after the initial injury; a Marcus-Gunn pupil at initial presentation is highly sensitive for vision tract injury and should be noted before fracture repair.[30] Patients with these findings, or other physical examination findings concerning for impending vision loss, should be considered corticosteroids and urgent optic nerve decompression.[31–33] Surgical repair of periorbital fractures around a damaged or only seeing eye should be carefully considered.

Complications associated with fractures of this region include the following:

- Septal hematoma
- Septal deviation
- Nasal deformity
- Nasal valve stenosis
- Synechiae between septum and turbinates
- Anosmia
- Cerebrospinal fluid (CSF) leak
- Maxillary sinusitis

Zygomaticomaxillary complex/orbital floor region

ZMC fractures can result in significant functional and esthetic derangement. The zygomatic nerve, cranial nerve V2, provides sensation to the midface via 3 main branches. The frontal branch of the facial nerve, cranial nerve VII, passes superficial to the zygomatic arch, deep to the superficial musculoaponeurotic system before transitioning deep to the temporoparietal fascia. Muscles of facial expression, zygomaticus major and minor, originate from the zygoma and can be disrupted by trauma or malpositioned with improper dissection during fracture repair. Finally, the lateral canthal tendon of the orbit inserts onto the lateral orbital tubercle (Whitnall's) on the orbital surface of the zygoma, below the ZF suture. Injury from trauma or improper dissection and malpositioning during fracture repair can result in abnormal palpebral fissure shape and orientation, possibly ectropion.[34] There is considerable discussion in the literature about delayed and nonoperative management of floor fractures. When they are deemed necessary, orbital floor implants must be carefully considered for necessity, material, size, and position. The most popular materials are titanium, porous polyethylene, and absorbable polymers. Their primary purpose is to restore orbital support returning orbital soft tissue back into the orbit. They must be large enough to cover the defect or strong enough to support by cantilever. If they are placed too low, they will not provide enough support. If placed too high, they can put pressure on the orbital contents leading to poor motility or even blindness. Postoperative CT verification of implant placement and eye examination are recommended. Navigation or intraoperative CT scanning is even better.

Complications associated with fractures of this region include the following:

- Cranial nerve V2 dysfunction, in particular infraorbital nerve dysfunction
- Facial nerve palsy/paralysis
- Poor malar projection with negative globe vector

- Facial asymmetry
- Trismus

Palate/alveolus/dentition region

The palate serves as a major horizontal buttress of the face and defines the occlusal plane, in conjunction with dentition. Thorough physical examination and review of imaging findings are essential to restoring premorbid occlusion and decreasing the risk of malocclusion, asymmetry, and dental disruption. It is important to recognize dental trauma to avoid the risk of aspiration and to determine acuity. Patients who have sustained isolated injury or are otherwise stable without the risk of aspiration can be considered for reimplantation of avulsed teeth, although this is typically successful only within the first hour from injury, with an intact periodontal ligament.

Examples of complications associated with fractures of this region include the following:

- Malocclusion
- Temporomandibular joint (TMJ) dysfunction
- Oronasal/oroantral fistula
- Dental trauma
  - Partially or completely avulsed teeth
  - Tooth fractures
  - Luxation

Mandible

The mandible is an arch osseous unit that articulates with the skull base at the glenoid fossae. In conjunction with the maxilla, it contributes to the occlusal plane via the lower dentition. The buccal surface of the mandible features the anterior and posterior ramus, the sigmoid notch, the condylar process and the coronoid. The lingual surface includes the medial sigmoid notch, lingula, and mandibular foramen. The inferior alveolar nerve (IAN) enters the foramen and traverses the lower ramus and body of the mandible, providing sensation to the dentition, lower lip, and chin. Isolated, single-segment mandible fractures commonly include the body, condyle, or angle. The lingual nerve is a branch of cranial nerve V3, often sharing a common tract with the IAN until it dives into the oral cavity at the medial ramus, near the third molar. The marginal mandibular nerve is typically 2 fingerbreadths below the mandibular border in the skeletally mature patient, as it descends from near the mandibular border in children. It is important to understand this anatomy to avoid inadvertent injury to these nerves when performing mandibular fracture repair. It is also important to document any preoperative dysfunction of these nerves.

A common combination fracture pattern observed is a parasymphyseal fracture with contralateral angle or subcondylar fracture. The unique geometry of the masticatory muscles insertions and their associated vectors of pull influence whether mandible fractures are "favorable" or "unfavorable." These vectors act to reduce or distract the fracture fragments depending on fracture orientation. Load-sharing fixation can be considered in simple, typically favorable fractures with minimal associated injuries. Comminution, multiple fractures, osseous defects, and comorbidities call for more rigidity. The atrophic and/or edentulous mandible presents a special situation because the loss of vertical mandibular height can make open reduction and internal fixation plating challenging,[35,36] often requiring load-bearing, heavy plates.

Complications associated with mandible fractures.

- Injury to IAN or, rarely, the lingual nerve
- Malocclusion
- Trismus
- Dental injury
- TMJ ankylosis

Stable, rigid fixation with precise anatomic reduction has been shown consistently to reduce the risk of malunion or nonunion, infection, and implant extrusion.[37–39] Motion across the fracture line leads to instability, hardware loosening and ultimately infection, loss of reduction, and fixation failure.

Panfacial fractures

Panfacial fractures require special consideration for management and risk reduction; these patients often require prolonged mechanical ventilation and treatment of concurrent central nervous system or other systemic injury. Generally, these are classified by concurrent fractures of the upper, middle, and lower thirds of the face. Organized fracture repair from stable to unstable in a stepwise fashion, either a top down, bottom up, centripetal, or centrifugal approach can help reduce complications by addressing complexity systematically.

SUMMARY

Midface and mandible fracture repair can be achieved safely by adhering to a systematic approach for early recognition of debilitating injuries, using advanced pharmacologic and imaging strategies for hemorrhage control, thorough knowledge of facial anatomy and early precise anatomic reduction and stable fixation. A consistently applied, systematic approach to the facial trauma patient in the acute, intraoperative and postoperative periods can reduce risks associated with midface and mandible fracture repair.

Surgeons must be aware of the intricate facial osseous and vascular anatomy and should familiarize themselves with maneuvers for rapid control of the airway and hemorrhage that may result from the inciting injury or during intraoperative repair.

FUNDING

Neha Datta is a fellow sponsored by the AO Foundation, specifically AO Craniomaxillofacial North America (AO CMF NA) which provides stipend support for fellow activities. For further information please visit https://www.aofoundation.org/aona/our-community/cmf/cmf-fellowships.

CLINICS CARE POINTS

- Use a systematic approach to initial patient stabilization and resuscitation, followed by thorough serial physical examinations to reduce the risk of missed injuries, evolving, or unexpected findings during operative repair of midface and mandibular fractures.

- Surgeons should maintain a high degree of suspicion for high-morbidity or mortality complications of facial trauma and sustained vigilance throughout the pre, intraoperative and postoperative period.

- Pharmacologic adjuncts such as TXA and 4F-PCC can significantly reduce hemorrhage and associated complications for patients with facial fractures, both in the acute and perioperative settings.

- High-resolution, multidetector CT imaging with 1-mm slices can assist with identifying subtle fractures and be used to create customized temporary dental splints and/or fixation plates. Intraoperative navigation can be used for precision fracture reduction and plate placement for complicated fractures, reducing the risk of malunion, malposition, or unsatisfactory outcomes.

- Early intervention with precise anatomic reduction is critical to minimizing the risk of acute and long-term complications. Guiding principles of rigid fixation, stabilizing unstable segments, immediate autogenous bone grafting, and early definitive soft tissue management all contribute to improved outcomes. For critically ill patients who are not stable for definitive repair, antibiotics, early soft tissue closure and temporary reduction, and fixation with MMF should be considered.

REFERENCES

1. Feldman JS, Farnoosh S, Kellman RM, et al. Skull base trauma: clinical considerations in evaluation and diagnosis and review of management techniques and surgical approaches. Semin Plast Surg 2017;31(4):177–88.
2. Färkkilä EM, Peacock ZS, Tannyhill RJ, et al. Risk factors for cervical spine injury in patients with mandibular fractures. J Oral Maxillofac Surg 2019 Jan;77(1):109–17.
3. Thomas JR, Kriet JD, Humphrey CD, editors. Facial plastic surgery clinics of North America30. Philadelphia: Elsevier; 2022. p. i–124. Issue 1, 2022-2031-31.
4. Kellman RM, Tatum SA. Principles in rigid fixation of the facial skeleton (78. In: Rosen CA, editor. Bailey's head and neck surgery-otolaryngology. 6th edition. Philadelphia: Lippincott-Raven Publishers; 2022. p. 1195–212.
5. Mundinger GS, Borsuk DE, Okhah Z, et al. Antibiotics and facial fractures: evidence-based recommendations compared with experience-based practice. Craniomaxillofac Trauma Reconstr 2015; 8(1):64–78.
6. Alpert B, Kushner GM, Tiwana PS. Contemporary management of infected mandibular fractures. Craniomaxillofac Trauma Reconstr 2008;1(1):25–9.
7. Battle WH. Three Lectures on Some Points Relating to Injuries to the Head. Br Med J 1890;2(1542): 141–7.
8. Kim DY, Biffl W, Bokhari F, et al. Evaluation and management of blunt cerebrovascular injury: a practice management guideline from the eastern association for the surgery of trauma. J Trauma Acute Care Surg 2020 Jun;88(6):875–87.
9. Sellers W, Bendas C, Toy F, et al. Utility of 4-factor prothrombin complex concentrate in trauma and acute-care surgical patients. J Am Osteopath Assoc 2018;118(12):789–97.
10. Jehan F, Aziz H, O'Keeffe T, et al. The role of four-factor prothrombin complex concentrate in coagulopathy of trauma: a propensity matched analysis. J Trauma Acute Care Surg 2018;85(1):18–24.
11. Zeeshan M, Hamidi M, Feinstein AJ, et al. Four-factor prothrombin complex concentrate is associated with improved survival in trauma-related hemorrhage: a nationwide propensity-matched analysis. J Trauma Acute Care Surg 2019;87(2):274–81.
12. Tanaka KA, Shettar S, Vandyck K, et al. Roles of four-factor prothrombin complex concentrate in the management of critical bleeding. Transfus Med Rev 2021;35(4):96–103.
13. Choi WS, Irwin MG, Samman N. The effect of tranexamic acid on blood loss during orthognathic surgery: a randomized controlled trial. J Oral Maxillofac Surg 2009;67(1):125–33.

14. Zahed R, Mousavi Jazayeri MH, Naderi A, et al. Topical tranexamic acid compared with anterior nasal packing for treatment of epistaxis in patients taking antiplatelet drugs: randomized controlled trial. Acad Emerg Med 2018;25(3):261–6.

15. Gharaibeh A, Savage HI, Scherer RW, et al. Medical interventions for traumatic hyphema. Cochrane Database Syst Rev 2013;12:CD005431.

16. Christabel A, Muthusekhar MR, Narayanan V, et al. Effectiveness of tranexamic acid on intraoperative blood loss in isolated Le Fort I osteotomies–a prospective, triple blinded randomized clinical trial. J Cranio-Maxillo-Fac Surg 2014;42(7):1221–4.

17. Zhang C, Tianjia Z, Lv H, et al. The possibility of internal carotid-cavernous fistula after maxillary fracture. J Craniofac Surg 2022;33(8):2586–8.

18. Hwang JH, Kim WH, Choi JH, et al. Delayed rupture of a posttraumatic retromaxillary pseudoaneurysm causing massive bleeding: a case report. Arch Craniofac Surg 2021;22(3):168–72.

19. DeLong MR, Gandolfi BM, Barr ML, et al. Intraoperative Image-Guided Navigation in Craniofacial Surgery: Review and Grading of the Current Literature. J Craniofac Surg 2019;30(2):465–72.

20. Ebker T, Korn P, Heiland M, et al. Comprehensive virtual orthognathic planning concept in surgery-first patients. Br J Oral Maxillofac Surg 2022;S0266-4356(22):00132–42.

21. Chin SJ, Wilde F, Neuhaus M, et al. Accuracy of virtual surgical planning of orthognathic surgery with aid of CAD/CAM fabricated surgical splint-A novel 3D analyzing algorithm. J Cranio-Maxillo-Fac Surg 2017 Dec;45(12):1962–70.

22. Marschall JS, Kushner GM. Point-of-care three-dimensional printing for craniomaxillofacial trauma. Plast Aesthet Res 2021;8:28.

23. Dolman RM, Bentley KC, Head TW, et al. The effect of hypotensive anesthesia on blood loss and operative time during Le Fort I osteotomies. J Oral Maxillofac Surg 2000 Aug;58(8):834–9. ; discussion 840.

24. Varol A, Basa S, Ozturk S. The role of controlled hypotension upon transfusion requirement during maxillary downfracture in double jaw surgery. J Cranio-Maxillo-Fac Surg 2010;38:345–9.

25. Zellin G, Rasmusson L, Palsson J, et al. Evaluation of haemorrhage depressors on blood loss during orthognathic surgery: a retrospective study. J Oral Maxillofac Surg 2004;62:662–6.

26. Chauncey J.M., Wieters J.S., Tranexamic Acid. [Updated 2022 Jul 25]. In: StatPearls [Internet]. Treasure Island (FL): StatPearls Publishing; 2022.

27. Nguyen M, Koshy JC, Hollier LH Jr. Pearls of nasoorbitoethmoid trauma management. Semin Plast Surg 2010 Nov;24(4):383–8.

28. Morris LM, Kellman RM. Complications in facial trauma. Facial Plast Surg Clin North Am 2013 Nov; 21(4):605–17.

29. Girotto JA, Gamble WB, Robertson B, et al. Blindness after reduction of facial fractures. Plastic and Reconstructive Surg 1998;102(6):1821–34.

30. Ord RA. Postoperative retrobulbar haemorrhage and blindness complicating trauma surgery. Br J Oral Surg 1981;19:202.

31. Levin LA, Joseph MP, Rizzo JF III, Lessell S. Optic canal decompression in Indirect optic nerve trauma. Opthalmology 1994;101:566.

32. Cook MW, Levin LA, Joseph MP, et al. Traumatic optic neuropathy: a meta-analysis. Arch Otolaryngol Head Neck Surg 1996;122:389.

33. Voss JO, Hartwig S, Doll C, et al. The "tight orbit": Incidence and management of the orbital compartment syndrome. J Cranio-Maxillo-Fac Surg 2016 Aug;44(8):1008–14.

34. Birgfeld CB, Mundinger GS, Gruss JS. Evidence-based medicine: evaluation and treatment of zygoma fractures. Plast Reconstr Surg 2017; 139(1):168e–80e.

35. Seu M, Jazayeri HE, Lopez J, et al. Comparing load-sharing miniplate and load-bearing plate fixation in atrophic edentulous mandibular fractures: a systematic review and meta-analysis. J Craniofac Surg 2021;32(7):2401–5.

36. Façanha de Carvalho E, Alkmin Paiva GL, Yonezaki F, et al. Computer-Aided Surgical Simulation in Severe Atrophic Mandibular Fractures: A New Method for Guided Reduction and Temporary Stabilization Before Fixation. J Oral Maxillofac Surg 2021;79(4):892.e1–7.

37. Chrcanovic BR. Open versus closed reduction: comminuted mandibular fractures. Oral Maxillofac Surg 2013;17(2):95–104.

38. Singh AK, Dahal S, Singh S, et al. Is manual reduction adequate for intraoperative control of occlusion during fixation of mandibular fractures? A systematic review and meta-analysis. Br J Oral Maxillofac Surg 2022;60(3):271–8.

39. Klatt J, Heiland M, Blessmann M, et al. Clinical indication for intraoperative 3D imaging during open reduction of fractures of the neck and head of the mandibular condyle. J Craniomaxillofac Surg 2011; 39(4):244–8.

Reducing Systemic Risks in a Traumatic Panfacial Injury Patient

Kendra Black, MD, Jay Doucet, MD, MSc, FRCSC, FACS, RDMS*

KEYWORDS

• Panfacial trauma • Critical care • Facial injury • Airway injury • Tracheostomy

KEY POINTS

• Panfacial trauma is caused by high-energy trauma and may include airway and ventilatory compromise, bleeding issues, and associated neurologic trauma such as cervical spine injury and trauma brain injury.
• Priorities for the initial management of panfacial trauma have been established by the Advanced Trauma Life Support Course (ATLS).
• Critical Care is frequently required for panfacial trauma, and a multidisciplinary approach is recommended, including the facial surgeon, the acute care surgery (ACS)/trauma surgeon, surgical intensivist, other surgeons, and the anesthesiologist along with the patient and family regarding the order and timing of procedures, and for postoperative management.
• A "damage control" approach may be required in unstable patients with multiple and associated injuries, following the "ABC's" of ATLS.

INTRODUCTION

Panfacial trauma refers to injuries caused by high-energy mechanisms to two or more regions of the craniofacial skeleton, including the frontal bone, the midface, and the occlusal unit. As with any trauma, Advanced Trauma Life Support protocols should be followed in unstable patients.[1] For the patient with panfacial traumatic injury, advanced perioperative care or critical care is frequently required in two scenarios. A patient may present to the trauma bay or emergency room with signs of a surgical emergency such as degloving scalp, facial injury, or direct airway injury, and an operation may be scheduled as soon as the patient leaves the emergency room (ER). Alternately, the choice to do surgery could be made when the patient is already receiving intensive care for concomitant injuries. Surgical critical care, a component of the acute-care surgery[2] model, is necessary for both scenarios to reduce systemic risks, improve the patient's condition and enable a successful surgical operation.[3]

TIMING OF SURGERY
Simultaneous Resuscitation and Surgery

Insufficient oxygen transport to the organs during shock causes cellular hypoxia, which, if not treated immediately, can cause organ failure and death.[4] Hypovolemia, dehydration, fluid shifts, hemorrhagic shock, and other categories of shock could all be present in a patient with ACS. Patients with cardiac tamponade, abdominal compartment syndrome, tension pneumothorax, pulmonary, or air embolism may also show obstructive shock. Patients who experience neurogenic shock, such as those who have suffered a cervical spinal cord injury, and septic shock may show distributive shock. Shock is most noticeable in those patients with hypotension, but in its early stages it can be subtle and only be picked up with small

Division of Trauma, Surgical Critical Care, Burns & Acute Care Surgery, University of California San Diego, 200 West Arbor Drive, #8896, San Diego, CA 92103, USA
* Corresponding author.
E-mail address: jdoucet@ucsd.edu

Facial Plast Surg Clin N Am 31 (2023) 315–324
https://doi.org/10.1016/j.fsc.2023.01.015
1064-7406/23/© 2023 Elsevier Inc. All rights reserved.

alterations in vital signs, organ function, laboratory findings, or particular imaging. Major trauma patients who are in shock and undergoing emergency surgery typically need simultaneous assessment, resuscitation, and initiation without necessarily having a full history, complete imaging, or complete laboratory results. Resuscitation starts immediately and may need to continue throughout the operation. The surgical team, anesthesiology providers, operating room (OR) nurses, and technicians must use effective communication and teamwork to reduce risks. Multiple sources of shock may be present at the same time in a trauma patient.

Rapid assessment of the preoperative facial trauma patient with shock includes evaluation of vital signs, available preoperative tests, and imaging, particularly point-of-care ultrasonography (POCUS) if uncertainty exists and time, skill, and equipment permit.[5–7] Changes in vital signs include tachycardia, hypertension, and rapid shallow respiration. In general, hypotension is defined as a systolic blood pressure of less than 90 mm Hg. Increases in peripheral vasoconstriction, cardiac output, and regional changes in circulation may delay the onset of hypotension despite significant hypovolemia in patients with physiologic reserve. The difference between the systolic and diastolic pressures defines pulse pressure. Before the onset of overt hypotension, the pulse pressure typically decreases due to vasoconstriction in hypovolemic states. Wide pulse pressure, in which the difference between systolic and diastolic blood pressures is greater than the diastolic blood pressure, may be indicative of vasodilation, which is observed in early distributive shock states such as septic shock. If time permits, placement of an arterial pressure line permits immediate assessment of blood pressure and facilitates blood gas and intraoperative laboratory testing. Any available preoperative test results should be reviewed. When a patient is hemodynamically unstable, additional testing should be limited to studies that influence intraoperative decision-making and do not place the patient at an undue risk of deterioration in inaccessible or poorly monitored settings, such as the computed tomography (CT) or MRI scanner. Blood gases, including base deficit and lactate, can detect respiratory or metabolic derangements. Blood counts can be used to help diagnose sepsis and anemia. Electrolytes can become deranged due to sepsis or excessive crystalloid administration. Laboratory markers for the heart, liver, and kidneys can detect organ dysfunction and ischemia.

Rapid point-of-care imaging at the bedside can help differentiate shock states. The source of shock states can be determined by a preoperative chest x-ray, such as massive hemothorax or tension pneumothorax. Although these are primarily clinical diagnoses, the chest x-ray is confirmatory and indicates the proper placement of a chest tube. Any simple pneumothorax seen on a chest x-ray requires attention as it may lead to subsequent deterioration, particularly after intubation and positive pressure ventilation, which would necessitate the placement of a chest tube. The anterior-posterior view (AP) pelvic x-ray detects pelvic fractures, which can cause hemorrhagic shock. The KUB can detect free air in a patient with abdominal trauma.

POCUS is a necessary skill set for surgical intensivists and a useful skill set for acute-care surgeons. POCUS permits the differentiation of shock states.[5–9] POCUS can detect hypovolemia if the inferior vena cava is small or collapsible, or if ventricular filling is inadequate. It can detect obstructive shock by identifying pneumothorax on chest views due to the absence of plural sliding. It can also detect cardiac tamponade by showing pericardial effusion or collapse of the right ventricle. In advanced septic shock, global myocardial dysfunction is observable. Congestive cardiomyopathy with dilated ventricles and poor performance is also highlighted. The abdominal section of focused assessment with sonography for trauma (FAST) can detect free abdominal fluid or hemoperitoneum.

Immediate Versus Delayed Surgery

Situations requiring immediate surgery to halt a life-threatening pathologic process necessitate rapid assessment, immediate resuscitative measures to correct shock states, prompt transfer to the OR, safe induction of anesthesia, and appropriate surgery. Before the onset of the "lethal triad" of hypothermia, metabolic acidosis, and coagulopathy, damage control surgery may be required. Damage control approaches must arrest hemorrhage, prevent contamination of clean tissues from hollow viscus injuries, and detect injuries that may require delay definitive management after stabilization from hypovolemic shock states such as trauma-related hemorrhage.[10]

Obstructive shock, such as caused by tension pneumothorax or cardiac tamponade, requires immediate surgical intervention. Although a chest tube or finger thoracostomy may be performed quickly to relieve tension pneumothorax, cardiac tamponade due to cardiac injury requires pericardiotomy, typically by median sternotomy although left anterior thoracotomy may be necessary during cardiac arrest or if sternotomy is not possible.

In intensive care unit (ICU) patients with multiple injuries a multidisciplinary approach is best; this involves the facial surgeon, ACS surgeon, surgical intensivist, other surgeons, and the anesthesiologist along with the patient and family. The team can then discuss the need, risks, and benefits of surgery, timing and order of procedures, and strategies to permit performance or delay of the procedure. Good preoperative communication of the agreed-upon plan of all team members with the patient and family is essential and is documentation of their level of understanding. A "damage control" approach may be required in unstable patients with multiple and associated injuries, especially in penetrating trauma, blast injuries, and conflict surgery.[11] This would prioritize those procedures stabilizing the "ABCs" of ATLS, before definitive fixation.

AIRWAY MANAGEMENT

Patients may arrive after major trauma with airway compromise or need for early ventilation. Airway obstruction, due to direct airway trauma or inability to clear blood or secretions, altered mental status, chest trauma, or cervical cord injury may require intubation during the initial trauma assessment. This requires the attendance of an airway provider with skills in emergency intubation and the judicious use of a rapid sequence induction for intubation. In some cases, a surgical airway, such as a surgical or needle cricothyrotomy may be necessary.

Induction of anesthesia and intubation are critical steps in the management of the panfacial trauma patient. To avoid exacerbating shock states and increasing the risk of intraoperative cardiac arrest, it is necessary to select agents with care and administer them at the proper time. Induction agents with minimal vasodilatory properties, such as etomidate or ketamine, are preferred. Etomidate is known to cause transient adrenocortical suppression, and this risk is weighed against the danger of hypotension posed by conventional agents.[2] Ketamine causes mild myocardial depression, and patients with severe shock and possibly depleted adrenergic reserves should take a lower dose. Owing to the lack of myocardial effects, high-opioid-dose anesthetics are frequently used in cardiac surgery. However, this should be avoided in shock states due to the patient's dependence on high catecholamine levels. Propofol should be avoided because it causes arterial and venous vasodilation, decreased cardiac contractility, and cardiac arrest in shock states after induction.

Understanding the effect of increased intrathoracic pressure during inadequate cardiac preload influences the timing of intubation in hypovolemic shock. Patients who are dependent on afterload because of inadequate left ventricular performance due to cardiogenic shock typically tolerate intubation, positive pressure ventilation, and PEEP quite well. However, in hypovolemic shock (or hypovolemic preload-deficient patients?), preload-deficient patients, intubation and high airway pressures or high PEEP may precipitate cardiac arrest. Typically, a fluid bolus is administered intravenously before induction, intubation, and positive pressure ventilation. In conscious, breathing shock patients, intubation can often be delayed until arrival in the OR, where the optimal combination of team members and equipment is available, sufficient time has passed to allow and evaluate fluid resuscitation, and severe hypotension or incipient cardiac arrest can be optimally managed.

The decision to perform early intraoperative tracheostomy can be aided by an algorithm shown in **Fig. 1**.[12] Submental intubation is a technique that involves passing an endotracheal tube (ETT) through the anterior floor of the mouth, and then down the airway, leaving the facial bones, mandible, and skull base untouched. The tube can be removed after recovery from anesthesia or left in place for a few days of ventilatory support.[13]

OPTIMIZING RESPIRATORY FUNCTION

The critically ill trauma patient may present multiple preoperative respiratory management challenges. Patients suffering from trauma may sustain thoracic injuries that affect ventilation and oxygenation. Multiple segmental rib fractures can impair ventilation by causing paradoxic respiratory motion in the flail segment during spontaneous breathing. Hemothorax and pneumothorax can also hinder ventilation by decreasing the available tidal volume and increasing intrathoracic pressures. Pain from rib fractures can also inhibit spontaneous respiration. Aspiration of blood and secretions from facial fractures may require repeat suctioning, intubation, and bronchoscopy. Pulmonary contusions cause direct alveolar injury and regional hypoxic pulmonary vasoconstriction, thereby worsening oxygenation. Intubation, mechanical ventilation, and appropriate chest tube placement are the most important preoperative tools for optimizing thoracic injury patients. Intubation and positive pressure ventilation will stop the paradoxic movement of the chest wall in the flail chest and reverse the hypoventilation caused by pain. The removal of air and blood from the pleural space by chest tubes permits full lung expansion.

Hypoventilation can cause atelectasis, lobar collapse, mucous plugging, hypercarbia, obtundation, aspiration, and respiratory and cardiac arrest in spontaneously breathing patients with facial

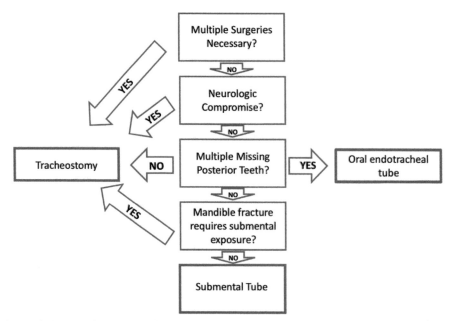

Fig. 1. Airway decision-making in panfacial fractures. (After Curtis W, Horswell BB. Panfacial fractures: an approach to management. Oral Maxillofac Surg Clin North Am. 2013 Nov;25(4):649-60.)

trauma. The bedside incentive spirometer is frequently used to encourage deep breathing and assess vital capacity at the bedside. Patients who have sustained head, facial or thoracic trauma are at risk for pulmonary deterioration and should undergo repeated chest physiotherapy.

Patients who are intubated in the ICU are monitored using arterial blood gas, chest x-ray, and ventilator parameters. Patients with thoracic trauma may require bronchoscopy to assess for tracheobronchial injury, to obtain washings and culture to detect pneumonia, or to remove mucus or clots obstructing bronchial airways. Even with appropriate chest tube drainage, a retained hemothorax may occur and may necessitate video-assisted thoracoscopic surgery (VATS).

For facial trauma patients who are in the ICU for several days, hypoxemia may result from adult respiratory distress syndrome (ARDS) or from hospital-acquired pneumonia. ARDS may necessitate advanced ventilatory modes like pressure-controlled inverse ratio ventilation (PCIRV) or airway pressure release ventilation (APRV), proning, inhaled broncho-vasodilators like nitric oxide, or extracorporeal membrane oxygenation (ECMO). Owing to the inability of many anesthesia machines to perform advanced ventilation modes such as PCIRV or APRV, abdominal incisions may prevent proning, and ECMO may necessitate continuous anticoagulation, such interventions may make surgical procedures difficult or impossible. Severe

hypoxemia in ARDS patients can also be precipitated by minor changes in patient position. During high levels of ventilatory support, exchanging the ETT or placement of a tracheostomy are high-risk procedures as rapid desaturation can occur during even brief interruptions of mechanical ventilation. This may lead to delays in planned definitive facial surgery.

INITIAL RESUSCITATION

All trauma patients who might have a shock state should receive supplemental oxygen. This may counter any hypoventilation and hypoxemia and extends the period of tolerable apnea should intubation become necessary.

Most patients suspected in shock usually initially receive a crystalloid boluses of 1000 mL as a diagnostic challenge. Patients with trauma and hemorrhagic shock should be quickly converted to blood products if hypotension does not resolve after 1 L of crystalloid in adults or 10 mL/kg in children.[14] A 1:1 ratio of packed cells to plasma is maintained. Plateletpheresis units are given every 4 to 6 units. A massive transfusion protocol (MTP) ensures adequate availability of products, mobilizes resources, and reminds practitioners to test for fibrinolysis, coagulopathies and when to administer calcium, tranexamic acid, fibrinogen, cryoprecipitate, and clotting factors. The existence of an MTP in the hospital improves patient outcomes.[15]

Vasopressors may be required preoperatively and intraoperatively in the trauma patient. They are often required to ensure organ perfusion in undifferentiated or nonhemorrhagic shock states but should be avoided in hemorrhagic shock states unless adequate blood and crystalloid administration has failed to correct the shock state.

Administration of vasopressors typically is done via a central venous catheter (CVC) due to the risk of tissue necrosis with extravasation at peripheral intravenous sites, although phenylephrine is commonly given via peripheral intravenous sites.

The target blood pressure in preoperative trauma patients is unknown. Higher target MAPs may be associated with decreased need for renal replacement therapy but an increased risk of arrythmias.[16,17] High doses of vasopressor raise concern for mesenteric ischemia and bowel necrosis. Typically, an MAP of 65 mm Hg is used.[18] Urine output of 0.5 mL/kg is desirable and decreasing base deficit or lactate on blood gases are evidence of adequate resuscitation.

MONITORING

Standard monitors used preoperatively include the electrocardiograph (EKG), saturation monitor, and blood pressure cuff. End-tidal capnography is useful in intubated patients. Invasive monitoring usually includes intra-arterial line blood pressure monitoring; however, this should not be allowed to delay urgent surgery and can be placed after induction and incision. The arterial line can also allow measurement of post-to-post? respiratory variation that can give stroke volume variation (SVV), stroke volume, and calculated cardiac output.[9,19] An SVV of $\geq$15% implies inadequate preload and fluid responsiveness. The arterial line also facilitates repeat laboratory testing, especially arterial blood gases.

The CVC allows the measurement of central venous pressure (CVP). Interpretation of the CVP with regard to fluid responsiveness should be performed with caution, as correlation is poor in many scenarios. If the actual need is access for rapid illustration of intravenous fluid, two large bore peripheral IVs, 18 gauge or larger will actually generate higher flows than a triple lumen 20 cm 7 French CVC. The CVC can also be used for blood and can obtain the superior vena cava oxygen saturation ($S_{cv}O_2$) by venous blood gas sampling or use of an oximetric catheter tip. $S_{cv}O_2$ can be used as a surrogate of oxygen consumption and cardiac output, a $S_{cv}O_2$ greater than 70% is usually considered an indicator of adequate oxygen delivery during resuscitation.

The PA catheter has not been shown to improve survival in critical care but is often used in specific scenarios where cardiac issues predominate such as right ventricular failure, pulmonary hypertension or embolism, and acute valvular disease. Transesophageal echocardiography (TEE) is increasingly used as an intraoperative monitoring technique in trauma patients.[20,21] Direct visualization and if the desired measurement of chamber sizes and flows allows rapid differentiation of shock states. TEE usually is only performed in the OR by a trained anesthesiologist, although indwelling disposable TEE probes are available, which can be placed intraoperatively and left in place postoperatively for up to 72 h in intubated patients.[22]

The Foley bladder catheter is placed preoperatively that allows for measurement of urine output, which can be reassuring of adequate renal perfusion with 0.5 mL/kg hourly. The Foley catheter can also be equipped with a temperature sensor to provide continuous core body temperature. The sampling port on most Foley catheters can also be used to provide bladder pressures, which can be used to diagnose intrabdominal hypertension and abdominal compartment syndrome.[23]

MANAGEMENT: HEMORRHAGE

Acute hemorrhage is a concern with panfacial injuries. Scalp lacerations may be associated with substantial blood loss, and operative disimpaction maneuvers may injure vessel walls or relieve an occlusion in the internal maxillary artery distribution or associated venous plexus, resulting in substantial bleeding.[12] In stable patients, consideration of induced intraoperative hypotension by anesthesia can help limit blood loss during these procedures.[24] Panfacial injuries may also cause disturbances in the facial vasculature or precipitate a pseudoaneurysm with delayed bleeding weeks after the injury and reduction.[25]

The primary strategy in the trauma patient in hemorrhagic shock is to control bleeding and to replace blood losses. Inadequate preload is the principal cause of hypotension, whereas efforts are underway to control bleeding, judicious intravenous fluid administration is used to increase preload, allow intubation and positive pressure ventilation when ready and allow improved organ perfusion. The current standard crystalloid bolus in the Advanced Trauma Life Support (ATLS) program is 1 L of crystalloid followed by blood product administration if vital signs are not normalized.[14] Current guidelines recommend a one-to-one packed red cells to plasma ratio.[26] Trials using whole blood, which contains one unit of packed cells, one unit of plasma, and one unit of platelets per bag are underway in prehospital and hospital environments.[27] Fluids should be infused by a warming device to avoid hypothermia. Avoidance of administration of large volumes of crystalloid prevents death and morbidity due to excess tissue edema, pulmonary edema, hypothermia, dilutional coagulopathy, and metabolic acidosis. Careful monitoring is required to avoid excess resuscitation and hypervolemia which can result in pulmonary edema, abdominal compartment syndrome and extremity compartment syndrome. Vasopressors are not used as a substitute for transfusion, although may be temporarily necessary in early phases of resuscitation.

TRANSPORT TO THE OPERATING ROOM

Facial trauma patients who require urgent surgery require an organized process to transport the patient and team to the OR with appropriate monitoring.[28] Having a dedicated OR immediately available for surgical emergencies such as trauma cases has been shown to reduce mortality. Trauma centers having a direct to OR capability also have decreased mortality in major trauma victims.[29] Hybrid OR/ER rooms with integrated imaging allow simultaneous resuscitation, surgical preparation, and operative procedures with a seamless transition between resuscitation and operative teams.[30] A formal handover process between the resuscitation team and the operative team should occur and a senior member of the surgical team should be present during the handover.

POSTOPERATIVE INTENSIVE CARE UNIT CARE

Patients with acute trauma surgical illness who are admitted to the ICU promptly have better outcomes. The 2016 ICU Admission, Discharge, and Triage Guidelines provide an excellent framework for the implementation of appropriate ICU admission criteria in adult ICUs.[31] In patients with panfacial trauma, especially with multisystem injury, we strongly recommend direct ICU admission from the OR or emergency department (ED) whenever possible, as this will allow the ICU team to quickly review the patient's clinical issues and physiology and initiate the most appropriate critical care treatment. It is essential that the transfer of care given in a "handoff" from the OR and trauma/ED team to the ICU team is comprehensive and thorough. Transporting critically ill patients to the post-anesthesia care unit (PACU) before their admission to the ICU is fraught with complications due to a lack of care transition from the primary surgical team.

The optimal ICU care model for patients with acute surgical illness and trauma is the "semi-open, collaborative care" model, in which the ICU is staffed with attending intensivists and an ICU team responsible not only for minute-to-minute critical care but also for coordination of ICU care and communication with primary surgeons' teams. The primary attending surgeon and surgical team retain ultimate responsibility for the patient, but ICU patient care is a collaborative effort under this model, which combines the benefits of critical care expertise for trauma and surgery patients with the primary surgical service's responsibility for overall patient management. This is consistent with the Guidelines for the Optimal Care of the Injured Patient recommended for Level 1 Trauma Centers by the American College of Surgeons Committee on Trauma.[32]

DAILY ROUNDING INTENSIVE CARE UNIT CHECKLISTS

It has been documented that daily goals checklists and the ABCDEF Bundle reduce the risk of patient harm and improve ICU progress and outcomes. The ICU Liberation Collaborative[33] is a large-scale, real-world quality improvement initiative designed to implement the Society of Critical Care Medicine (SCCM) peripheral artery disease (PAD) Guidelines in 76 ICUs using the ABCDEF Bundle.[34] For every 10% increase in total or partial bundle compliance, implementation of the ABCDEF Bundle in 6064 patients across seven community hospitals was associated with significantly improved outcomes and significantly increased hospital survival. These results were even more striking when ICU patients receiving palliative care were excluded (12% and 23% higher odds of survival per 10% increase in bundle compliance, respectively, $P < .001$). Total or partial bundle compliance was also associated with longer survival and freedom from delirium and coma.[35]

A recent prospective multicenter cohort study (15,226 ICU adult patients, 68 ICUs, 20-month period) from a national quality improvement collaborative reported that ABCDEF Bundle performance was associated with a decreased likelihood of seven adverse types of outcomes.[36] (maybe a table showing those adverse outcomes?)

INTENSIVE CARE UNIT GOALS OF RESUSCITATION

The primary objective of critical care support for patients with acute surgical illness is the restoration of oxygen delivery, maintenance of hemodynamic stability, and improvement of organ function. It is important to recognize that no single endpoint of resuscitation is optimal for all ICU patients, and that it is best to assess all potential endpoints with the goal to adequately resuscitate, but NOT over-resuscitate patients, as over-resuscitation is associated with increased pulmonary complications, including the need for mechanical ventilation.

Resuscitation hemodynamic endpoints include adequate MAP without vasopressors, transthoracic echocardiography confirming inferior vena cava diameter and compressibility and cardiac function, normal mixed or central venous oxygen saturation, and other monitoring invasive or noninvasive devices.

POSTOPERATIVE TRANSFUSION STRATEGY

The vast majority of red blood cell (RBC) transfusions in the ICU are administered to treat anemia, not bleeding. Critically ill patients should generally adhere to a restrictive RBC transfusion strategy (ie, consider RBC transfusion when Hb < 7 g/dL). The use of RBC transfusion to treat anemia does not improve outcomes for the most of the critically ill patients, with the exception of those with acute-coronary syndrome. The decision to transfuse RBCs should not be based solely on the patient's hemoglobin level, but also on clinical factors, alternative treatments, and patient preferences.[37]

An updated systematic review with trial sequential analysis included 31 trials comparing restrictive versus liberal transfusion strategies in adults or children, with a total of 9813 randomized patients.[38] Restrictive transfusion strategies were associated with a decrease in the number of RBC units transfused and the number of patients transfused, whereas mortality, overall morbidity, and myocardial infarction were not affected. A review of seven randomized controlled trials (RCTs) involving 5558 high-risk patients confirmed noninferiority, safety, and a significant decrease in RBC transfusions in the restrictive group.[39]

POSTOPERATIVE INFECTION

Early infections are typically caused by contamination from the injury and may demand a surgical washout and the administration of antibiotics. The most common cause of late infections is hardware loosening, which results in micromotion at the fracture site and can lead to necrotic bone and nonunion.[40]

Sepsis is usually the result of infections of concomitant traumatic injuries. Sepsis is a medical emergency and is common in the surgical ICU,

particularly in abdominal trauma. Early recognition and knowledge of the current evidence-based sepsis definitions and guidelines is required. The 2021 Surviving Sepsis Campaign Guidelines uses the Sepsis-3 definitions, and a 1-h Sepsis Bundle.[41] The 1-h bundle is composed of the following five elements: measuring the lactate level, obtaining blood culture before administration of antibiotics, administering broad-spectrum antibiotics, beginning rapid administration of 30 mL/kg crystalloid fluid for hypotension or lactate ≥ 4 mmol/L, and administering vasopressors if the patient is hypotensive during or after fluid resuscitation to maintain mean arterial pressure (MAP) at ≥ 65 mm Hg within 1 h from sepsis recognition.

POSTOPERATIVE RESPIRATORY FAILURE

Panfacial trauma patients may have respiratory failure postoperatively and require ventilatory support. Not all patients with hypoxemia will require intubation and initiation of invasive mechanical ventilation. Noninvasive ventilation with noninvasive positive pressure ventilation (NIPPV) or heated high-flow nasal cannula (HFNC) can be used in an attempt to prevent the need for intubation in some patients with hypoxemia. HFNC is a novel method of oxygen therapy to deliver heated and humidified oxygen at a rate of up to 60 L/min. HFNC has a widely proven clinical efficacy, easier application, and better patient tolerance in critically ill patients.

However, panfacial trauma patients are typically unsuitable for NIPPV due to the fact that the interface may not fit properly, cause discomfort, and/or destabilize fractures or cause pneumocephalus. Similarly, patients with facial deformities may be unable to achieve an adequate interface fit, resulting in air leaks that reduce the effectiveness of NIPPV. Depending on the location of the deformity or the severity of the injury; however, some patients may tolerate NIPPV if the optimal interface is selected. For instance, a patient with only a soft tissue injury may be able to tolerate a nasal mask or HFNC whereas NIPPV should be avoided in patients with multiple facial fractures or those requiring zygomatic wiring.

LIBERATION FROM MECHANICAL VENTILATION

Liberation from mechanical ventilation involves three steps: readiness testing, weaning, and extubation. Patients who have been mechanically ventilated for more than 24 h should undergo a daily ventilator liberation protocol evaluation. Protocols for liberation include instructions for weaning readiness as well as subsequent weaning trials and extubation. Support for daily protocolized liberation strategies is derived from the observation that clinicians consistently underestimate the capacity of patients to breathe independently from the ventilator and from randomized trials showing the superiority of protocol use over standard care.[42] As a result, ICUs have incorporated liberation protocols into routine care for patients who are mechanically ventilated. To be considered ready for weaning, patients should have all of the following: improvement in the underlying cause of respiratory failure, adequate oxygenation, an arterial pH > 7.25, hemodynamic stability, and the ability to take spontaneous respirations. Other criteria, such as awake status and lack of fever, are often included. The rapid shallow breathing index (RSBI; the ratio of respiratory frequency to tidal volume (f/VT)) is the most widely used and extensively studied predictor. Patients who have an acceptable RSBI without contraindications are candidates for the extubation protocol. Extubation protocols typically include an ETT cuff leak test, as an indicator of airway edema and possible post-extubation stridor. However, a cuff leak does not need to be performed unless risk factors for post-extubation stridor from laryngeal edema are present (eg, prolonged period of intubation, traumatic intubation, large ETT, aspiration). In questionable cases of airway edema in panfacial trauma, video laryngobronchoscopy can be used to examine the tissues outside the ETT for excess edema, and the ETT can be removed over the videoscope to assess for stridor and immediate reinsertion and reintubation if required. Panfacial trauma patients who fail extubation and require reintubation may be candidates for tracheostomy if not readily reversible factors for airway edema or hypoventilation are present. Typically, a brief course of intravenous glucocorticoid therapy is also administered.

NUTRITION

During panfacial trauma reconstructive procedures, providing early enteral feeding access should be taken into consideration. Placement of an enteral feeding tube in patients with panfacial trauma may be difficult or impossible if delayed until the ICU phase of care, particularly if interdental wire immobilization is present. An initial assessment of nutrition is crucial for all critically ill surgical patients. The 2022 ASPEN/SCCM Guidelines suggest starting feeding between 12 and 25 kcal/kg in the first 7 to 10 days of ICU stay. These guidelines also found no significant difference in clinical outcomes between early exclusive parenteral nutrition (PN) and enteral nutrition (EN) during the first week of critical illness. As PN was not found to be superior to EN and no differences in harm were identified, either PN or EN is acceptable.[43]

CLINICS CARE POINTS

- Panfacial trauma is caused by high-energy trauma to two or more regions of the craniofacial skeleton, including the frontal bone, the midface, and the occlusal unit. Advanced Trauma Life Support Course priorities and a multidisciplinary approach may be required. Damage control techniques may be required in unstable patients.
- Preoperative planning may require careful consideration of airway management, including protocols for immediate or delayed endotracheal intubation, urgent surgical airway, planned tracheostomy, submental airway, or planned postoperative extubation.
- Postoperative critical care is frequently required using a semi-closed collaborative intensive care unit team model to manage issues such as respiratory failure, ongoing bleeding, shock, anemia and transfusion protocols, nutrition, and management of infection. Standardized communications, checklists, and team models reduce postoperative complications and errors.

DISCLOSURE

The authors have no significant disclosures for this content.

REFERENCES

1. Massenburg BB, Lang MS. Management of Panfacial Trauma: Sequencing and Pitfalls. Semin Plast Surg 2021;35(4):292–8.
2. Bruder EA, Ball IM, Ridi S, et al. Single induction dose of etomidate versus other induction agents for endotracheal intubation in critically ill patients. Cochrane Database Syst Rev 2015;1:CD010225.
3. To KB, Kamdar NS, Patil P, et al. Acute Care Surgery Model and Outcomes in Emergency General Surgery. J Am Coll Surg 2019;228(1):21–8. e7.
4. Vincent JL, De Backer D. Circulatory shock. N Engl J Med 2013;369(18):1726–34.
5. Kanji HD, McCallum J, Sirounis D, et al. Limited echocardiography-guided therapy in subacute shock is associated with change in management and improved outcomes. J Crit Care 2014;29(5):700–5.

6. Shokoohi H, Boniface KS, Pourmand A, et al. Bedside Ultrasound Reduces Diagnostic Uncertainty and Guides Resuscitation in Patients With Undifferentiated Hypotension. Crit Care Med 2015; 43(12):2562–9.

7. Ferrada P. Image-based resuscitation of the hypotensive patient with cardiac ultrasound: An evidence-based review. J Trauma Acute Care Surg 2016;80(3):511–8.

8. Meisinger QC, Brown MA, Dehqanzada ZA, et al. A 10-year restrospective evaluation of ultrasound in pregnant abdominal trauma patients. Emerg Radiol 2016;23(2):105–9.

9. Bentzer P, Griesdale DE, Boyd J, et al. Will This Hemodynamically Unstable Patient Respond to a Bolus of Intravenous Fluids? JAMA 2016;316(12):1298–309.

10. Waibel BH, Rotondo MF. Damage control for intra-abdominal sepsis. Surg Clin North Am 2012;92(2): 243–57, viii.

11. Fawaz R, Dagain A, Pons Y, et al. Head Face and Neck Surgeon Deployment in the New French Role 2: The Damage Control Resuscitation and Surgical Team. Mil Med 2022;usac329.

12. Curtis W, Horswell BB. Panfacial fractures: an approach to management. Oral Maxillofacial Surg Clin N Am 2013;25(4):649–60.

13. Shetty PM, Yadav SK, Upadya M. Submental intubation in patients with panfacial fractures: A prospective study. Indian J Anaesth 2011;55(3):299–304.

14. Henry SM. Advanced trauma life support course student manual. 10th edition. Chicago, IL, USA: American College of Surgeons; 2018.

15. Bawazeer M, Ahmed N, Izadi H, et al. Compliance with a Massive Transfusion Protocol (MTP) Impacts Patient Outcome. Injury 2014;46. https://doi.org/10.1016/j.injury.2014.09.020.

16. Poukkanen M, Wilkman E, Vaara ST, et al. Hemodynamic variables and progression of acute kidney injury in critically ill patients with severe sepsis: data from the prospective observational FINNAKI study. Crit Care 2013;17(6):R295.

17. Hylands M, Moller MH, Asfar P, et al. A systematic review of vasopressor blood pressure targets in critically ill adults with hypotension. Can J Anaesth 2017;64(7):703–15.

18. Rochwerg B, Hylands M, Møller MH, et al. CCCS-SSAI WlkiRecs clinical practice guideline: vasopressor blood pressure targets in critically ill adults with hypotension and vasopressor use in early traumatic shock. Intensive Care Med 2017;43(7):1062–4.

19. Jozwiak M, Monnet X, Teboul JL. Pressure Waveform Analysis. Anesth Analg 2018;126(6):1930–3.

20. Porter TR, Shillcutt SK, Adams MS, et al. Guidelines for the use of echocardiography as a monitor for therapeutic intervention in adults: a report from the American Society of Echocardiography. J Am Soc Echocardiogr 2015;28(1):40–56.

21. Reeves ST, Finley AC, Skubas NJ, et al. Special article: basic perioperative transesophageal echocardiography examination: a consensus statement of the American Society of Echocardiography and the Society of Cardiovascular Anesthesiologists. Anesth Analg 2013;117(3):543–58.

22. Maltais S, Costello WT, Billings FT, et al. Episodic monoplane transesophageal echocardiography impacts postoperative management of the cardiac surgery patient. J Cardiothorac Vasc Anesth 2013; 27(4):665–9.

23. Kirkpatrick AW, Sugrue M, McKee JL, et al. Update from the Abdominal Compartment Society (WSACS) on intra-abdominal hypertension and abdominal compartment syndrome: past, present, and future beyond Banff 2017. Anaesthesiol Intensive Ther 2017;49(2):83–7.

24. Choi WS, Samman N. Risks and benefits of deliberate hypotension in anaesthesia: a systematic review. Int J Oral Maxillofac Surg 2008;37(8):687–703.

25. Alonso N, de Oliveira Bastos E, Massenburg BB. Pseudoaneurysm of the internal maxillary artery: A case report of facial trauma and recurrent bleeding. Int J Surg Case Rep 2016;21:63–6.

26. Holcomb JB, Tilley BC, Baraniuk S, et al. Transfusion of plasma, platelets, and red blood cells in a 1:1:1 vs a 1:1:2 ratio and mortality in patients with severe trauma: the PROPPR randomized clinical trial. JAMA 2015;313(5):471–82.

27. Spinella PC, Gurney J, Yazer MH. Low titer group O whole blood for prehospital hemorrhagic shock: It is an offer we cannot refuse. Transfusion 2019;59(7): 2177–9.

28. Warren J, Fromm RE, Orr RA, et al. Guidelines for the inter- and intrahospital transport of critically ill patients. Crit Care Med 2004;32(1):256–62.

29. Deree J, Shenvi E, Fortlage D, et al. Patient factors and operating room resuscitation predict mortality in traumatic abdominal aortic injury: a 20-year analysis. J Vasc Surg 2007;45(3):493–7.

30. Watanabe H, Shimojo Y, Hira E, et al. First establishment of a new table-rotated-type hybrid emergency room system. Scand J Trauma Resusc Emerg Med 2018;26(1):80.

31. Nates JL, Nunnally M, Kleinpell R, et al. ICU Admission, Discharge, and Triage Guidelines: A Framework to Enhance Clinical Operations, Development of Institutional Policies, and Further Research. Crit Care Med 2016;44(8):1553–602.

32. Committee on Trauma, American College of Surgeons. Resources for optimal care of the injured patient (2014 standards). Chicago, IL, USA.: American College of Surgeons; 2014.

33. Pun BT, Balas MC, Barnes-Daly MA, et al. Caring for Critically Ill Patients with the ABCDEF Bundle: Results of the ICU Liberation Collaborative in Over 15,000 Adults. Crit Care Med 2019;47(1):3–14.

34. Ely EW. The ABCDEF Bundle: Science and Philosophy of How ICU Liberation Serves Patients and Families. Crit Care Med 2017;45(2):321–30.

35. Barnes-Daly MA, Phillips G, Ely EW. Improving Hospital Survival and Reducing Brain Dysfunction at Seven California Community Hospitals: Implementing PAD Guidelines Via the ABCDEF Bundle in 6,064 Patients. Crit Care Med 2017;45(2):171–8.

36. Pun BT, Balas MC, Barnes-Daly MA, et al. Caring for Critically Ill Patients with the ABCDEF Bundle: Results of the ICU Liberation Collaborative in Over 15,000 Adults. Crit Care Med 2019;47(1):3–14.

37. Napolitano LM, Kurek S, Luchette FA, et al. Clinical practice guideline: red blood cell transfusion in adult trauma and critical care. J Trauma 2009;67(6): 1439–42.

38. Holst LB, Petersen MW, Haase N, et al. Restrictive versus liberal transfusion strategy for red blood cell transfusion: systematic review of randomised trials with meta-analysis and trial sequential analysis. BMJ 2015;350:h1354.

39. Spahn DR, Spahn GH, Stein P. Evidence base for restrictive transfusion triggers in high-risk patients. Transfus Med Hemother 2015;42(2):110–4.

40. Ricketts S, Gill HS, Fialkov JA, et al. Facial Fractures. Plast Reconstr Surg 2016;137(2):424e–44e.

41. Evans L, Rhodes A, Alhazzani W, et al. Surviving sepsis campaign: international guidelines for management of sepsis and septic shock 2021. Intensive Care Med 2021;47(11):1181–247.

42. Girard TD, Alhazzani W, Kress JP, et al. An Official American Thoracic Society/American College of Chest Physicians Clinical Practice Guideline: Liberation from Mechanical Ventilation in Critically Ill Adults. Rehabilitation Protocols, Ventilator Liberation Protocols, and Cuff Leak Tests. Am J Respir Crit Care Med 2017;195(1):120–33.

43. Compher C, Bingham AL, McCall M, et al. Guidelines for the provision of nutrition support therapy in the adult critically ill patient: The American Society for Parenteral and Enteral Nutrition. JPEN (J Parenter Enteral Nutr) 2022;46(1):12–41.

Reducing Risk for Perioperative Anesthesia Complications

Sara Meitzen, MD[a],*, Jessica Black, MD[b]

KEYWORDS

- Anesthesia complications • Facial plastic surgery complications • Ambulatory surgery
- Office-based anesthesia

KEY POINTS

- Success within the outpatient setting relies on suitable patient selection, allowing for safe care and discharge to home following recovery.
- The crucial anesthetic components for facial plastic surgery include a still surgical field, perioperative normotension, smooth and rapid emergence, avoidance of postoperative nausea and vomiting, and fast-track discharge.
- Monitored anesthesia care provides numerous benefits when performed well and safely yet requires the scrupulous patient selection and provider vigilance.
- The lack of institutional backup within the outpatient setting hinders emergency management, highlighting the need for preparedness.

GENERAL CONSIDERATIONS

For some time, the growth of facial plastic surgery has swelled, pushing beyond hospital facilities and into ambulatory centers and offices.[1] Of the 560,000 cases performed in 2021,[2] approximately 80% were performed in outpatient settings.[3] These shifts have accommodated demand and contained cost while also introducing new challenges. Within these outpatient facilities, it is the facial cosmetic surgery patient seemingly suffering a higher proportion of significant anesthetic complications.[4] Meanwhile, the specialty is seeing more comorbidities as older patients increasingly pursue esthetic surgery.[3,5] Hearteningly, since the last review,[6] increasing awareness and improvements in patient selection may now be driving the more recent improvements.[1] Here, we highlight certain anesthetic considerations for optimal outcomes.

PRACTICE GUIDELINES FOR OUTPATIENT SURGERY

Steps to ensure standard quality of care in outpatient settings include the following:[5,7–9]

- Facility accreditation
- Surgical safety checklists
- Availability of emergency equipment, medications, and protocols, including transfers protocols to a prespecified facility
- Physical presence of personnel with training in advanced cardiac life support until all patients are discharged home

Cost-saving measures are quickly lost when unexpected complications occur. While acknowledging practical limitations, given the lack of institutional backup, the American Society of Anesthesiologists (ASA) believes that anesthesiologist participation in all office-based surgery is the

[a] UCSD Advanced Airway Management Program, Department of Anesthesiology, University of California San Diego School of Medicine, 200 West Arbor Drive, San Diego, CA 92103, USA; [b] Department of Anesthesiology, University of California San Diego School of Medicine, 200 West Arbor Drive, San Diego, CA 92103, USA
* Corresponding author.
E-mail address: Smeitzen@health.ucsd.edu

Facial Plast Surg Clin N Am 31 (2023) 325–332
https://doi.org/10.1016/j.fsc.2023.01.016
1064-7406/23/© 2023 Elsevier Inc. All rights reserved.

best means to achieve the safest anesthesia care.[10]

BASIC ANESTHESIA OBJECTIVES IN FACIAL PLASTIC SURGERY

- A quiet surgical field
- Hematoma prevention
- Timely return to wakefulness
- Prevention of postoperative nausea and vomiting (PONV)
- Efficient post-anesthesia care unit (PACU) discharge

Preoperative Considerations

Safety outcomes and cost containment rely on proper patient selection and prescreening, with referral out when preexisting conditions impart unjustifiable risk. The anesthesiologist should ensure that the planned procedure falls within the facility and practitioner's scope of practice and is of a duration and complexity predictive of PACU discharge to home.[1,6,10]

With caveats, these conditions are generally unfavorable for outpatient procedures.[1]

- Active infection
- Cardiovascular disease
- Coagulopathy
- Insulin-dependent diabetes
- Obesity
- Obstructive sleep apnea (OSA)
- Poorly controlled hypertension
- Thromboembolic disease

Special considerations for obstructive sleep apnea

OSA elevates perioperative risk,[10–15] including opioid-induced respiratory depression and post-discharge death,[11] and is frequent with obesity. Severe OSA is largely inappropriate for outpatient surgery. Significantly underdiagnosed, reliance on validated preoperative screening tools, such as STOP-BANG, is emphasized.[16] Specific perioperative care strategies remain controversial,[12,13,15] although careful consideration for outpatient surgery can be carefully considered if all the following apply.[14]

- Body mass index (BMI) < 50
- Optimized comorbid conditions
- Continuous positive airway pressure (CPAP) therapy compliance, with postoperative use not disallowed by nature of procedure, or planned nonopioid management of postoperative pain

Positioning and monitoring

Careful positioning avoids nerve traction and pressure point injuries. A rotated operating table can impair respiratory intervention during monitored anesthesia care (MAC) and general anesthesia (GA), emphasizing the routine use of alarm monitors and adherence to ASA standard monitoring guidelines.[10] A moderate or deep sedation anesthetic now calls for continuous observation of ventilation adequacy *in conjunction with* continuous capnography, unless disallowed by the nature of the procedure.[10]

Deep vein thrombosis (DVT) prophylaxis

The incidence of venous thromboembolism (VTE) in facial plastic surgery is low. Most patients require only noninvasive prophylaxis using sequential compression devices, reserving chemical prophylaxis for high-risk patients.[17]

Multimodal analgesia and enhanced recovery after surgery

Enhanced recovery after surgery (ERAS) protocols with multimodal analgesia improve patient satisfaction, facilitate early ambulation, and decrease postoperative pain while reducing undesirable side effects, such as drowsiness, PONV, and constipation within the cosmetic surgery patient population.[18] Single-dose dexamethasone is associated with shorter PACU stays and lower pain scores up to 48 h postoperatively with minimal side effects.[18,19] Gabapentinoids decrease pain scores and opioid consumption with no difference in PACU stay despite increases in sedation.[20] Other adjunct analgesics such as acetaminophen, ketamine, and alpha-2 agonists have also shown evidence of efficacy in the perioperative setting and should be used on an individual basis. A recent meta-analysis suggests that ibuprofen, a nonsteroidal anti-inflammatory drug (NSAID), provides equivalent pain control to narcotics in plastic surgery patients without an increased risk of bleeding.[21] Ketorolac also shows evidence of superior pain control without evidence of adverse events or significant increases in bleeding.[22]

Intraoperative Considerations

Local anesthetics

Local anesthesia is a common component of facial cosmetic surgery.[6] As such, it must be recognized that LAST can occur anytime LA is used,[23] even well below recommended dosing limits, sometimes with tragic consequences. Maximum dosage recommendations carry several limitations,[23] with numerous factors affecting toxicity thresholds. The large doses used with tumescent lidocaine techniques, up to 21 mg/kg in facial plastics,[24] seem relatively safe though risk mitigation and preparedness constitute responsible practice.[25]

Risk factors for LAST should prompt decreased dosing, and include impaired metabolic and clearance capabilities (**Table 1**) as well as[26]

- Hypoxia and acidosis
- Cardiac disease (especially ischemia, arrhythmias, conduction abnormalities, and low ejection fraction)
- Extremes of age
- Mitochondrial dysfunction (eg, carnitine deficiency)
- Low muscle mass
- Low BMI
- Female > male
- Renal disease

Whenever LA is used, an established LAST treatment plan should be available and implemented early at prodrome onset (**Box 1**), to halt deleterious progression. Treatment focuses on reversing toxicity with the administration of 20% lipid emulsion as well as airway management, cardiopulmonary resuscitation as needed, and seizure control to manage hypoxia and acidosis, as both exacerbate LAST.[26]

Any LA can induce LAST, and severe cases can rapidly deteriorate. Early intervention can prevent or delay progression. Increasingly, published cases describe the rapid reversal of LAST with lipid therapy, including cardiac arrest,[27] thus justifying the availability of lipid emulsion anywhere large LA doses are administered. Resuscitation can be prolonged, necessitating cardiopulmonary bypass in refractory cases and underscoring the importance of a preformulated transfer protocol.

Conscious sedation
MAC provides worthwhile benefits, removing malignant hyperthermia (MH) and PONV triggers while avoiding invasive airway instrumentation and tumultuous emergence phenomena.[6] PACU time is shortened, and overall efficiency and patient satisfaction are improved.[6,28] However, the risk of unrecognized hypoventilation with an unsecured airway is exacerbated in any head and neck procedure, which limits airway access and visibility.

Given these factors, it may come as no surprise that MAC is no less hazardous than GA.[4] 48% of MAC malpractice claims involve death or permanent brain damage,[29] with 21% citing respiratory depression as the mechanism of injury, and over a quarter composed of facial plastic surgery cases.[30] Substandard care was determined causative in half, whereas 34% were deemed preventable with better monitoring, vigilance, and audible alarms.[29]

Table 1
Local Anesthetic Systemic Toxicity (LAST) risk increases with impaired metabolic and clearance capabilities

Decreased LA Plasma Clearance	Decreased LA Metabolism

• Low cardiac output
• SIRS, sepsis, and shock
• Any decrease in hepatic blood flow
	• Hepatic disease
	• Cytochrome P450 3A4 inhibition
	  ○ Ritonavir and delavirdine
	  ○ Clarithromycin and erythromycin
	  ○ Sertraline and fluoxetine
	  ○ Verapamil and diltiazem
	  ○ Steroids

Listing of CYP3A4 inhibitors is not exhaustive.
Data from Ref.[25]

Given this, it seems a little stretch to assert that a monitoring mechanism of ventilation is mandatory for any MAC case, and especially so when direct airway visualization is impaired by the anesthesia provider. All monitors will inevitably have their limitations,[30] yet deliberate omission of ventilatory monitoring with continuous capnography deserves serious consideration.

Fire risk during monitored anesthesia care
Absent attentive care, the fire triad (oxidizer, fuel, and heat source) is readily manifested in facial plastic surgery. Total MAC claims involving fires on-the-patient have increased to 31%,[31] with 64% of these involving plastic surgery procedures on the face.[31]

Risk mitigation calls for oxygen concentrations below 30% during open oxygen delivery near a heat source,[32] and endotracheal tube (ETT) or LMA utilization for procedures above the T7 dermatome anticipated to require higher oxygen

Box 1
LAST presenting signs and symptoms

- Vertigo
- Tinnitus
- Metallic taste
- Perioral numbness
- Tachycardia
- Hypertension

LAST early signs and symptoms.
Data from Ref.[26]

supplementation.[33] Challenging conventional practice beliefs, perifacial oxygen concentrations beyond 60% are achieved with low flow nasal cannula rates ($\leq$3 L/min) in sedated patients.[34] Oxygen delivery and capnography measurement with tubing advanced through an in situ nasal airway have been described, achieving local oxygen levels less than 30%.[34] The ASA delineates other prevention strategies,[10] and the authors also recommend local oxygen concentration measurement when feasible. Absent this capability, unsafe oxygen supplementation should be discontinued for 1 to 3 min before energy use.[10]

Intravenous anesthetics for monitored anesthesia care

A successful MAC requires adequate local anesthesia. Patient discomfort or movement with initial infiltration can be prevented by bolus of ultra-short-acting opioids, such as alfentanil (7 to 10 mcg/kg), briefly "stunning" the patient and with low likelihood of apnea.[6] Otherwise, anxiolysis with midazolam (1 to 3 mg IV) and hypnosis with propofol infusion (loading dose of 0.5 to 1 mg/kg, then 25 to 100 mcg/kg/min) is common practice.

Opioid-sparing approaches can use dexmedetomidine or ketamine to lessen the risk of ventilatory depression. Dexmedetomidine (loading dose of 0.5 to 1 mcg/kg over 10 min, then 0.2 to 1.0 mcg/kg/h) has a delayed onset of 15 min and peak effect within 1 h, somewhat hampering ease of titration.[6]

Pretreatment with propofol or midazolam before ketamine (loading dose of 0.5 mcg/kg then 3 to 10 mcg/kg/min),[6] avoids unpleasant hallucinations, whereas glycopyrrolate lessens secretions. Ketamine's dissociative amnestic effect can render a deep sedative state in an awake appearing patient, masking the potential for airway compromise.[6,10]

Minimal postoperative pain, characterizing most facial plastic procedures, is suited to ultra-short-acting opioids, which facilitate fast-track recovery.[35] Remifentanil (loading dose 1 to 2 mcg/kg then 0.05 to 0.08 mcg/kg/min) rapidly produces a short-acting, easily titratable, and dense analgesia, rendering it ideal in the outpatient facial plastics setting.[6] Fentanyl (0.5 to 1 mcg/kg) can be reserved and dosed at the conclusion of the surgery, or omitted entirely, when appropriate.

Polypharmacy with synergistic agents risks apnea and airway obstruction, warranting careful attention and close monitoring.[10,30] Given a decreased volume of distribution as well as limited physiologic reserves and clearance capabilities, the elderly are more prone to develop circulatory and respiratory compromise after sedation.[30] Doses should be decreased accordingly.[6]

General anesthesia

Still a common preference among patients and practitioners, a GA provides a reliable airway and stationery surgical field.

Airway management: endotracheal tube versus laryngeal mask airway (LMA) When feasible, LMA utilization avoids neuromuscular blockade and reversal, reduces operating time, and facilitates a quick and smooth emergence. Careful assessment of seal adequacy and leak pressure, gastric auscultation to confirm the absence of insufflation, and spontaneous ventilation or minimization of driving pressures constitute safe practice.[6]

Anesthetic maintenance An inhalational agent allows ease of titration and continuous measurement of mean alveolar concentration. Sevoflurane shows less PONV and postoperative drowsiness than isoflurane with less coughing and postoperative agitation than desflurane.[36] Nitrous oxide has analgesic properties and allows for rapid recovery, though increased exposure (>1 h) increases PONV risk.[37]

Total intravenous anesthesia (TIVA) with propofol decreases PONV risk[36,37] and pain scores, mitigates the inflammatory stress response to surgery, and consistently rates higher in quality of recovery studies.[38] TIVA also improves discharge times,[38] perioperative hemodynamics,[6] and intraoperative blood loss.[39]

Highlighted safeguards against awareness of TIVA include the following:[40]

- Standardized drug concentrations
- Avoidance of mixing agents
- Infusion lines fitted with Luer-locks and anti-reflux valves with dead space minimized
- Intravenous cannula visibility, whenever possible
- Utilization of processed electroencephalogram with paralysis
- A loading dose to better ensure expected plasma concentrations when initiating or increasing infusion rates

Remifentanil is common in the ambulatory setting and provides rapid, titratable hemodynamic and pain control[40] and decreases PACU times.[6] However, dexmedetomidine avoids hyperalgesia and reduces postoperative pain, PONV, shivering, and hypotension.[37,41,42] A slow time to effect and variable context-sensitive half time may hamper a full embrace within the ambulatory setting until familiarity with the drug is optimized.[41]

When neuromuscular blockade is required, reversal with sugammadex leads to earlier tracheal extubation and reduces the incidence of postoperative residual muscle paralysis.[35]

Intraoperative hematoma prevention

Elevated blood pressure is associated with an increased incidence of hematoma[43] and traditionally, purposeful induction of intraoperative hypotension sought to decrease such risk.[6]

Controlled hypotension may mask inadequate hemostasis, and newer reports indicate that intraoperative normotension improves hematoma rates. Newer practice emphasizes the preoperative treatment of chronic hypertension, avoidance of intraoperative systolic blood pressure (SBP) less than 100 mm Hg, and postoperative treatment of SBP greater than 139 mm Hg.[44] Specific perioperative medical management regimens have been reported,[6,43] though comparative studies are absent in the literature. Currently, it seems that no specific antihypertensive medication has a correlative effect on hematoma rate in facelifts.[44]

In addition, new evidence supports TXA administration for improving hemostasis and reducing operative time in facial plastic procedures. Further study may help delineate optimal dosing and administration routes.[45]

Emergence

For patients with underlying hypertension, the longer-acting labetalol can circumvent postoperative hypertension. Sincere consideration to potential laryngospasm following a deep extubation, and necessitating undesirable airway manipulation around delicate surgical tissue, is a must. Extubation of a fully awake patient with intact protective airway reflexes seeks to avoid such intervention.

A smooth emergence Peri-extubation remifentanil infusion (0.05 to 0.06 mcg/kg/min)[6,46] provides hemodynamic stability, suppresses cough response, and avoids emergence agitation.[47] Dexmedetomidine (single dose ranging from 0.5 to 1.0 mcg/kg over 10 min or continuous infusion 0.1 to 1.2 mcg/kg/h) shows numerous benefits, including decreased coughing, agitation, hypertension, tachycardia, shivering, pain, and PONV without a delay in extubation,[42,47,48] prolongation of PACU stay,[42] or residual sedation or bradycardia in the PACU.[42]

Less stimulating than an ETT, an LMA offers a smoother and more efficient emergence profile.[6,49] The Bailey maneuver is a method of inserting an LMA behind a patient's existing ETT under a deep plane of anesthesia, just before emergence, thus aiding in a smooth emergence by replacing ETT for LMA.[49]

Malignant hyperthermia

A patient with known or suspected susceptibility can undergo outpatient surgery with a non-triggering anesthetic following proper preparation of the anesthesia machine. This entails flushing the machine, removing vaporizers, replacement of all disposables, and the placement of charcoal filters.[50]

Exposing a susceptible patient to succinylcholine or volatile anesthetics can trigger MH. Outcome hinges on early initiation of intravenous dantrolene before transfer, as every 30-min delay doubles the risk for serious complications,[51–53] thus justifying the financial burden of stocking dantrolene. Up to 10 mg/kg may be necessary for initial stabilization, translating to 700 mg for the average size male,[51,52] or approximately three 250 mg vials of Ryanodex (dantrolene sodium). The cost is half that of former formulations and reconstitution far simpler (Box 2).

Postoperative Considerations

Postoperative nausea and vomiting

PONV is distressing for the patient and prolongs PACU stays, whereas forceful emesis elevates hematoma risk. Risk factors for PONV include the following:[37]

- Female sex
- Volatile anesthesia, dose-dependent
- Nitrous oxide exposure > 1 h
- General versus regional anesthesia
- History of PONV or motion sickness
- Nonsmoking
- Long procedures
- Age < 50
- Postoperative opioids, dose-dependent

Post-discharge nausea vomiting

Affecting 17% of ambulatory surgery patients, PDNV is three times more likely with[37]

- Females
- Age < 50
- PACU opioids
- PONV in the PACU
- PDNV history

Box 2
Key indicators of stability signaling transfer to receiving hospital can proceed

- Intravenous (IV) dantrolene administration has begun
- End-tidal C02 is declining or normal
- Heart rate is stable or decreasing with no signs of life-threatening dysrhythmias
- Temperature is declining
- If present, generalized muscular rigidity is resolving

Data from Ref.[52]

Multiagent prophylaxis is commonly justified in the presence of just a single risk factor[37] with additional agents for high-risk patients (eg, aprepitant, scopolamine). Palonosetron shows improved efficacy over ondansetron with a longer half-life.[37] Amisulpride, a new dopamine receptor antagonist, may fill the gap created with the black box warning attached to droperidol.[54]

Other prevention strategies include the following:[37]

- Multimodal analgesia and opioid minimization
- Propofol infusion as the primary anesthetic (antiemetic effect limited to immediate postoperative period 53)
- Perioperative dexmedetomidine
- Volatile avoidance
- Adequate hydration

Antiemetic treatment with prophylaxis failure

Within a 6-h window, rescue medications should be of a different class from previously administered medications. Combination therapy may be more effective for treating established PONV.[37]

Obstructive sleep apnea

Observation of adequate respiratory function on room air and in an unstimulated environment, preferably while asleep, signals potential suitability for discharge.[10] OSA coincides with longer PACU stays and may stress limited resources in the outpatient setting.

Women taking oral contraceptives

Sugammadex and aprepitant decrease hormonal contraceptive efficacy for 7 and 28 days, respectively, necessitating alternative, nonhormonal contraceptives.[55,56] Written and verbal instructions should be provided before discharge.

SUMMARY

Demand within the facial plastic specialties continues to grow, and as patient age shifts up and operating sites shift out to ambulatory settings, thoughtful anesthetic care is pivotal to safety. Appropriate regulation, care team and facility preparation, careful patient selection, and attentive anesthetic care will improve patient and surgical outcomes.

CLINICS CARE POINTS

- Facility accreditation
- Safety checklists and emergency protocols
- Proper patient selection
- Aging patients require consideration

- Deliberate exclusion of continuous capnography, a standard means of ventilatory monitoring via measurement of expired carbon dioxide, during monitored anesthesia care (MAC) warrants sincere consideration of risks
- Multimodal analgesia and opioid reduction
- Special attention to fire risk during MAC cases
- Large local anesthetic (LA) dosing regimens should require lipid emulsion availability
- LAST risk factors should prompt decreased LA dosing
- Dantrolene availability wherever triggering anesthetics are administered
- Preference for total intravenous anesthesia while taking awareness preventative measures
- Smooth emergence strategies, including LMA utilization and peri-extubation anesthetic infusion
- Intraoperative normotension and tranexamic acid (TXA) for hematoma prevention
- Multimodal postoperative nausea and vomiting and post-discharge nausea vomiting prevention
- Alternative, nonhormonal contraceptive counseling following aprepitant or sugammadex in females
- Fast-tracking patient discharge

DISCLOSURE

The authors have nothing to disclose.

REFERENCES

1. Seligson E, Beutler SS, Urman RD. Office-based anesthesia: an update on safety and outcomes (2017-2019). Curr Opin Anaesthesiol 2019;32(6): 756–61.
2. Aesthetic Plastic Surgery National Databank Statistics. 2021. Available at: http://www.surgery.org/media/statistics. Accessed August 28, 2022.
3. American Society of Plastic Surgeons. Plastic surgery statistics report. 2020. 2020 Plastic Surgery Statistics Report. Available at: https://www.plasticsurgery.org/news/plastic-surgery-statistics. Accessed August 29, 2022.
4. Starling J 3rd, Thosani MK, Coldiron BM. Determining the safety of office-based surgery: what 10 years of Florida data and 6 years of Alabama data reveal. Dermatol Surg 2012;38(2):171–7.
5. Osman BM, Shapiro FE. Safe anesthesia for office-based plastic surgery: Proceedings from the PRS

Korea 2018 meeting in Seoul, Korea. Arch Plast Surg 2019;46(3):189–97.

6. Nekhendzy V, Ramaiah VK. Prevention of perioperative and anesthesia-related complications in facial cosmetic surgery. Facial Plast Surg Clin North Am 2013;21(4):559–77.

7. Rosenberg NM, Urman RD, Gallagher S, et al. Effect of an office-based surgical safety system on patient outcomes. Eplasty 2012;12:e59.

8. Shapiro FE, Punwani N, Rosenberg NM, et al. Office-based anesthesia: safety and outcomes. Anesth Analg 2014;119(2):276–85.

9. Gupta V, Parikh R, Nguyen L, et al. Is Office-Based Surgery Safe? Comparing Outcomes of 183,914 Aesthetic Surgical Procedures Across Different Types of Accredited Facilities. Aesthet Surg J 2017;37(2):226–35.

10. American Society of Anesthesiologists: Guidelines, Statements, Clinical Resources. Guidelines, Statements, Clinical Resources (asahq.org). Available at: https://www.asahq.org/standards-and-guidelines. Accessed August 26, 2022.

11. Weinger M, Lee L. No patient shall be harmed by opioid-induced respiratory depression. Anesth Patient Saf FoundNewslett 2011;26:21–8.

12. Rothfield KP. Read the fine print: updated sleep apnea guidelines and risk stratification. Anesthesiology 2014;121(3):665–6.

13. Grewal G, Joshi GP. Obesity and Obstructive Sleep Apnea in the Ambulatory Patient. Anesthesiol Clin 2019;37(2):215–24.

14. Joshi GP, Ankichetty SP, Gan TJ, et al. Society for Ambulatory Anesthesia consensus statement on preoperative selection of adult patients with obstructive sleep apnea scheduled for ambulatory surgery. Anesth Analg 2012;115(5):1060–8.

15. Rodriguez LV. Anesthesia for Ambulatory and Office-Based Ear, Nose, and Throat Surgery. Otolaryngol Clin North Am 2019;52(6):1157–67.

16. Chung F, Abdullah HR, Liao P. STOP-Bang Questionnaire: A Practical Approach to Screen for Obstructive Sleep Apnea. Chest 2016;149(3):631–8.

17. Pannucci CJ. The Vast Majority of Aesthetic Surgery Patients are at Low Risk for Venous Thromboembolism and Do Not Require Chemical Prophylaxis. Aesthet Surg J 2017;37(9):NP109–10.

18. Bartlett EL, Zavlin D, Friedman JD, et al. Enhanced Recovery After Surgery: The Plastic Surgery Paradigm Shift. Aesthet Surg J 2018;38(6):676–85.

19. Waldron NH, Jones CA, Gan TJ, et al. Impact of perioperative dexamethasone on postoperative analgesia and side-effects: systematic review and meta-analysis. Br J Anaesth 2013;110(2):191–200.

20. Mishriky BM, Waldron NH, Habib AS. Impact of pregabalin on acute and persistent postoperative pain: a systematic review and meta-analysis. Br J Anaesth 2015;114(1):10–31.

21. Kelley BP, Bennett KG, Chung KC, et al. Ibuprofen May Not Increase Bleeding Risk in Plastic Surgery: A Systematic Review and Meta-Analysis. Plast Reconstr Surg 2016;137(4):1309–16.

22. Gobble RM, Hoang HLT, Kachniarz B, et al. Ketorolac does not increase perioperative bleeding: a meta-analysis of randomized controlled trials. Plast Reconstr Surg 2014;133(3):741–55.

23. Weinberg G. Local Anesthetic Systemic Toxicity and Liposuction: Looking Back, Looking Forward. Anesth Analg 2016;122(5):1250–2.

24. Ramon Y, Barak Y, Ullmann Y, et al. Pharmacokinetics of high-dose diluted lidocaine in local anesthesia for facelift procedures. Ther Drug Monit 2007;29(5):644–7.

25. Klein JA, Kassarjdian N. Lidocaine toxicity with tumescent liposuction. A case report of probable drug interactions. Dermatol Surg 1997;23(12):1169–74.

26. Weinberg G, Rupnik B, Aggarwal N, et al. Local anesthetic systemic toxicity (LAST) revisited: a paradigm in evolution. APSF Newsletter 2020;35:1–32.

27. Weinberg GL, Riou B. Lipid Emulsion Infusion: Resuscitation for Local Anesthetic and Other Drug Overdose. Anesthesiology 2012;117(1):180–7.

28. Jumaily JS, Jumaily M, Donnelly T, et al. Quality of recovery and safety of deep intravenous sedation compared to general anesthesia in facial plastic surgery: A prospective cohort study. Am J Otolaryngol 2022;43(2):103352.

29. Metzner J, Posner KL, Lam MS, et al. Closed claims' analysis. Best Pract Res Clin Anaesthesiol 2011;25(2):263–76.

30. Bhananker SM, Posner KL, Cheney FW, et al. Injury and liability associated with monitored anesthesia care: a closed claims analysis. Anesthesiology 2006;104(2):228–34.

31. Jones TS, Black IH, Robinson TN, et al. Operating Room Fires. Anesthesiology 2019;130(3):492–501.

32. Lampotang S, Gravenstein N, Paulus DA, et al. Reducing the incidence of surgical fires: supplying nasal cannulae with sub-100% O_2 gas mixtures from anesthesia machines. Anesth Analg 2005;101(5):1407–12.

33. Emergency Care Research Institute. Surgical Fire Prevention. Available at: https://www.ecri.org/Accident_Investigation/Pages/SurgicalFire-Prevention.aspx. Accessed May 3, 2018.

34. Meneghetti SC, Morgan MM, Fritz J, et al. Operating room fires: optimizing safety. Plast Reconstr Surg 2007;120(6):1701–8.

35. White PF, Eng M. Fast-track anesthetic techniques for ambulatory surgery. Curr Opin Anaesthesiol 2007;20(6):545–57.

36. Gupta A, Stierer T, Zuckerman R, et al. Comparison of recovery profile after ambulatory anesthesia with

propofol, isoflurane, sevoflurane and desflurane: a systematic review. Anesth Analg 2004;98(3):632–41.

37. Gan TJ, Belani KG, Bergese S, et al. Fourth consensus guidelines for the management of post-operative nausea and vomiting. Anesth Analg 2020;131(2):411–48 [published correction appears in Anesth Analg. 2020 Nov;131(5):e241].

38. McIlroy EI, Leslie K. Total intravenous anaesthesia in ambulatory care. Curr Opin Anaesthesiol 2019; 32(6):703–7.

39. Lu VM, Phan K, Oh LJ. Total intravenous versus inhalational anesthesia in endoscopic sinus surgery: A meta-analysis. Laryngoscope 2020;130(3):575–83.

40. Nimmo AF, Absalom AR, Bagshaw O, et al. Guidelines for the safe practice of total intravenous anaesthesia (TIVA): Joint Guidelines from the Association of Anaesthetists and the Society for Intravenous Anaesthesia. Anaesthesia 2019;74(2):211–24.

41. Grape S, Kirkham KR, Frauenknecht J, et al. Intraoperative analgesia with remifentanil vs. dexmedetomidine: a systematic review and meta-analysis with trial sequential analysis. Anaesthesia 2019; 74(6):793–800.

42. Sin JCK, Tabah A, MJJ Campher, et al. The effect of dexmedetomidine on postanesthesia care unit discharge and recovery: a systematic review and meta-analysis. Anesth Analg 2022;134(6):1229–44.

43. Ramanadham SR, Costa CR, Narasimhan K, et al. Refining the anesthesia management of the face-lift patient: lessons learned from 1089 consecutive face lifts. Plast Reconstr Surg 2015;135(3):723–30.

44. Trussler AP, Hatef DA, Rohrich RJ. Management of hypertension in the facelift patient: results of a national consensus survey. Aesthet Surg J 2011; 31(5):493–500.

45. Tiourin E, Barton N, Janis JE. Methods for Minimizing Bleeding in Facelift Surgery: An Evidence-based Review. Plast Reconstr Surg Glob Open 2021;9(8):e3765.

46. Lee JH, Choi SH, Choi YS, et al. Does the type of anesthetic agent affect remifentanil effect-site concentration for preventing endotracheal tube-induced cough during anesthetic emergence? Comparison

of propofol, sevoflurane, and desflurane. J Clin Anesth 2014;26(6):466–74.

47. Polat R, Peker K, Baran I, et al. Comparison between dexmedetomidine and remifentanil infusion in emergence agitation during recovery after nasal surgery: A randomized double-blind trial. Anaesthesist 2015; 64(10):740–6.

48. Aouad MT, Zeeni C, Al Nawwar R, et al. Dexmedetomidine for improved quality of emergence from general anesthesia: a dose-finding study. Anesth Analg 2019;129(6):1504–11.

49. Nair I, Bailey PM. Review of uses of the laryngeal mask in ENT anaesthesia. Anaesthesia 1995; 50(10):898–900.

50. Bilmen JG, Hopkins PM. The use of charcoal filters in malignant hyperthermia: have they found their place? Anaesthesia 2019;74(1):13–6.

51. Larach MG, Gronert GA, Allen GC, et al. Clinical presentation, treatment, and complications of malignant hyperthermia in North America from 1987 to 2006. Anesth Analg 2010;110(2):498–507.

52. Larach MG, Dirksen SJ, Belani KG, et al. Special article: Creation of a guide for the transfer of care of the malignant hyperthermia patient from ambulatory surgery centers to receiving hospital facilities. Anesth Analg 2012;114(1):94–100.

53. Kumar G, Stendall C, Mistry R, et al. A comparison of total intravenous anaesthesia using propofol with sevoflurane or desflurane in ambulatory surgery: systematic review and meta-analysis. Anaesthesia 2014;69(10):1138–50.

54. Smyla N, Koch T, Eberhart LH, et al. An overview of intravenous amisulpride as a new therapeutic option for the prophylaxis and treatment of postoperative nausea and vomiting. Expert Opin Pharmacother 2020;21(5):517–22.

55. U.S. Food and Drug Administration. 207865lbl.pdf (fda.gov). Available at: https://www.fda.gov. Accessed September 1, 2022.

56. Lazorwitz A, Dindinger E, Aguirre N, et al. Pre- and post-operative counseling for women on hormonal contraceptives receiving sugammadex at an academic hospital. J Anesth 2020;34(2):294–7.

Reducing Legal Risks and Social Media Issues for Cosmetic Surgery

Tyler Marion, MD, MBA[1], Tyler Werbel, MD, MS[1], Abel Torres, MD, JD, MBA*

KEYWORDS

• Social media • Risk management • Informed consent • Medical malpractice • Adverse events

KEY POINTS

• Most physicians can expect to have at least one malpractice lawsuit in their career.
• Appropriate informed consent and accurate documentation in the medical records helps protect physicians from malpractice lawsuits and improves patient care.
• Implementing checklists helps prevent medical errors and root cause analysis can help identify a problem and prevent the same error from occurring again.
• Good communication helps prevent adverse events and is imperative when dealing with patients after an adverse event.
• When using a patient's photo for social media, informed consent must include the details of the photo's use, who will see the photo, and the risk that complete anonymity may be unachievable.

INTRODUCTION

Most physicians can expect to be sued at least once during their career by age 65, approaching 99% in high-risk specialties like plastic surgery.[1] Regardless of the outcome, these litigations have a significant impact on physicians, both professionally and emotionally. Does this mean one should be concerned to the point of avoiding cosmetic procedures? Not necessarily. In the authors' opinion, it means physicians performing cosmetic procedures should be aware of the risk of malpractice and they should take steps to minimize adverse events and interactions that can increase the likelihood of a lawsuit. The following sections can help address key areas where physicians are likely to run into problems and will discuss actions one can take to reduce legal risk.

LEGAL RISKS

Litigation with cosmetic procedures can be the result of a variety of events ranging from complications/adverse events or inadequate informed consent. One commonly reported reason for unhappiness by the cosmetic patient is an unfavorable result, which can ultimately drive the desire for a malpractice suit.[2] Halepas and colleagues[2] describe essentially three ways in which a doctor can be at risk for malpractice by failing to adhere to the standard of care in: (1) performing an improper procedure, (2) improper execution of a procedure, and (3) failing to provide sufficient information to a patient negating the informed consent.

Consent

When informed consent is not obtained or is obtained improperly, negligence can be alleged. Negligence is defined as the failure to meet a standard of behavior established to protect people against unreasonable risk. Medical negligence is a type of professional negligence and requires four things. There needs to be a duty established by the physician, a breach of that duty by that

Department of Dermatology, University of Florida College of Medicine, Gainesville, FL, USA
[1] These authors contributed equally to this work.
* Corresponding author. Department of Dermatology, University of Florida College of Medicine, 4037 Northwest 86 Terrace, 4th Floor, Gainesville, FL 32606.
E-mail address: abeltorres@dermatology.med.ufl.edu

Facial Plast Surg Clin N Am 31 (2023) 333–340
https://doi.org/10.1016/j.fsc.2023.01.017

physician, a closely linked connection between the conduct and resulting injury, and a true injury.[3] Professional negligence is judged by peers or a judge but with guidance from a professional as to what that duty, also known as the standard of care, is (expert testimony).

Consent can be either implied or expressed. Implied consent is when the conduct of the patient indicates awareness and understanding of the planned action with the patient having the opportunity to withdraw.[4] The gray area with implied consent is that it can be difficult for a physician to prove proper consent was given. Ordinarily, except in emergency situations, physicians should not rely on implied consent. The act of laying hands on the patient to examine them is a type of implied consent but it is prudent to ask the patient for permission before performing the examination, especially in cases where sensitive areas may be involved. It is wise to document that consent was obtained.

Express consent is obtained either orally or written. Oral consent can become problematic as it can be difficult to prove if witnesses to the consent are not available. Written express consent provides more tangible proof and may provide the most protection. It is important to distinguish simple consent from informed consent. In simple consent, a medical patient is agreeing to be touched in some way either physically or via medications, etc. Failure to obtain this consent can result in an allegation of assault, which is fear of a harmful or offensive touching, or an allegation of battery, which is an actual harmful or offensive touching. An assault or battery can leave the physician liable for civil or criminal penalties, for which the physician would not be protected by malpractice insurance. It is important to understand that the fear of and actual perception of a harmful or offensive touching is ordinarily based on a reasonable person's standard, but if the physician knows or has reason to know that an individual has heightened, even if unreasonable, perceptions, the physician can be liable. It is not rare when dealing with cosmetic patients that perceptions can be distorted, and thus physicians performing cosmetic procedures should be especially aware of the importance of proper simple consent as well as informed consent.

As noted above, obtaining simple consent may prevent a claim of a battery or assault, but the physician still needs to obtain informed consent for treatment or procedures.[5] Informed consent consists of helping a patient to make an informed decision before the treatment/procedure by providing adequate information, including a discussion of the risks, benefits, and alternatives, so they can decide on the treatment or procedure that is in their best interest.[6]

A legitimate concern that can arise is whether one is disclosing enough information to adequately obtain informed consent. There are two standards that the courts ordinarily use as a guide. The first is the Professional Standard which is, if a physician provides information that other physicians would disclose in a same or similar circumstances.[7] The second standard is the Legal Standard, which implies that a physician should provide information that a reasonable person would consider important when deciding to undergo a treatment or procedure.[8]

Informed consent is especially important with cosmetic procedures, when you consider that these are elective procedures that a patient doesn't have a medical necessity to undergo. The courts have ruled that it is imperative to explain the benefit of the given procedure, reasonable alternatives, and the realistic results the patient should expect. For example, are the results permanent or are the results temporary as is the case with botulinum toxin. When disclosing the risks of performing the procedure a physician performing soft-tissue filler in the glabellar region should ordinarily disclose to the patient that there is a risk of permanent blindness. If the physician accidently injects into a branch of the facial artery with anastomosis to branches of the ophthalmologic artery leading to blindness, the physician may be found liable if they did not provide information regarding the possibility of a serious risks with the procedure.

Although supporting staff can help obtain consent, the responsibility ultimately falls upon the physician. Therefore, when staff is assisting, it is prudent for the physician to properly train the staff and ask patients to either recount what they understood or ask the patients questions to ascertain their understanding and document it.

Medical Records

In addition to helping physicians in the management of their patients, the medical record becomes important if a physician is faced with a malpractice lawsuit, as it often serves as the only credible evidence for malpractice defense.[9] Hence, physicians need to maintain accurate and complete documentation. It is also important to be mindful when modifying the record as it can negatively impact the credibility of the physician and the credibility of the record.[10] Therefore, if a change needs to be made (eg, an important medication was not documented in the history), we suggest including a signature and date next to the updated change to make it clear when the change was done. Fortunately, electronic medical records for the most part are able to record these changes automatically. Regardless, physicians should still be mindful of any changes as they can still undermine credibility in the record. Thus, a nice rule of thumb is to make changes because they are likely to benefit patient care.

The record should include all important discussions with the patient or related third parties. Informed consents, diagnostic considerations, plan of care, and any patient details specific to that encounter should be documented. In the case of cosmetic procedures, it is often prudent to take before and after photos to include in the medical record. *As we know, symmetry is an important component of beauty, and pre-existing asymmetry is very common and not immediately perceived by many patients. Post-surgery, a patient is now focused on the results and may mistakenly think that any asymmetry was caused by the procedure. Photographs can help mitigate this problem.* Similarly, when adverse events or complications do happen, they should be documented objectively, avoiding opinionated statements or premature conclusions.[10]

RISK MANAGEMENT TECHNIQUES
Checklists

Checklists have been increasingly advocated as a method to prevent medical errors, thus helping patients and protecting physicians.[11] Checklists can help ensure that tasks are completed in proper order to avoid overlooking key steps. Checklists can be incorporated into different aspects of every day practice including the process of obtaining informed consents, medical records, and implementing surgical safety measures. Their effectiveness is abundantly supported in the medical literature. For instance, Haynes and colleagues[11] found surgical safety checklists were associated with reductions in mortality rates and complications in patients undergoing noncardiac surgery.

Root Cause Analysis

Unfortunately, mistakes and adverse events are inevitable in an imperfect world. When an error does occur, responding promptly and creating systems to avoid repeated mistakes is imperative. Root cause analysis (RCA) is a problem-solving technique used to find the root cause of problems when they occur to prevent them from recurring. Briefly, the events of a given problem are analyzed considering the unique circumstance of the case. Once the mistake is identified, the physician can then develop a system to prevent this same error

from happening again in the future. When a medical error does occur, self-evaluation is encouraged in the form of morbidity and mortality peer review activities as these activities are often protected from legal discovery. It should be mentioned that RCAs may be federally protected from legal discovery under the 2005 Patient Safety and Quality Improvement Act (PSQIA), as an RCA is classified as a patient safety work product. Of note, the privilege and confidentiality protections ordinarily only apply to an RCA that is developed by providers for reporting to a federally listed patient safety organization (PSO) or is developed by a PSO.[12]

Communication

Communication is a skill set we as physicians should master to best treat our patients. This skill set becomes even more critical when managing adverse events because how a situation is handled can commonly determine whether the adverse event results in litigation. We propose the following mnemonic to enhance communication when dealing with an adverse event. We call it *the three Cs of communication:*

Compassion: Patients want to know their doctor cares. Showing compassion and being empathetic can help develop trust and increase the likelihood of patients listening to what the physician has to say.

Clarification: Clarifying the patient's concern and possible misperceptions can help the physician understand what may have happened and how to proceed.

Coordinate: Coordinating a course of action with the patient and their support group can help both the physician and patient and avoid unwanted interventions by others.

Unique Considerations for the Cosmetic Patient

In addition to the techniques and strategies that should be used in ordinary patient care, there are unique factors to consider when dealing with the facial plastic or cosmetic patient. First, the relationship between the facial plastic surgeon and patient differs from the traditional physician-patient relationship, as cosmetic procedures are primarily elective.[13] Although cosmetic improvement can also lead to patient well-being, satisfaction often depends on the opinion of the patient. The inherent issue with subjective results is that the patient's expectations can dictate how the outcome is perceived.

Managing patient expectations is thus, a very important aspect when performing cosmetic/aesthetic surgeries. If the patient has unrealistic expectations from the beginning, they are unlikely to be satisfied with the results. Given the often rewarding financial compensation for cosmetic procedures, physicians face a conflict of interest to provide realistic expectations that can risk the patients not moving forward with the procedures. Yet, honest conversations lead to greater trust and satisfaction for all parties. It's the ethical approach and in turn reduces the risk of malpractice.

Surgeons are trained extensively on how to operate, but the concept of when not to operate is just as important and sometimes not given the same importance.[14] It is the physician's duty to listen to the patient and discern the desired outcome. The next step for the physician is to determine if the desired outcome can be achieved by the cosmetic procedure or potentially cause more harm. If the physician does not feel comfortable proceeding, they should stop and try to educate the patient as to a better choice. Physicians understand that they should not perform a cosmetic procedure they opine will not provide the desired outcome or could be harmful to the patient but patients can be persuasive.

This ties in with the importance of awareness of body dysmorphic disorder (BDD) as the prevalence of these patients increases significantly in aesthetic medicine.[15] In the fifth edition of Diagnostic and Statistical Manual of Mental Disorders (DSM-5), BDD is defined as the preoccupation with perceived flaws in physical appearance that are not observable or appear slight to others.[16] Performing cosmetic surgeries on a patient with BDD can cause harm and opens the physician up to risk of a lawsuit. Knowing when to have a suspicion of BDD and how to screen for it is imperative for facial plastic surgeons and for risk management. The Dysmorphic Concern Questionnaire and the BDD Questionnaire-Dermatology version are two validated screening tools used in the dermatology setting and can be easily used in any specialty.[17]

SOCIAL MEDIA

Whether we like it or not, social media is increasingly the norm in our society. Platforms such as Facebook, Instagram, Twitter, Snapchat, and now TikTok are ubiquitous and used frequently. In fact, 72% of Americans use some form of social media platform.[18] Thus, it should come as no surprise that many physicians, especially those focusing on cosmetic/aesthetic procedures, have taken to social media to advertise and build their personal brand. In a recent survey, individuals seeking cosmetic procedures were found to be among the group of people who valued social media platforms the most when choosing a cosmetic practice.[19] Although providers can benefit from increased visibility, physicians must also consider the increased risk of liability with social media interactions, especially Health Insurance Portability and Accountability Act (HIPAA) violations.[20]

Clinical photographs have historically been used to capture images, to communicate with other physicians, monitor treatment progress, or for publication purposes. Earlier in this article, we encouraged the value of photographs in the cosmetic surgery process. We explained that informed consent should be obtained, but it is imperative to understand the nuances involved when it relates to photography. Informed consent related to photography best includes the details of the photo's use, who will see the photo, and the risk that complete anonymity may be unachievable. McG Taylor and colleagues espouse that photography consent should be discussed with patients at three levels: (1) the image is for the medical record, (2) the image can be used as a teaching modality, and (3) the image can be used for publication and thus can be accessible within the public domain.[21,22]

Using photos for social media introduces a tricky fourth variable because the image is not only accessible to the public, but it is also often being marketed and actively introduced to the public. Therefore, when using a patient's photo on social media, the use of the photo should be explicitly explained, and the patient should understand that their identity may not remain anonymous.

Soliciting Reviews and Review Moderation

Online reviews increasingly serve as a starting point for businesses to attract patients, and patients frequently use them to help decide what service to use or what practice to join. Consumers should be able to trust that online reviews represent honest opinions of users of a product or service, but unfortunately, some companies abuse that trust by paying for fake or inflated reviews and/or review filtering. Although asking for reviews from patients who have used your service can support the health of your business, it is important to adhere to Federal Trade Commission (FTC) guidelines on this subject. The FTC recommends that practices should (1) avoid asking family, friends, or staff for reviews, at least without disclosing your relationship to them, (2) avoid asking for reviews from only people who you suspect will write positive ratings or from people who have not used your services, (3) disclose any incentive offered for completing a review and disclose all reviews including unfavorable ones. Any incentive should not be conditional on a positive review being written.[23] A plastic surgeon in New York faced the consequences of deviating from these recommendations when he paid employees for positive online reviews and subsequently faced a $300,000 penalty.[24]

When accumulating online reviews, a practice is often faced with how to moderate falsified information or prohibited content, such as obscenity. Either human moderators, automated systems, or both may be used depending on the scale and resources of the practice. In addition, although the FTC explicitly recommends having a reasonable process in place to moderate reviews after publication, a system that examines reviews before publication (on a practice's website, for example) offers the advantages of catching issues before they are viewed by the general public. Although there are many credible review moderation systems available, the FTC recommends that practices (1) have a reasonable and consistent process in place that can identify fake or suspicious reviews, (2) avoid editing reviews to alter the message, and (3) treat positive and negative reviews in a similar fashion. One should not attempt to bury unfavorable reviews to preferentially display positive ones. Finally, the FTC recommends disclosing how reviews are collected, moderated, and displayed.[25]

How to Handle a Bad Review

Unfortunately, negative reviews are probably inevitable when practicing medicine. It is reasonable to be concerned about negative reviews as they can affect the livelihood of your business. For example, a survey found that a single negative review of a plastic surgeon would deter 22% of patient respondents from seeing that physician and would prompt 55% of respondents to do additional research before making a decision.[26] So how do you handle a bad review? Although each case is unique and should be handled on an individual basis, there are several rules of thumb that can help: What should you not do?

1. You should not respond impulsively, as doing so may come across as defensive and angry.
2. You should not disclose any information about the patient or even acknowledge that the reviewer was a patient in your office, to maintain compliance with HIPAA.
3. You should not ignore negative reviews. Criticism, if looked at objectively, can offer the opportunity for improvement.
4. You should not bribe or intimidate patient into removing their negative reviews.

5. You should not selectively delete negative comments just because they are negative.

So what can you do?

1. You should consider if it is even worth responding to the negative review. Often, the risk of an HIPAA violation or escalating emotions may outweigh the benefits of any potential resolution. Should you decide to contact a patient regarding a negative review, you should consider discussing the matter with the patient offline. This will minimize the risk of an HIPAA violation. In addition, it may offer the opportunity to empathize with the patient, to allow them to vent, and to politely ask for the removal of the negative review if a reasonable resolution is met.[27]
2. If you decide to respond to reviews online, you should only respond with general policies. For example, one may thank the reviewer for the feedback, make them aware that you cannot respond freely online due to HIPAA, and invite them to call your office with any questions and concerns.
3. You may assess if the review violates the platform's community guidelines, terms of service, or policies. For example, Healthgrades user agreement prohibits "material that is false, factually inaccurate or misleading, material that is defamatory, libelous, deceptive or fraudulent, … [and] material that is obscene or derogatory."[28] If you determine that the review violates the platform's terms of service, you should consider flagging the review for removal. In addition, you may contact their relevant customer service department to explain in the platform's own language how the review violates the terms of service. Remember, you should avoid including any information that can violate HIPAA in these explanations.
4. For additional guidance with reviews that you are very concerned about or which recur, you may consider hiring an experienced attorney.
5. When all else fails, you may consider legal action for defamation. In one case, a plastic surgeon sued a patient for defamation after she posted complaints on several websites about the results of her recent cosmetic surgery. However, the court ruled that the patient's comments were protected opinion,[29] a result which has been reported to occur most of the time. That same publication also noted that most, if not all, suits against review sites were dismissed.[30]

Ownership of Content

Under US intellectual property law, photographers and videographers ordinarily own the copyrights to the content they create with one main exception being work for hire. In the former cases, the subject of such photos and videos has no right to ownership. Once registered with the US Copyright Office, copyright protection typically lasts for the duration of the life of the creator plus an additional 70 years, at which time the content enters the Public Domain. Once in the public domain, photos or videos can no longer be owned and are thus not protected by intellectual property laws. Therefore, anyone can use the photo or video without obtaining permission. Photographs and videos may also enter the Public Domain if the copyright owner designated the content as such or if the content did not meet the requirements for copyright protection. Finally, there are situations referred to as fair use where content can be used without permission despite being under copyright protection. Fair use includes the use of copyright-protected works for educational purposes, which is defined as non-commercial, non-entertainment instruction using already published works.[31]

Special consideration is given to content that is posted on social media platforms. Although ownership of content is typically retained by the user for many social media services, such as Twitter and Instagram, these companies are frequently granted a royalty-free, worldwide license (with the right to sublicense) to use such content however they see fit. In addition, there is considerable variation in the duration of such licenses. Whereas Facebook's and Instagram's licenses usually end when you fully delete the content or your account, Twitter's content licenses last forever.[32,33] Therefore, it is highly recommended that physicians read the fine print and fully understand each platform's terms of service agreement before posting.

How to Properly Remove Photographs

For legal reasons or otherwise, you may find yourself in the situation of needing to remove medical photographs from social media platforms. Unfortunately, it is not as simple as pressing the delete button. Although each social media platform has different rules regarding the process of deleting a user's data, typically deleted content is first transferred to a temporary location, such as a "Recently Deleted" or "Trash" folder. In the case of Instagram, these files are housed in the Recently Deleted folder for 30 days before the deletion process begins. One can expedite the deletion process earlier by deleting the content from the Recently Deleted folder, at which point the content is no longer visible to other users. However, the deletion process can take up to 90 days to fully

delete the data and another 90 days to remove the content from backup systems.[32] Although this process will remove the content from future access, unfortunately everything that is posted on the Internet can potentially be saved by social media users and thus can be permanent. Therefore, it is a good rule of thumb to take great care when uploading medical photographs to social media platforms, websites, or other online forums.

Social Media as an Advertising Platform

As previously discussed, images are usually owned by the photographer or, in the case of work for hire, the relevant employer.[31] However, when those photographs are used for business purposes, such as advertising or promotion, one can potentially run into the problem of misappropriation. Misappropriation is typically defined as the use of name and likeness for an exploitive purpose, such as financial gain.

There is no definitive conclusion on who owns the copyright of a medical image. However, some sources state that the institution or physician owns the copyright if the medical image is unidentifiable, but the patient retains the rights if the image has identifiable features.[34,35] Therefore, to use a medical image for commercial interest, the physician must obtain consent to use protected health information and the patient should understand that the photos will be used for the physician's benefit.[34] To protect yourself from patient claims that they are entitled to compensation from using their images, it should be specified in the consent form that they understand the photo will be used for promotional purposes and they will not be compensated for the use of their photo.[34] Morse v. Studin[36] represents a good example of failure to specify the uses of the medical photographs. In this case, a plastic surgeon used before and after photos in a newsletter mailed to patients for the sole purpose of soliciting their services. However, the consent form only covered educational use of the medical images, and the non-educational newsletter was not covered by the written consent.[36]

SUMMARY

It is important to understand legal malpractice risks and strategies to reduce risks in plastic surgery. In addition to the financial burden of a lawsuit, the stress a physician undergoes can be significant, occasionally leading to the medical malpractice stress syndrome (MMSS), a condition characterized by many symptoms seen in major depressive disorder and generalized anxiety disorder. If left unchecked, MMSS can at best lead to physician stress and dissatisfaction with their work and at worse lead to adverse events such as physician suicide.[37]

Therefore, plastic surgeons should put emphasis on proper patient selection, obtaining appropriate informed written consent, maintaining a consistent accurate medical record, and using checklists.

When using social media platforms for business purposes, it pays to carefully review the terms of service and how to remove content. Also, when obtaining informed consent to use a patient's photos on social media, you should explicitly explain how the photo will be used and emphasize that their identity may not remain anonymous. If using the photos for advertising purposes, more explicit information should be provided to the patient as to the intent for the use and, when appropriate, a compensation agreement with the patient can be considered. As is often said, "to err is human." Mistakes are inevitable, but by understanding the legal malpractice risks and carefully using the strategies discussed, physicians can minimize the likelihood of adverse events or at least minimize the negative sequelae of malpractice lawsuits.

Clinics Care Points

1. Appropriate informed consent and accurate medical documentation improves patient care and protects the physician from malpractice lawsuits.

2. Prompt communication with the patient following an adverse event can minimize the likelihood of litigation.

3. When handling a bad review, in most cases it is prudent to respond with general policies and/or a request for the patient to call your office in order to avoid violating HIPAA regulations.

4. When considering the use of patient photos on a social media platform, informed consent should include the specific details of the photos' use, who will see the pictures, and an explanation of how photos are removed from the relevant social media platform.

CLINICS CARE POINTS

- Appropriate informed consent and accurate medical documentation improves patient care and protects the physician from malpractice lawsuits.

- Prompt communication with the patient following an adverse event can minimize the likelihood of litigation.

- When handling a bad review, in most cases it is prudent to respond with general policies and/or a request for the patient to call your office in order to avoid violating HIPAA regulations.

- When considering the use of patient photos on a social media platform, informed consent should include the specific details of the photos' use, who will see the pictures, and an explanation of how photos are removed from the relevant social media platform.

ACKNOWLEDGMENTS

The authors gratefully acknowledge the contributions of Captain Star Q. Lopez, USAF (Ret.) JD, LLM, MBA, MA. Who is currently a US medical student and contributed research in the areas of Medutainment, consent, copyright and other social media issues some of which we have incorporated into this publication.

DISCLOSURE

The information provided is for academic purposes only and should not be construed as legal advice.

REFERENCES

1. Jena AB, Seabury S, Lakdawalla D, et al. Malpractice risk according to physician specialty. N Engl J Med 2011;365(7):629–36.
2. Halepas S, Muchemi F, Higham ZL, et al. The past decade in courts, what oral-maxillofacial surgery should know about facial cosmetic surgery. J Oral Maxillofac Surg 2021;79(8):1743–9.
3. Thornton RG. Utilizing causation. Proc (Bayl Univ Med Cent) 2001;14(4):455–7.
4. Flannery F. Consent to treatment, legal medicine: legal dynamics of medical encounters. St Louis (MO): CV Mosby Company; 1988.
5. Waltz J, Scheuneman T. Informed consent to therapy. Northwest Univ Law Rev 1970;64(5):628.
6. Cobbs v. Grant , 23 Cal.App.3d 313, 100 Cal. Rptr. 98 (Cal. Ct. App. 1972).
7. Redden E, and Baker B. Medicolegal problems in the management of patients with skin cancer, In: Friedman R, Rigel D, Kopf A, et al. Cancer of the Skin, Ch 41, 1991, Philadelphia:WB Sanders, 603–610.
8. Natanson v. Kline , 187 Kan. 186, 354 P.2d 670 (Kan. 1960).
9. Holder AR. The importance of medical records. JAMA 1974;228(1):118–9.

10. Tennenhouse J, Kasher M. Risk prevention skills. San Rafael: Tennenhouse Professional Publications.1988:69.

11. Haynes AB, Weiser TG, Berry WR, et al. A surgical safety checklist to reduce morbidity and mortality in a global population. N Engl J Med 2009;360(5):491–9.

12. Patient Safety and Quality Improvement Act, 42 §299b-21 to 299b-26 (2005).

13. Verwey H., Carstens P., Cosmetic surgery and responsible patient selection - does a legal duty to screen patients exist? De Sure Law Journal. 46(2), 2013, 432-450.

14. Sykes JM. Managing the psychological aspects of plastic surgery patients. Curr Opin Otolaryngol Head Neck Surg 2009;17(4):321–5.

15. Ribeiro RVE. Prevalence of body dysmorphic disorder in plastic surgery and dermatology patients: a systematic review with meta-analysis. Aesthetic Plast Surg 2017;41(4):964–70.

16. Association AP. Diagnostic and statistical manual of mental disorders: DSM-5. Washington D.C.: American Psychiatric Publishing; 2013.

17. Sun MD, Rieder EA. How we do it: body dysmorphic disorder for the cosmetic dermatologist. Dermatol Surg 2021;47(4):585–6.

18. Social Media Fact Sheet. Pew Research Center, Available at: https://www.pewresearch.org/internet/fact-sheet/social-media/. Accessed July 26, 2022.

19. Murphy EC, Nelson K, Friedman AJ. The influence of dermatologists' use of social media on attracting patients. J Drugs Dermatol 2020;19(5):532–8.

20. Galadari HI. Social media and modern dermatology. Int J Dermatol 2018;57(1):110–1.

21. McG Taylor D, Foster E, Dunkin CS, et al. A study of the personal use of digital photography within plastic surgery. J Plast Reconstr Aesthet Surg 2008; 61(1):37–40.

22. Terms of Service. Twitter. Available at: https://twitter.com/en/tos. Accessed July 25, 2022.

23. Soliciting and Paying for Online Reviews: A Guide for Marketers. Federal Trade Commission. Available at: https://www.ftc.gov/business-guidance/resources/soliciting-paying-online-reviews-guide-marketers. Accessed July 26, 2022.

24. Attorney General Cuomo Secures Settlement With Plastic Surgery Franchise That Flooded Internet With False Positive Reviews. New York State Office of the Attorney General Website. Available at: https://ag.ny.gov/press-release/2009/attorney-general-cuomo-secures-settlement-plastic-surgery-franchise-flooded. Accessed July 26, 2022.

25. Featuring Online Customer Reviews: A Guide for Platforms. Federal Trade Commission. Available at: https://www.ftc.gov/business-guidance/resources/featuring-online-customer-reviews-guide-platforms. Accessed July 26, 2022.

26. Fan KL, Graziano F, Economides JM, et al. The public's preferences on plastic surgery social media engagement and professionalism: demystifying the impact of demographics. Plast Reconstr Surg 2019;143(2):619–30.

27. Powell D, Stebbins A. How medical providers can remove & respond to negative medical reviews. Available at: https://www.minclaw.com/how-doctors-can-respond-to-negative-online-reviews/. Accessed July 26, 2022.

28. Healthgrades Limited License and User Agreement. Available at: https://www.healthgrades.com/content/user-agreement. Accessed July 26, 2022.

29. Lotus v. Nazarifroshani, 21 F. Supp. 3d 849 (E.D. Ky. 2014).

30. Vanderpool D. What can I do about a negative online review? Innov Clin Neurosci 2017;14(5–6):31–2.

31. Copyright Act, Pub. L. No. 94-553, 17 §101-810 (1976).

32. Terms of Use. Instagram. Available at: https://help.instagram.com/581066165581870. Accessed July 25, 2022.

33. Twitter Terms of Service. Twitter. Available at: https://twitter.com/en/tos. Accessed July 25, 2022.

34. Hodge SDJ. A picture may be worth a thousand words but they may not always be appropriate in a medical context. Illinois: DePaul Law Review; 2021. p. 465–96.

35. Hawkins S. Copyright Fair Use and How it Works for Online Images, Soc. Media Exam'R. 2011. Available at: https://www.socialmediaexaminer.com/copyright-fair-use-and-how-it-works-for-online-images/. Accessed July 26, 2022.

36. Morse v. Studin , 283 A.D.2d 622, 725 N.Y.S.2d 93 (N.Y. App. Div. 2001).

37. Reyes R, Reyes C. At your defense: medical malpractice stress syndrome takes its toll. Emerg Med News 2017;39(2):19.

Moving?

Make sure your subscription moves with you!

To notify us of your new address, find your **Clinics Account Number** (located on your mailing label above your name), and contact customer service at:

Email: journalscustomerservice-usa@elsevier.com

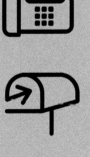

800-654-2452 (subscribers in the U.S. & Canada)
314-447-8871 (subscribers outside of the U.S. & Canada)

Fax number: 314-447-8029

Elsevier Health Sciences Division
Subscription Customer Service
3251 Riverport Lane
Maryland Heights, MO 63043

*To ensure uninterrupted delivery of your subscription, please notify us at least 4 weeks in advance of move.

9780323938792